Discursive Perspectives in Therapeutic Practice

International Perspectives in Philosophy and Psychiatry

Series editors: Bill (K.W.M.) Fulford, Katherine Morris, John Z. Sadler, and Giovanni Stanghellini

Volumes in the series:

Maladapting Minds
Adriaens and De Block (eds.)

Portrait of the Psychiatrist as a Young Man: The early writing and work of R.D. Laing, 1927–1960
Beveridge

Mind, Meaning, and Mental Disorder 2e
Bolton and Hill

What is Mental Disorder?
Bolton

Delusions and Other Irrational Beliefs
Bortolotti

Postpsychiatry
Bracken and Thomas

Philosophy, Psychoanalysis, and the A-rational Mind
Brakel

Unconscious Knowing and Other Essays in Psycho-Philosophical Analysis
Brakel

Psychiatry as Cognitive Neuroscience
Broome and Bortolotti (eds.)

Free Will and Responsibility: A guide for practitioners
Callender

Reconceiving Schizophrenia
Chung, Fulford, and Graham (eds.)

Nature and Narrative: An introduction to the new philosophy of psychiatry
Fulford, Morris, Sadler, and Stanghellini (eds.)

Oxford Textbook of Philosophy and Psychiatry
Fulford, Thornton, and Graham

The Mind and its Discontents 2e
Gillett

Thinking Through Dementia
Hughes

Dementia: Mind, meaning, and the person
Hughes, Louw, and Sabat (eds.)

Talking Cures and Placebo Effects
Jopling

Philosophical Issues in Psychiatry II: Nosology
Kendler and Parnas (eds.)

Discursive Perspectives in Therapeutic Practice
Lock and Strong (eds.)

Schizophrenia and the Fate of the Self
Lysaker and Lysaker

Responsibility and Psychopathy
Malatesti and McMillan

Body-Subjects and Disordered Minds
Matthews

Rationality and Compulsion: Applying action theory to psychiatry
Nordenfelt

Philosophical Perspectives on Technology and Psychiatry
Phillips (ed.)

The Metaphor of Mental Illness
Pickering

Mapping the Edges and the In-between
Potter

Trauma, Truth, and Reconciliation: Healing damaged relationships
Potter (ed.)

The Philosophy of Psychiatry: A companion
Radden

The Virtuous Psychiatrist
Radden and Sadler

Autonomy and Mental Disorder
Radoilska (ed.)

Feelings of Being
Ratcliffe

Values and Psychiatric Diagnosis
Sadler

Disembodied Spirits and Deanimated Bodies: The psychopathology of common sense
Stanghellini

Essential Philosophy of Psychiatry
Thornton

Empirical Ethics in Psychiatry
Widdershoven, McMillan, Hope, and van der Scheer (eds.)

The Sublime Object of Psychiatry: Schizophrenia in clinical and cultural theory
Woods

Discursive Perspectives in Therapeutic Practice

Edited by

Andy Lock
Professor of Psychology
Massey University
New Zealand

and

Tom Strong
Professor, Educational Studies in Counselling Psychology
University of Calgary
Canada

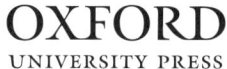

OXFORD
UNIVERSITY PRESS

Great Clarendon Street, Oxford, OX2 6DP,
United Kingdom

Oxford University Press is a department of the University of Oxford.
It furthers the University's objective of excellence in research, scholarship,
and education by publishing worldwide. Oxford is a registered trade mark of
Oxford University Press in the UK and in certain other countries

© Oxford University Press, 2012

The moral rights of the authors have been asserted

First Edition published in 2012

Impression: 1

All rights reserved. No part of this publication may be reproduced, stored in
a retrieval system, or transmitted, in any form or by any means, without the
prior permission in writing of Oxford University Press, or as expressly permitted
by law, by licence or under terms agreed with the appropriate reprographics
rights organization. Enquiries concerning reproduction outside the scope of the
above should be sent to the Rights Department, Oxford University Press, at the
address above

You must not circulate this work in any other form
and you must impose this same condition on any acquirer

British Library Cataloguing in Publication Data

Data available

Library of Congress Cataloguing in Publication Data

Data available

ISBN 978–0–19–959275–3

Printed and bound by
CPI Antony Rowe, Chippenham, Wiltshire

Whilst every effort has been made to ensure that the contents of this work
are as complete, accurate and-up-to-date as possible at the date of writing,
Oxford University Press is not able to give any guarantee or assurance that
such is the case. Readers are urged to take appropriately qualified medical
advice in all cases. The information in this work is intended to be useful to the
general reader, but should not be used as a means of self-diagnosis or for the
prescription of medication

Links to third party websites are provided by Oxford in good faith and
for information only. Oxford disclaims any responsibility for the materials
contained in any third party website referenced in this work.

Acknowledgements

This volume has its origins in the Discursive Therapies postgraduate programme at Massey University, New Zealand. This programme took advantage of Massey's history of distance education to develop a wholly on-line programme in which not only were students 'at a distance', but so too were the teachers. The programme began as a collaboration in 2004 between the Massey School of Psychology and the 'Just Therapy' team at the Family Centre in Lower Hutt, New Zealand. Later, a partnership was developed with the Taos Institute centred in the United States, brought about through a synergy of ideas, participants, and structure—Taos also being a 'virtual' Institution.

This web-based programme had roots going back another 10 years to 1994, when the web was in its infancy. Its birth can be dated very precisely: an evening in May during a lecturing visit to Massey by Rom Harré, and about half-way down a second bottle of a rather good 1992 Coonawarra Cabernet Sauvignon. Quite how the idea came up that maybe the web offered a way to reinvent the nature of tertiary education is difficult to reconstruct, but the thought that it might be possible to build an academic department that no traditional university could possibly afford to physically instantiate was in itself intoxicating. Propelled by Rom's legendary levels of energetic enthusiasm and encouragement, we had, by the end of the week, talked Mick Billig, John Shotter, and Ken Gergen into 'coming out to play', and in those early days of the web we constructed a 'virtual faculty' (traces of which can still be found through a judicious choice of search terms). A great debt is owed to Rom and everyone else: none of us knew quite what we were doing or where things would lead, and the whole exercise became one of social constructionism in practice. It was within this nexus that we editors first 'met' and began to collaborate, and the programme that underpins this volume was conceived.

This volume is more of a joint collaborative production than many edited books. An apt analogy would be with an orchestra. There are many themes and variations here, but they are all played out around one particular motif: a dialogue between theory and practice. To all who contributed the chapters that make up this book, many thanks for your hard work, humour, and great teaching and writing. May the conversations and emails that went into your chapters keep us in dialogue for years to come. But it is not only the work of the contributors to the programme that finds a voice here, but those of our students are woven through all the chapters. A remarkable bunch of people: thanks, guys for your pioneering spirits, and for braving cyberspace in the days before Facebook, YouTube, Skype, and other such applications gave the web its current social persona.

This book owes much to support provided by colleagues at Massey University's School of Psychology, most notably Ian Evans and Mandy Morgan. Their support helped translate the Virtual Faculty into a Discursive Therapies Postgraduate programme where many of this book's contributors played roles as instructors and course developers. Helen Page has been a godsend, for her proofing skills, keeping track of numerous revisions of chapters, and countless other forms of assistance. At Calgary we have benefited from the support of many colleagues and students, especially, Sally St George, Dan Wulff, Karl Tomm, Olga Sutherland, Shari Couture, Don Zeman, and Ottar Ness. We are grateful to both universities resources and brief periods of leave that have enabled us to get together on a number of occasions in both New Zealand and Canada, working on this volume and our recently published joint-authored book on social constructionism. Thanks are due to our families and friends who were willing to indulge us for where the many conversations that went into this book took us. And to Charlotte Green at Oxford University Press, thank you for your patience, tact, advice, and support.

The Discursive Therapies Programme was recommended for closure in 2010 as part of Massey's Academic Reform project, making this both a valedictory volume and an opportunity to put the clock back to the 1990 to pursue again the same, exciting challenge: where do we go from here?

Contents

Contributors ix

1. Discursive therapy: why language, and how we use it in therapeutic dialogues, matters 1
   Andy Lock and Tom Strong

2. Talking to listen: its pre-history, invention, and future in the field of psychotherapy 23
   Lois Shawver

3. Positioning theory, narratology, and pronoun analysis as discursive therapies 45
   Rom Harré and Mirjana Dedaić

4. Therapeutic communication from a constructionist standpoint 65
   Kenneth J. Gergen and Mary Gergen

5. Ontological social constructionism in the context of a social ecology: the importance of our living bodies 83
   John Shotter

6. Narrative therapy: challenges and communities of practice 106
   Susanna Chamberlain

7. Collaborative therapy: performing reflective and dialogical relationships 126
   Sue Levin and Saliha Bava

8. Solution-focused brief therapy: listening in the present with an ear toward the future 143
   Maureen Duffy

9. From Wittgenstein, complexity, and narrative emergence: discourse and solution-focused brief therapy 163
   Gale Miller and Mark McKergow

10. Activity and performance (and their discourses) in social therapeutic method *184*
    Lois Holzman and Fred Newman

11. Developing a 'just therapy': context and the ascription of meaning *196*
    Charles Waldegrave

12. Māori expressions of healing in 'just therapy' *212*
    Maria Maniapoto

13. A systematic narrative review of discursive therapies research: considering the value of circumstantial evidence *224*
    Ronald J. Chenail, Melissa DeVincentis, Harriet E. Kiviat, and Cynthia Somers

14. Problematizing social context in evidence-based therapy evaluation practice/governance *245*
    Robbie Busch

15. The body, trauma, and narrative approaches to healing *269*
    Maureen Duffy

16. Narrative, discourse, psychotherapy—neuroscience? *288*
    John Cromby

17. Conversation and its therapeutic possibilities *308*
    Tom Strong

    Author Index *323*

    Subject Index *331*

Contributors

Saliha Bava, Ph.D. is an Associate Professor of Marriage and Family Therapy (MFT) at the School of Social and Behavioral Sciences, Mercy College, Dobbs Ferry. She is the former Associate Director of Houston Galveston Institute, an internationally renowned Family Therapy training centre and the home for Collaborative Therapy. As the Director of Research with the International Trauma Studies Program, affiliated with Columbia University, she is researching performance (theatre) as research and psychosocial practices within the context of post-political violence. She is also an online faculty member at Massey University, New Zealand and doctoral advisor at the Taos-Tilburg's Social Sciences Program, Netherlands. For the past 20 years, she has been a consultant and designer of performative and dialogic processes within human systems—organizational, community, family, learning, and research systems. She is a couples and family therapist and coach for generative professional and personal relationships. She is the co-founding editor of the *International Journal for Collaborative Practices,* on the advisory editorial board of *Family Process*, and the associate editor of *The Qualitative Report.*

Dr Bava received her Masters in Social Work from Tata Institute of Social Sciences, Mumbai, India; Ph.D. in Human Development with specialization in MFT from Virginia Tech; and completed the Executive Program for Nonprofit Leaders from Stanford University's Business School. She lives in New York City and is interested in the performance of (complex) relationships among people, the systems we create, and the construction of our social lives and realities.

Robbie Busch is a Curriculum Development Facilitator at the School of Psychology, Massey University where has been teaching for the past 6 years. He also tutored critical human geography at the University of Canterbury while completing his master's degree in the Geography and Journalism Departments. Robbie's academic interests are in narrative therapy, critical theory, psychotherapy evaluation, qualitative methodologies, the media and identity, environmental psychology, and teaching and learning in psychology. He is currently finishing his doctoral thesis on the relationship between narrative therapy and evidence-based psychotherapy evaluation.

Susanna Chamberlain was a Family Therapist for two decades, closely involved with Narrative Therapy and the Dulwich Centre. She has also taught in universities in Australia since 1991, and obtained a Ph.D. on the nature of the Self. She is currently preparing her thesis for publication as a book, entitled *Which Self?*. Susanna works for Griffith University in Brisbane, Australia, convening the Social Enterprise core stream in the School of Humanities. She has been instrumental in developing this innovative programme which enables students to explore potential careers in the third sector while challenging them to consider issues of social justice. Her research interests include the pedagogy of learning and teaching, human rights and governmentality.

Ronald J. Chenail, Ph.D., is Professor of Family Therapy, Vice President for Institutional Effectiveness, and Director of the Graduate Certificate in Qualitative Research Program at Nova Southeastern University located in Fort Lauderdale, Florida, USA. He is also editor of two journals—*The Qualitative Report* and the *Journal of Marital and Family Therapy*. He has written over 100 journal articles, book chapters, and books, given over 170 conference presentations, and secured and worked on grants and contracts totalling over $700,000. His books include *Medical Discourse and systemic frames of comprehension, practicing therapy: Exercises for growing therapists* (with Anne Rambo and Anthony Heath [Ablex, 1991]), *The talk of the clinic: Explorations in the analysis of medical and therapeutic discourse* (with Bud Morris [Erlbaum, 1995]), and *Qualitative research proposals and reports: A guide* (with Patricia Munhall [3rd ed., Jones & Bartlett, 2007]).

John Cromby is in the School of Sport, Exercise and Health Sciences at Loughborough University; previously, he has worked in mental health, drug addiction, and intellectual impairment services. He is interested in the character of experience, and in the way that it is jointly constituted at the intersection of social influence and the body. He is examining this intersection by engaging with topics such as feeling, emotion, 'depression', and paranoia, and by experimenting with methods of jointly analysing textual data and embodied activity.

Mirjana Dedaić (Ph.D., Georgetown University) is a critically oriented sociocognitive linguist. She is currently teaching in the Georgetown's Communication, Culture & Technology's Master's Program. Her research interests are interdisciplinary, applying pragmatics, critical theory, discursive psychology, and critical discourse analysis on topics concerning identity construction, gender, and politics. She has taught at several universities in the United States and Croatia and published in leading linguistic journals. Her books include *At war with words* (Mouton de Gruyter, 2003) and *South Slavic discourse particles* (Benjamins, 2010).

Melissa DeVincentis is the behaviour specialist for one of the largest preschools in the country for children with autism. She is a licensed marriage and family therapist (LMFT) and board certified behaviour analyst (BCBA). She is working on her dissertation in order to complete the Ph.D. Family Therapy programme at Nova Southeastern University. Her concentration is on supporting families who have children on the autism spectrum. She has been involved in a number of research projects including solution-focused couple's therapy for families who have a child with autism and improving social referencing in children with autism. She also co-developed a parent training series for parents who have children with high magnitude behaviours. She has presented locally and nationally on various topics including providing home and school support. Additionally, she has consulted in school systems and trained professionals both nationally and internationally on best practice techniques when working with families and children on the autism spectrum.

Maureen Duffy, Ph.D., is a practising family therapist, consultant, educator, and author with over 25 years of experience. Maureen has published over 40 book chapters and journal articles and has presented her work nationally and internationally. She is the co-author of a forthcoming book, *Mobbing: Causes, consequences, and solutions,* to be published by Oxford University Press. She is on the editorial boards of *The Journal of Marital and Family Therapy, The Journal of Systemic Therapies,* and *The Family Journal,* and is an editor of *The Qualitative Report.* Maureen has won awards for outstanding achievement in education. She enjoys spending time with her family, living in Miami, continuing to improve her Spanish, and trips to Ireland.

Kenneth J. Gergen is a Senior Research Professor at Swarthmore College, and President of the Taos Institute, a non-profit educational organization. He has served as president of two divisions of the American Psychological Association, and the Associate Editor of both the *American Psychologist,* and *Theory and Psychology.* Gergen has been a major contributor to social constructionist theory and practice. Among his major works are *Realities and relationships: Soundings in social construction* (Harvard University Press, 1995), *The saturated self* (Basic Books, 1991), *An invitation to social construction* (Sage, 1999), and *Relational being, beyond self and community* (Oxford University Press, 2009). With Mary Gergen, he is a co-editor of the *Positive Aging Newsletter,* an online journal.

Mary Gergen is Professor Emerita, Penn State University, Brandywine, in Psychology and Women's Studies, and a founder and board member of the Taos Institute. She is also an advisor to doctoral students in the Institute's programme with Tilburg University, The Netherlands. She locates herself at the crossroads of feminist theory and social constructionism. Among her major works are *Feminist thought and the structure of knowledge* (New York University Press, 1988), *Social construction: Entering the dialogue* (with K. J. Gergen [Thomson Learning, 1981]); *and Feminist reconstructions in psychology: Narrative, gender, and performance* (Sage, 2000). She has also written numerous pieces for journals and books relating feminist ideas to relational theory, qualitative methods, and narrative. She is also a pioneer in performative social science, which she began creating during her fellowship year at the Netherlands Institute for Advanced Study in 1988. The Gergens have recently completed a new book, *Do you love me? Adventures in performative social science.*

Rom Harré graduated in mathematics and philosophy from Auckland University. He subsequently did graduate work at Oxford and returned to Oxford as the University Lecturer in Philosophy of Science. His contacts with the psychology of the time shocked him for their pseudo-scientific character. With like-minded people he began a reforming crusade. In 1988 he joined Georgetown University in Washington DC as Distinguished Research Professor of Psychology. He has also taught in Pakistan, Australia, Japan, Spain, and Denmark. He has continued to work in philosophy of natural science, recently publishing *Pavlov's dogs and Schrodinger's cat* on experimental method. He has also published a number of psychological studies in which language use has taken the centre stage. He combines his work in the United States with

Directorship of the Centre for the Philosophy of Natural and Social Science at the London School of Economics, and with the presidency of the International Society for the Philosophy of Chemistry.

Lois Holzman is co-founder and director of the East Side Institute for Group and Short Term Psychotherapy—for 30 years an independent research, training, and organizing centre at the forefront of new approaches to human development, learning, therapeutics, and community building. Lois travels extensively, meeting with grassroots innovators and organizations, and university scholars and researchers, introducing them to the social therapeutic/performance approach to human development pioneered by the Institute, and to each other. Among her books are *Vygotsky at work and play* (Routledge, 2009), *Schools for growth: Radical alternatives to current educational model* (Lawrence Erlbaum, 1997), and *Postmodern psychology: A postmodern culture of the mind* (Routledge, 2002). She received her Ph.D. in developmental psychology from Columbia University.

Harriet E. Kiviat, MA, LMHC, NCC, is a doctoral candidate in the Nova Southeastern University Marriage and Family Therapy program located in Fort Lauderdale, Florida, USA. She also maintains a private clinical practice in Boynton Beach, Florida. A licensed clinician and clinical supervisor, Harriet utilizes Ericksonian hypnotherapy in her practice and has presented on that subject. She has published two chapters in the area of solution-focused therapy, has participated as a co-researcher and presenter in qualitative and quantitative studies related to MFT, and has provided ad hoc reviews for a national journal. Harriet's doctoral research focuses on the lived experiences of older students in MFT training and supervision and she plans to teach and supervise new therapists in a university setting.

Sue Levin, Ph.D. is the executive director of the Houston Galveston Institute (HGI). Having been with HGI for more than 25 years, she has been mentored by the creators of Collaborative Therapy, Harry Goolishian and Harlene Anderson. In addition to clinical practice, training, and administration for HGI, Sue is on the faculty of Our Lady of the Lake University, Masters psychology programme, is an Associate of the Taos Institute, is an Online Adjunct Faculty of Massey University, and is past-president of the Board of Directors of the Texas Association for Marriage & Family Therapy. Sue has authored more than 15 publications and presented at conferences and workshops in Europe, Scandinavia, Mexico, and all over North America. Among other achievements, Sue led HGI during its outstanding service to the community, in disaster mental health, following Hurricanes Katrina, Rita and Ike.

Andy Lock is Professor of Psychology at Massey University, Palmerston North, New Zealand. His main interest is in how speaking is constructed, and the constructive consequences of speaking. He has pursued these interests in the contexts of development (*Action, gesture and symbol: The emergence of language* [Academic Press, 1978], *The guided reinvention of language* [Academic Press, 1980]; culture (*Indigenous psychologies*, with Paul Heelas [Academic Press, 1991]; evolution (*Handbook of human symbolic* *evolution*, with Charles Peters [Clarendon Press, 1996]; and social constructionism (*Social constructionism: Sources and stirrings in theory and practice*, with Tom Strong [Cambridge University Press, 2010]. He can be contacted by email: A.J.Lock@massey.ac.nz.

Mark McKergow, Ph.D., MBA is Director of the Centre for Solutions Focus at Work based in London, UK. He has pioneered the use of the solution-focused approach in organizational and business coaching and consulting and is working to develop connections between this approach and other philosophical, academic, and practice traditions. He is the author of three books including *The solutions focus* (Nicholas Brealey 2nd ed., 2007) which is in eleven languages, is a board member of SFCT (the professional body for SF practitioners in organisations) and edits the SFCT academic journal *InterAction*.

Skype: mark.mckergow. Email: mark@sfwork.com. Websites: http://www.sfwork.com (SF consulting, training, coaching); http://www.hostleadership.com (free download of Mark's latest ground-breaking work); http://www.asfct.org (SF professional body and *InterAction* journal).

Maria Maniapoto, DipMāori/Tohu Māori, BA, MEd (VUW) is of Māori descent, she is Ngai Tuhoe and Ngati Paretekawa. She graduated from Victoria University of Wellington (VUW) in 2004, with a Masters in Education, Bachelor of Arts and Diploma of Māori Studies. Maria has been recently working in social policy research, and community development work at the Family Centre in Lower Hutt, Wellington, New Zealand. Maria's passion in the education of indigenous peoples at tertiary level has brought her to the Cape York Institute, Cairns, Australia to work on the Higher Expectations Program for Indigenous Tertiary students.

Gale Miller is Professor of Sociology and Research Professor of Social and Cultural Sciences, Marquette University. He has long-standing research interests in the Sociology of Troubles and Social Problems, Social Theory and Institutions. His research has focused on how troubles and problems are defined in human service institutions, such as work to welfare programmes (*Enforcing the work ethic* [State University of New York Press, 1991]) and solution-focused brief therapy (*Becoming miracle workers* [AldineTransaction, 1997]). His current research deals with individuals and families coping with such enduring crises as having a family member imprisoned for sex offenses in the United States and managing drug addiction and methadone treatment in Denmark.

Fred Newman is the creator of social therapy and co-founder of the East Side Institute for Group and Short Term Psychotherapy and the All Stars Project, Inc., both in New York City. He received his Ph.D. in analytic philosophy/foundations of mathematics from Stanford University, and throughout his 40-year career as therapist, playwright, director, community organizer and political strategist, he has brought a philosophical expertise and sensibility to engage issues of development, learning and human growth. His books include *Performance of a lifetime: A practical-philosophical* *guide to the joyous life* (with Phyllis Goldberg, Castillo International 1996) and, with Lois Holzman, *The end of knowing: A new developmental way of learning* (Routledge, 1997), *Lev Vygotsky: Revolutionary scientist* (Routledge, 1993), and *Unscientific psychology* (Greenwood Press, 1996).

Lois Shawver is a clinical psychologist. She is best known as the founder and host of 'PMTH', a large active online group of therapists who are interested in postmodern therapy. However, she has published widely, including professional articles, book chapters, and two books, many building on the writing of Ludwig Wittgenstein. Her most recent book, *Nostalgic postmodernism* (Paralogic Press, 2006), has been translated into Spanish by Karin Taverniers, a multi-lingual therapist who has accepted Dr Shawver's invitation to become the future host of PMTH.

If you wish to join PMTH, write Dr Taverniers at: ktaverniers@gmail.com. You can follow Dr Shawver on Twitter at @jolanza.

John Shotter is Emeritus Professor of Communication in the Department of Communication, University of New Hampshire. His long-term interest has been, and still is, in the social conditions conducive to people having a voice in determining the conditions of their own lives, i.e. in the development of participatory democracies and civil societies. He is the author of *Social accountability and selfhood* (Blackwell, 1984); *Cultural politics of everyday life: Social constructionism, rhetoric, and knowing of the third kind* (Open University, 1993); *Conversational realities: the construction of life through language* (Sage, 1993); *Conversational realities revisited: Life, language, body, and world* (Taos Publications, 2008); *Social construction on the edge: Withness-thinking and embodiment* (Taos Publications, 2010); *Getting it: Withness-thinking and the dialogical... in practice* (Hampton Press, 2011). He calls his current approach to social theory a *social ecological* approach. His current interest is in the role of *dynamic stabilities* within turbulent, flowing realities, and the use *descriptive concepts* in picking out crucial aspects of what occurs 'in between', i.e. within our dynamically unfolding, practical relations with our surroundings.

Cynthia Somers, B.Sc., M.B.A., is a Ph.D. candidate in the Family Therapy department at Nova Southeastern University in Florida. She taught chemistry and integrated science at the high school level prior to entering the business world where she served as head of purchasing and export departments for over 10 years. As a family therapy student, she co-authored two published marriage and family therapy articles and presented at conferences internationally, nationally, and locally. Cynthia has significant interest in the area of domestic violence which is the subject of her dissertation. She desires to be an educator and a clinician who specializes in domestic violence.

Tom Strong is a Professor, therapist and counsellor-educator at the University of Calgary who writes on the collaborative, critically reflective, and generative potentials of discursive approaches to psychotherapy. Author or co-author of over 70 articles and chapters, and co-author (with Andy Lock) of *Social constructionism: Sources and stirrings in theory and practice* (Cambridge University Press, 2010), he has also co-edited (with David Paré) *Furthering talk: Advances in the discursive therapies* (Kluwer Academic/Plenum, 2003).

Charles Waldegrave is a psychologist and social policy researcher. He leads the Family Centre Social Policy Research Unit based in Lower Hutt, Wellington, New Zealand and is a joint leader of the New Zealand Poverty Measurement Project (NZPMP) and the New Zealand Longitudinal Study on Ageing (NZLSA) research programmes.

Along with colleagues at the Family Centre, he helped develop an internationally recognized approach to contextualizing therapeutic work around cultural, gender, and socioeconomic equity, known as 'just therapy'. He has published extensively in all these areas and is regularly contracted to run therapeutic and applied social policy workshops throughout the world.

Chapter 1

Discursive therapy: why language, and how we use it in therapeutic dialogues, matters

Andy Lock and Tom Strong

The background to the present

Western science has massively transformed human life over the past few centuries. This is particularly true of medical science's assault on illnesses. Consider, for example, the case of smallpox. The British physician Edward Jenner demonstrated an immunizing effect against the contraction of smallpox by vaccinating people with cowpox in 1798. For the century prior to that demonstration, Behbehani (1983) estimates that smallpox killed 400,000 people a year in Europe. It is a particularly virulent disease, with a mortality rate between 20–60%, and up to 80% in children (Riedel 2005). In the 20th century, Koplow (2003) estimates world smallpox deaths of 300–500 million; the World Health Organization (WHO) has estimated there were 50 million cases worldwide in 1950; and 15 million cases, with 2 million deaths, as recently as 1967 (World Health Organization 2011). The numbers here are clearly reducing, as a result of vaccination campaigns, and in 1979 WHO certified the eradication of smallpox, it being the first (and only) major human disease to have been eliminated (De Cock 2001). The subsequent debate has been around whether the virus itself, stocks of which are securely held in two laboratories in the USA and Russia, should be destroyed. This is a great achievement for medical science.

Allied to Robert Koch's discovery that bacteria played a role in the transmission of disease (1880), the discovery of antibiotics, particularly penicillin, in the early 20th century, and even DDT (dichlorodiphenyltrichloroethane; which, while now banned, certainly prevented millions from contracting malaria), biomedical science has massively impacted on human life. Life expectancy has improved from 35 to 77 years in the industrial nations since Jenner's day, and since 1952 to today, from 38 to 64 in India, and 41 to 73 in China. Other medical problems have been shown to have genetic origins, and the biochemical processes at the root of most illnesses have been largely worked out, with a consequent growth in research to discover effective restorative drug treatments. These are spectacular achievements, and the canons of medical practice that underpin them are warranted by their effectiveness, leading to the enshrinement of principles of best practice, and the development of manuals, for example, Coulehan and Block (2005), that guide initial diagnostic procedures for identifying what illness a patient is presenting, and then the procedures to be followed in pursuit of the best possible prognosis.

We do not intend looking at the details of medical history and its concepts in any detail. We merely note the view of Fulford, Thornton, and Graham that 'until the 1960s, when the debate about mental illness was getting going, there was little in the way of concern about conceptual problems in medicine' (2006, p. 18). Medicine was striving to cure diseases: 'That such conditions were indeed *diseases* was not in question: and what was *meant* by calling these conditions diseases seemed all too self-evident' (ibid). What we suggest, in hindsight, is that with this ethos it was inevitable that departures from behavioural norms should come to be unreflectively viewed as 'mental illnesses', and that given the successes of medicine in dealing with illness, progress in curing and alleviating these mental illnesses was most likely to come about by applying a medical model to them. People thus present with symptoms, rather than problems or concerns, or what Szasz (1960, p. 113) was terming 'problems of living'. On the face of it, then, for the powers that were, mental illness had a clear similarity to physical illness: it has an identifiable site of diagnosis and treatment—an individual human being; and what that individual is exhibiting is clearly a departure from the naturally-given normal state of affairs. This view is not uncommon. For example, the National Alliance on Mental Illness in the USA is very clear on the issue:

> Mental illnesses are medical conditions that disrupt a person's thinking, feeling, mood, ability to relate to others and daily functioning. Just as diabetes is a disorder of the pancreas, mental illnesses are medical conditions that often result in a diminished capacity for coping with the ordinary demands of life (2011).

In the early medical era, the classification of mental deviance was a major goal, much in the same vein as reliably distinguishing one disease from another as for physical medicine. 'Psychiatry' was coined by Johann Reil in 1808 as the term for the endeavour: 'medical treatment of the mind' (*psych-*: mind; *-iatry*: medical treatment; from Greek *iātrikos*: medical, *iāsthai*: to heal). Subsequent 19th-century psychiatric work was synthesized by Emil Kraepelin in his 1887 text on clinical psychiatry. His major contribution was to distinguish two distinct forms of mental illness: affective disorders and cognitive disorders. These categories have subsequently been refined into separate varieties—bipolar disorder versus schizophrenia, paranoia, etc., along with further regroupings to produce various personality disorders. Language, in this way, becomes a tool with a use in diagnosis. Questions elicit answers which allow disorders to be determined. While diagnosis, for many reasons, remains as much an art as a science (see, for example, Rosenhan 1973), the discovery in 1948 of the stabilizing effect of lithium chloride for bipolar sufferers, and the identification in 1952 of the drug chlorpromazine as being effective in treating schizophrenia, helped cement the biomedical conception of mental disorder. A parallel history can be essayed cementing the role of genetic factors in mental disorders, and if there turns out to be 'a gene for everything', and gene influences can be established, then the problems caused can perhaps be fixed, because genes are expressed via chemical pathways, and where these are out-of-sync they may be able to be remediated. Again, if we shift to psychological or behavioural disturbances, then these can be conceived of as being based in inappropriate or conflicting beliefs, or on the acquisition of bad habits. Since psychology provides a scientific basis for understanding cognition and behaviour, these disturbances should, in theory, be able to be fixed, and as more studies are conducted, best practice can be arrived at and standardized (or manualized).

The most succinct statement of this general view is contained in the American Psychiatric Association's *Diagnostic and Statistical Manual of Mental Disorders* (2000). The DSM-IV-TR indicates that '. . . what are being classified are disorders that people *have*' (emphasis added, p. xxxi).

> . . . each of the mental disorders is conceptualized as a clinically significant behavioural or psychological syndrome or pattern that occurs *in an individual* and is associated with present distress (eg, a painful symptom) or disability (ie, impairment in one or more important areas of functioning. . . . Whatever its original cause, it must currently be considered a manifestation of a behavioural, psychological, or biological dysfunction *in the individual l.* . . Neither deviant behaviour (eg, political, religious, or sexual), nor conflicts that are primarily between the individual and society are mental disorders unless the deviance or conflict is a symptom of a dysfunction *in the individual* (emphasis added, p. xxxi).

This, then, is the current orthodoxy.

On the face of it, it appears a well-founded and motivated orthodoxy. Adopting a scientific perspective ensures that knowledge and practice can be aligned with reality. Given that all living humans have the same biological nature, then mental disorders, like physical illnesses, will exhibit discrete, universal categories. Western scientific understandings of illness are better founded than those they have replaced in the history of our own culture, and are therefore more likely to be effective in treating disorders in other cultures, as opposed to indigenous practices of spirit-healing, witchcraft, shamanism, and the like. After all, it stands to reason. It is against this background that the discursive therapies we introduce in this book have developed. We will look first at the general intellectual landscape that has contributed to this development.

'Culture wars' revisited

> Technology is [. . .] a queer thing. It brings you gifts with one hand, and stabs you in the back with the other
>
> C. P. Snow (1960), *The two cultures*.

C.P. Snow's characterization of a breakdown in communication between the sciences and the humanities in the mid-20th century came back in the 1990s in the guise of 'the culture wars'. While dichotomies are always crude, this one is perhaps reflective of a wider change occurring during that period, and continuing up to the present, in Western intellectual circles. Within the arts, Higgins (1978, p. 101) points to a historical change—he dates it as occurring in 1958—from cognitive to post-cognitive questions:

> The Cognitive Questions
> (asked by most artists of the 20th century, Platonic or Aristotelian till around 1958):
> 'How can I interpret this world of which I am a part? And what am I in it?'
> The Postcognitive Questions
> (asked by most artists since then):'Which world is this? What is to be done in it? Which of my selves is to do it?'

McHale (1992) suggests that the terms 'epistemological' and 'ontological' should preferably be used to construct the division between these two eras, and Higgins' questions indicate why: that is they shift from epistemological questions of how we can *know* the world to ontological ones of what world(s) we *exist* in, what we can do, etc. This shift in stance was not confined to the arts (and humanities), but can be noticed across most social science disciplines. Epistemological questions refer to knowledge about the world. To the basic ones stated by Higgins, McHale adds some more:

> What is there to be known?; Who knows it?; How do they know it and with what degree of certainty?; How is knowledge transmitted from one knower to another, and with what degree of reliability? What are the limits of the knowable?
>
> (McHale 1987, p. 9).

Ontological questions are those about being and modes of existence. McHale's additions here are:

> What is a world?; What kinds of worlds are there, how are they constituted, and how do they differ?; What happens when different kinds of worlds are placed in confrontation, or when boundaries between worlds are violated?; What is the mode of existence of a text, and what is the mode of existence of a world (or worlds) it projects?
>
> (McHale 1987, p. 10).

The behavioural sciences have not been immune to these shifts. The norms of psychological science emerge in a similar fashion to those of other sciences:

> the gradual elimination of the subjectivity and personal history of the investigators, and the gradual production of a description of nature in the ahistorical terms of form and structure
>
> (Bazeman 1988, quoted by Shotter 1993, p. 157).

This trajectory characterises that period of intellectual modernity referred to as the Enlightenment, starting from Descartes' *Discourse on Method* in which he crystallized the view that the world was open to rational, objective explanation. Embedded in this view were Descartes' fundamental arguments as to how certainty in our knowledge could be established. In making these arguments Descartes provided a celebration of individuality from which doubt could be dispelled and truth established—his conclusion 'cogito ergo sum'; I reason therefore I am; I cannot doubt that I am the one who doubts. But it is this foundational move that has been put under scrutiny again in the 50 or so years since Higgins' watershed. Descartes' foregrounding of individuality as undoubtedly given has become increasingly doubted (or contested), such that we might seem to be in a soup of uncertainty again. These doubts form the central planks of what has come to be called, for shorthand, 'postmodernism'. From these doubts, the project of the social sciences, in general, has shifted. This shift is very much centred in our 'grasp' of language, how it is used—for what purposes—and the problems that we have faced in coming to terms with how, as we used to think, language related to reality; and thus it is linked to our understanding of 'reality'; and finally, to our understanding of 'ourselves'. The project has shifted from an attempt to

> locate an already determined real world beyond the social and historical, and to attempt to discover this world in the depths of either people's organic or psychic nature. [Once] it was the task of language to represent the reality of these [hidden] worlds. But now, many

take seriously Foucault's claim (1972: 49) that our task 'consists of not—of no longer—treating discourses as a group of signs (signifying elements referring to contents or representations) but as practices that systematically form the objects of which we speak

(Shotter 1993, p. 38).

Our understanding of 'language' has itself shifted from the idealized pole of Saussure's (1916/1977) distinction—langue—to the reality of performance—parole. And the term 'language' has been gradually replaced by that of 'discourse'. And we find that

> discourse is not the possession of a single individual. Meaningful language is the product of social interdependence. It requires the coordinated actions of at least two persons, and until there is mutual agreement on the meaningful character of words, they fail to constitute language. If we follow this line of argument to its ineluctable conclusion, we find that it is not the mind of the single individual that provides whatever certitude we possess, but relationships of interdependency. If there were no interdependence—the joint creation of meaningful discourse—there would be no 'objects' or 'actions' or means of rendering them doubtful. We may rightfully replace Descartes's [sic] dictum with **communicamus ergo sum**
>
> (Gergen 1994, p. viii).

We communicate, therefore I am: and

> I am conscious of myself and become myself only while revealing myself for another, through another, and with the help of another . . . every internal experience ends up on the boundary . . . The very being of man (both internal and external) is a profound communication. To be means to communicate . . . To be means to be for the other; and through him, for oneself. Man has no internal sovereign territory; he is all and always on the boundary . . .
>
> (Bakhtin 1984, p. 287).

In this communicational view of ourselves, then, the current view we have of persons, is an illusion, maintained by the institution between us of certain special forms of communication. There has emerged a major shift, in some quarters at least, that: *human reality is a conversational one.* For example:

> The primary human reality is persons in conversation
>
> (Harré 1983, p. 58).

> Conversation, understood widely enough, is the form of human transactions in general
>
> (MacIntyre 1981, p. 197).

> If we see knowing not as having an essence, to be described by scientists or philosophers, but rather as a right, by current standards, to believe, then we are well on the way to seeing conversation as the ultimate context within which knowledge is to be understood
>
> (Rorty 1980, p. 389).

> The actual reality of language-speech is not the abstract system of linguistic forms, not the isolated monologic utterance, and not the psychophysiological act of its implementation, but the social event of verbal interaction implemented in an utterance or utterances. Thus, verbal interaction is the basic reality of language
>
> (Voloshinov 1973, 94).

If we pursue recent work further, then we find that a lot of the ground has been cleared in charting the characteristics of de Saussure's delineation of '*la parole*' as it has been transformed into a notion of discourse.

Language and reality

Let us start with a non-reflective, commonsense statement: 'language names things'. At first sight, this is a statement of an obvious truth. What you are reading at the moment is contained in a thing called a book. Its contents were originally written on a thing called a computer, and that computer rested on a thing called a desk. At this level of commonsense, language has nothing to do with the creation of the things it names. The things pre-exist the naming of them. The same holds for a commonsense view of what science is about: it is a process that seeks to isolate things that exist in reality that, for various reasons, we are unable to perceive with the naked eye, and once isolated—that is, established as having an existence in reality—give a name to. We are not going to dispute this obvious truth at the commonsense level. However, there is more to language than this, and just as physics has gone beyond having 'the thing' as its basic unit, so, too, have people who study language come to realize that there is more to it than just naming things. For example, saying some words can 'do things' (technically, language has a performative aspect): thus, 'I pronounce thee husband and wife' doesn't name something, it *does* something. In a similar way, a number of the differentiated 'things' that physicists trade in were not discovered so as to be labelled: Newton did not discover either 'momentum' or 'gravity', for example. He constructed both as conceptual ways of capturing regularities that were measurable between observable events. A third characteristic of language is that it deals with meanings. That it does so is wonderful, but this also creates problems for the commonsense view, because where science can work away to reveal causal relations amongst elements of the world, meanings don't have causal relations between them. As a consequence of this, one cannot cause someone to change their view, for example, by telling them to. Language doesn't work like that: being pronounced married does not causally result in one's being married; naming a dog doesn't cause other animals to become non-dogs—it certainly implies that there are animals of that non-dog status, but implication is not causation. Words are not in an independent existence of each other, as things can be, but are intimately related to each other, in the sense that no word can exist in isolation. Fourth, implicit in the previous points, is that 'language' doesn't actually exist in reality. We can observe acts of speaking, conversation, monologue, ranting and raving, etc., but we cannot observe 'language'. However, we can construct 'language' as an object, and talk about, and investigate it within that discursive frame of reference.

Fifth, when we observe language in use, we need to recognize that what is said cannot be taken in independence of the context in which it is said. There are a number of important components of context. One of these is situational, because we very often use our surroundings as props to get our meanings across: 'That one over there'. We can also use words that have dictionary meanings in ways that don't match those definitions: 'no?'. And we need to remember that speech is used by people with intonations, inflections, all manner of non-verbal accoutrements, timings, etc., that play a major part in the process of making meanings with each other. Voloshinov (1976, p. 99) gives an example which illustrates this: 'Two people are sitting in a room. They are both silent. Then one of them says "Well!" The other does not respond.' As Voloshinov says,

'For us outsiders this entire "conversation" is utterly incomprehensible': is it even a conversation, we might wonder. It is not just that we cannot hear the intonation with which the word 'Well!' is pronounced, but we lack also the extra-verbal context. In this particular case, we lack the knowledge that the two people were looking out the window as it began to snow, even though it was already May. Both had been expecting spring for some time and were bitterly disappointed by the late snowfall. This extra-verbal context comprises both their physical situation and their shared history, which needs to be known so as to distinguish between their being disappointed that this interminable winter re-intrudes into their hopes of spring as contrasted with ruing the fact that they dusted off and packed their skis last week because they didn't think they could have some fun with them until next winter.

This leads us into the last point we want to make here. Conversations are highly nuanced performances that draw on the discursive resources—sets of ideas and practices—available in a community, and unfold in real time. A conversation is more than an exchange of words, but involves embodied participants intimately responsive to each other in subtle ways that we are only just coming to appreciate (see Shotter, Chapter 5, for an extended treatment). It is unlikely that the second participant in Voloshinov's vignette made no response—at least a slight exhale of resignation is likely—but even if he or she made no overt response, that not-responding, paradoxically will constitute a response. It could be a sharing of dispirited despondency, or a resignation of 'there he/she goes again'. And as such, it will influence where things go next. Conversations have an element of improvisational jazz to them.

Having set the scene here as to why the commonsense view that language names 'things in reality' is obviously true at one level, but that there is more to language than just that, we turn in the next section to considering language as a discursive phenomenon in a little more detail, with an eye to making clear why a discursive perspective is central to understanding the treatment of mental 'illness'.

Discourse

Imagine giving someone directions to a party at your house. You would say something like: 'take the main road towards Littletown; turn left at the third crossroads, and then the third left; go over the bridge, and there are two houses on your left. Ours is the one on the right'. If, however, you were a speaker of Guugu Yimithirr, an Aboriginal language used in north-east Queensland, you would give different directions: 'go north on the Littletown road; turn west at the third crossroads, and then the third south; south of the bridge there are two houses to the east. Ours is the one to the south'. English speakers use an egocentric frame of reference for describing spatial relations; Guugu Yimithirr speakers use an absolute one based on cardinal points. Now, most English speakers can use the absolute system when they go hiking, using a map and compass, but certainly don't in everyday usage; Guugu Yimithirr speakers don't use maps and compasses, and don't have the option of the egocentric frame. If, then, a native English speaker were to attempt to teach a speaker of Guugu Yimithirr to dance a waltz, it is easy to imagine how difficult they might find the task, as specifying which leg to move next, and in which direction, continuously changes as the dancers twirl.

What we have here are two different discourses, in this case spatial ones, which orient their users to features of their world in different ways. These discourses work for their users as a form of 'second-nature', in that a speaker of Guugu Yimithirr is no more able to explain how they know where north is than you would be able to explain how you know this page you are reading is in front of you.

We can select any number of 'real-world objects' and find that they enter into different discourses that construct them as different 'subjects' for their community of users. Consider, for example, the Amazonian rainforest. It can be the subject of an ecological discourse that values it as fundamental to the health of the planet, and therefore must be preserved. It can be the subject of an economic discourse, whereby it is taking up space that could otherwise put to profitable purposes, and therefore it should be destroyed. Again, the way it is taken by the indigenous people who live in it will be quite different. There are a number of points about discourses that are implicit in this example.

First, as Lessa (2006, p. 285), following Foucault (1972), puts it, discourses are 'systems of thoughts composed of ideas, attitudes, courses of action, beliefs and practices that systematically construct the subjects and the worlds of which they speak'.

Second, the '. . .individual elements of a [discursive] system only have significance when considered in relation to the structure as a whole, and that structures are to be understood as self-contained, self-regulated, and self-transforming entities' (Howarth 2000, p. 17).

Third, discourses have the remarkable ability to become 'second nature'. From a biological point of view, whether one is male or female is a naturally-given distinction. However, at the cultural level:

> Being a man/woman involves appropriating gendered behaviours and making them part of the self that an individual presents to others. Repeated over time, these behaviours may be internalized as 'me'—that is, gender does not feel like a performance or an accomplishment to the actor, it just feels like her or his 'natural' way of behaving
>
> (Cameron 2001, p. 17).

It 'feels like' being 'male or female' is 'the way things are meant to be', whereas the norms of gendered behaviour are constructed during socialization out of the possibilities provided by the discourses in which the cultural practices of socialization are embedded. This is not to say that, at root, there may be forces that have acted to bias these practices in particular directions, but that is now somewhat beside the point in present times. 'Real (Western) men' don't eat yogurt, wear eye-shadow, wigs, codpieces, or skirts, but they have in the past, and they could in the future. Appropriateness is normative, not given.

Fourth, a number of these discourses can coexist within a culture at any one point in time. Some may be regarded as orthodox and consequently superior to others. Fifth, and allied to this, different discourses are not rationally distinct from each other, but can be rationally muddled, because they are subject to the powers of rhetorical argument and manipulation in real time, along with the 'naturally-felt rights' that have historically been accorded to some, dominant, discursive constellations at the expense of other, marginalized, ones. This plurality of discourses and their entanglements in modern society is indicative of how complex human activity can be, and why Foucault's coupling of 'power/knowledge' is such an insight into discourse dynamics.

In illustration of these last three points we will take two examples of the treatment of pregnancy as a reason for and against grounds for freedom or imprisonment that have recently been reported in the New Zealand media, and the way these have been treated from different discursive positions. On 25 November 2010, *The Timaru Herald* reported that a 19-year-old woman had pleaded guilty to 'nine charges of ill-treating animals and failing to prevent suffering' in the Oamaru District Court, and sentencing was set for 3 February 2011. *The Timaru Herald*'s reporting of her sentencing is reproduced in Box 1.1.

Box 1.1 *The Timaru Herald*

Pregnancy saved an Oamaru woman who left malnourished and emaciated dogs to starve to death from being sent to jail.

[The defendant] 19, was sentenced to two months' home detention and 100 hours' community work for ill-treating animals and failing to prevent suffering when she appeared in the Oamaru District Court yesterday.

[The defendant] is six months pregnant.

'That fact alone has saved you by the narrowest margin from a sentence of imprisonment,' Judge Paul Kellar said.

The veterinarian who dealt with the case said it was the worst case of animal neglect she had seen in her 19 years in the job, he said. She believed the dogs had been neglected for at least four months.

The abuse occurred when [the defendant] was living in Riversdale, Southland. Police and the SPCA were called to her address on June 8 following complaints from neighbours.

They found several dogs of different ages and breeds in such poor condition that some were barely able to move.

[The defendant] said she had arrived home from visiting Oamaru to find her partner, who was meant to be caring for the dogs, had left.

She found a dead puppy and buried it before heading to Gore to look for her partner.

Police also discovered a small sleepout where five small puppies were housed. It was littered with faeces and urine and had no food or water available.

Nine dogs were located and required urgent veterinarian care.

A Staffordshire pitbull cross was extremely thin with protruding ribs, spine and hip bones and had to be put down.

Two six-week-old puppies were described as 'close to death' from dehydration and hypothermia.

An autopsy on the dead puppy showed it had no food in its stomach or intestines and there were indications it had not been wormed for some time.

The cause of death was attributed to starvation and hypothermia. A second puppy found dead at the address was found to have died of the same causes.

> **Box 1.1 *The Timaru Herald* (continued)**
>
> 'The facts make for somewhat disturbing reading,' Judge Kellar said.
>
> 'There is a photo attached to the summary of facts (that) I wouldn't wish on anybody.'
>
> He said if [the defendant] could not afford to care for the dogs there were other options available.
>
> 'It's perhaps trite that pets depend on their owners to take responsibility for them ... [therefore] owners have got a responsibility to provide at least some of [their basic needs].'
>
> The sentence should highlight 'under no uncertain terms' the abuse was completely unacceptable, he said.
>
> [The defendant] had shown little remorse for the abuse except until Tuesday when she made a $100 donation to the SPCA, he said.
>
> She was disqualified from owning a dog for 10 years.
>
> www.stuff.co.nz/timaru-herald/news/4611437/Pregnant-woman-avoids-jail

Note that the justification as to why she avoided a jail sentence, and thus maintained her liberty, was her pregnancy. It subsequently emerged this was her third conviction stemming from her behaviour in the previous 11 months: the first for assaulting her then partner, the second for drunk driving. In the second example (Box 1.2), reported by the *Sunday Star-Times* on 30 January 2011, pregnancy is used as the justification for remanding the defendant rather than granting her bail. As the Government welfare agency 'Child, Youth and Family Service' noted, they had previously 'removed two children from her care and we don't believe she is capable of caring for this child either', and given 'her history of serious drug abuse, mental health issues and transience' they 'have grave concerns about the wellbeing of her unborn child'.

> **Box 1.2 *Sunday Star-Times***
>
> A lawyer who refused to seek bail for a drug-addicted pregnant client assigned to him is being hailed as a hero.
>
> Child advocate Christine Rankin said lawyer Tony Bouchier's actions were heroic, after he contacted Child, Youth and Family about the case.
>
> Six months pregnant [the defendant], 35, who is on a methadone programme, was charged with possessing instruments for methamphetamine use, and appeared in court last week, after police found her living rough in a garden shed in the Auckland suburb of Glen Innes.
>
> Rotting food, beer bottles, a petrol can and, according to police, needles littered the floor near where she was sleeping. Barefoot and filthy, her urine-soaked trousers allegedly had a rusty razorblade and a used hypodermic needle in the pockets.
>
> She would have been released on bail last Monday but for the efforts of her assigned counsel, Bouchier, who was upset the police declined to apply for detention under the Alcoholism and Drug Addiction Act.

Box 1.2 *Sunday Star-Times* (continued)

'I'm supposed to go and get her bail but I know where she's going to go,' he said. 'I know I'm sticking my neck out to a degree, but morally, I think I'm right.'

'Morally, I think looking out for [the defendant] is looking out for the baby. [The defendant] is not concerned with the baby. [The defendant] is concerned about [the defendant].'

[The defendant] was remanded in custody and Bouchier contacted Child, Youth and Family over the case, but was told that until the baby was born, it was out of their jurisdiction. They would, however, take the baby as soon as it was born.

'We've got 12 agencies under investigation over a horrific child abuse case in West Auckland. This baby is being abused too, but because it's inside her, I couldn't get anyone interested,' Bouchier said.

Rankin said Bouchier's courage in standing up for what was right was 'heroic'. 'That baby will be born an addict,' she said. 'Children seem to be at the end of the line of so many people we protect, and he should be put up as a hero—that he's got the courage to say something.'

On Friday police reapplied for detention under the Alcoholism and Drug Addiction Act, which has a clause that an addict can be detained if they are 'a source of harm, suffering, or serious annoyance to others'.

Bernadine McKenzie, head of Child, Youth and Family, said the agency welcomed the court decision to remand the woman in custody while consideration was given to granting a detention order.

'Her history of serious drug abuse, mental health issues and transience means we have grave concerns about the wellbeing of her unborn child.'

'We have previously removed two children from her care and we don't believe she is capable of caring for this child either. We will lodge an order with the Family Court giving us the ability to remove the child as soon as it is born.'

McKenzie said CYF had been actively working with a number of parties including the police and mental health agencies to do what it could to protect the unborn child. A meeting with the woman's family had been arranged to discuss what support they could provide.

'The safety of the baby is always the paramount consideration. In this case, because of the woman's history, the baby is expected to be removed.'

McKenzie said that unless she was under the age of 17, CYF did not have the legal power to detain a pregnant woman with drug addiction and mental health problems but could work with other agencies to have her detained.

Residents near the shed where [the defendant] was living said she would be straight back on drugs if she was released. A man, who declined to be named, said they noticed her living in the shed around Christmas.

'You could tell she was on something. She could hardly walk. She just looked like a veteran of alcohol abuse.'

[The defendant] returns to court on Tuesday to reapply for bail.

http://www.stuff.co.nz/national/4598137/Lawyer-acts-to-aid-unborn-baby
http://www.stuff.co.nz/sunday-star-times/news/4597591/Lawyer-acts-to-aid-unborn-baby

These two cases have led commentators to bring a number of competing discourses into public debate. We will consider primarily the discourses of 'rights' and 'responsibilities' here as they are invoked by these commentators, but we will also comment on some of the ways the examples of these discourses accomplish their goals. We will thus be concerned with illustrating both macro- and micro-aspects of the particular statements given in invoking these discourses.

With respect to the first case, under the headline 'Produce the licence or forget about reproducing', Michael Laws, a former MP and local authority mayor, puts the view in the *Sunday Star-Times* on 6 February 2011 with respect to the first judgement that:

> in the Oamaru District Court last week a new wrinkle was added to the old question: what is more important—a human life or that of an animal? On this occasion, the animal won . . . She is deemed unworthy to own a dog but a kid is just fine.

He then goes on to use the second case to consolidate his view that:

> in these excessively libertarian times, our society allows rights to people who should not have them in the first place and who are not in a position to exercise them responsibly . . . Having a child should require a test . . . Instead we work on the opposite tangent: have as many kids as you like. But if you want that dog? Prove yourself.

The way out of this dilemma, in Law's' view, is to either 'involuntarily sterilise these pathetic wretches' or to 'offer financial inducements for them not to have children'. He puts forward as part of his argument the case of adoption in New Zealand:

> The adoptive parents are put through a series of tests to determine whether they would be worthy parents. It is a searching examination of not simply the physical environment that will be provided to any child, but the psychological fitness.

Note that there is a surface rhetoric here that has an immediate appeal: being judged fit to have children while being judged unfit to own a dog because of one's serious level of maltreatment of animals is somewhat contradictory. Note also that there is no necessary connection between how one has treated a dog in the past and how one might treat a future child. Note again, then, that once we go beyond the surface of the rhetoric that we are faced with major questions. Who might decide that someone qualifies for involuntary sterilization or financial inducements to that end? On what evidence could such a decision be made?

The second case provides us with additional dilemmas. Who makes decisions? Under New Zealand law, a defence lawyer is obliged to act on behalf of his or her client. It is unusual, then, for a defence lawyer to argue against the release on bail of his client because of concerns for the safety of another individual—even if that other is the client's unborn child. One might expect in such a situation that it is the duty of the Crown Prosecutor or Police to oppose bail. However, since the Justice Department has limited facilities to deal with pregnant addicts, and since the other individual potentially at risk is not, at this point, an independent individual but an intimately dependent responsibility of the accused, there are grounds for their decision not to oppose bail.

What comes out of these cases is that there is little hope of arriving at a distinct, manualized, set of rules for making decisions as to what should be done in what, at a prime facie level, are similar problems: should a pregnant woman be incarcerated or not? It also follows here that there is a difference between making decisions and formulating judgments (a point discussed fully by Shotter, Chapter 5, this volume).

These cases also raise a further concern: the relation between states and the sense that can be made of them. While we have focused on the issue of how the meaning of pregnancy can be judged differently with respect to its meaning in particular situations, this doesn't detract from the categorical determination of whether someone is pregnant or not. The state of pregnancy is clearly determined: a woman either is or is not pregnant, and it is possible to make a mistaken diagnosis. This is the position also taken up by the orthodoxy of treating categories of mental disturbance. That is, there are discrete categories of mental illness that will be universally characteristic of humans. Here we enter something of a minefield. The crucial question is the extent to which the presentation and consequent classification of mental problems is culturally-specific as opposed to universal. Consider, for example, the case of hysteria. Charcot, for example, wrote to Freud in 1888 (cited by Micale, 1993, p. 496) that 'Rest assured, hysteria is coming along, and one day it will occupy gloriously the important place it deserves in the sun'. But by the mid 1970s, the editors of the *British Medical Journal* (1976) described hysterical neuroses as 'a virtual historical curiosity in Britain'. The same might be said of dromomania, or travelling fugue, an uncontrollable psychological urge to wander. Only a handful of cases of such behaviour have been documented, nearly all in France in the late 19th century. The philosopher Ian Hacking (1998), in his study 'Mad Travellers' quotes the notes of the French doctor Philippe Tissie on the case of Albert Dadas:

> It all began one morning last July when we noticed a young man of twenty-six crying in Dr Pitre's ward. He had just come from a long journey on foot and was exhausted, and wept because he could not prevent himself from departing on a trip when the need took him; he deserted his family, work and daily life to walk as fast as he could, straight ahead, sometimes doing 70 km a day on foot until, in the end, he would be arrested for vagrancy and thrown into prison.

Hacking uses these cases to make the case for the manifestation of many mental disorders to be an ecological one, drawing on the metaphor of the ecological niche. Cooper (1999) summarizes his position thus:

> Like biological organisms, Hacking suggests, transient mental disorders can only flourish within a particular environment. While organisms depend on food supplies and breeding sites, mental disorders need a medical community that will recognise them, and a contemporary culture that creates space for them between healthy, virtuous activities on the one hand, and vicious, criminal ones on the other. In the 1890s France provided the perfect environment for fugue. Police controls meant that wandering men would soon be picked up, and the medical community was happy to recognise fugue as a sub-type of either epilepsy or hysteria. At the same time cultural fascination with tourism and vagrancy allowed fugue to thrive in the ambiguous space between.

A similar line has been argued for by the medical historian Edward Shorter (1992). Shorter proposes the notion of 'symptom pools'. Shorter's thesis is that psychosomatic symptoms vary over time as cultures change so as to match the medical diagnoses of the day. If we translate 'symptom pools' into 'discourse resources' then we can see the link to our concern here: that 'anxiety', for example, may at first present itself in an inchoate way, and then take up particular forms as the sufferer takes up the prevalent meanings from the concepts and practices circulating in their particular cultural milieu. Watters (2010) draws on Shorter's formulation with respect to case studies of the relatively recent appearance of anorexia in Hong Kong, and the recent construction of 'depression' in Japan, amongst others, to similarly argue for this cultural moulding and hence presentation of mental problems. We find here, then, a reflection of Whorf's (1956, p. 212) conception of the role of language in cultural life: 'We dissect nature along lines laid down by our native language . . . Language is not simply a reporting device for experience but a defining framework of it.' This is a strong social constructionist thesis: the claim would be that whereas the DSM-IV-TR devotes only a few pages at the end under the heading 'Culture-Bound Syndromes', the preceding 800 plus pages of the major classifications of mental illness should be under the same heading.

A weaker constructionist view has been offered by Guillain (1949, cited by Micale, 1993, p. 496), that, with respect to hysteria, for example, 'in reality, the patients have not changed since Charcot; it is the words to describe them that have changed'. In one sense, this is trivially true: what was 'hysteria' is now divided into the dissociative and somatoform disorders. But even in this weaker sense, there has been a decline in the modern equivalent of hysteria–conversion disorder. The annual incidence of conversion disorders seen by psychiatrists is approximately 22 cases per 100,000 in the mid-20th century (Stephansson et al. 1976), which is a far cry from the 25% of all women claimed by one practitioner in 1859 (Briggs 2000). Tseng (2001) notes that these disorders are mostly associated with cultures that have strict taboos on the direct expression of the emotions in social situations. Conversion symptoms may thus arise as a more acceptable form of non-verbal communication of a forbidden idea or feelings (Schwartz et al. 2001). Conversely, in modern, developed cultures, where there is more open 'psychobabble' and emotional expression, there is less scope for symptoms to develop. This is a 'socio-ecological' point, but one that doesn't challenge the underlying reality of the disorder. The disorder is real, as with smallpox, but the conditions under which it is engendered have been reduced. This notion is likely to be reinforced by studies such as those of Marshall et al. (1997) that demonstrate deviations in brain function for those diagnosed with conversion disorders: it must be real if brains 'have it', mustn't it? But this is where the situation gets quite complex.

Watters (2010) provides, inter alia, a review of the development of a market in Japan by GlaxoKlineSmith, Eli Lilly, and other Western drug companies for selective serotonin reuptake inhibitors (SSRIs). These antidepressant drugs generated massive sales during the 1990s, largely in the USA. Drawing on the work of Kirmayer (e.g. 2001, 2002, 2005) on cross-cultural psychiatry, and his doctoral student Kitanaka (2008), Watters builds an account of the development of a framework in Japanese society of the discursive resources that would align the way the population and its psychiatric profession could reconceive and revalue 'unhappiness' as 'depression', building his case around Kirmayer's point that:

> The clinical presentation of depression and anxiety is a function not only of patients' ethnocultural backgrounds, but of the structure of the healthcare system they find

themselves in and the diagnostic categories and concepts they encounter in mass media and in dialogue with family, friends, and clinicians (2001, cited by Watters 2010, p. 197).

Once these—what we are calling discursive resources—are in place, then, and only then, was it possible for the Japanese to have 'depression' in the sense of a framework that constructs it as something that can be treated as such. The logic here is similar to the phenomenological philosopher Hubert Dreyfus (1967) develops for the role of the body in guiding 'learning'. What a behaviourist would cast as response shaping through reward, Dreyfus (1967, p. 25) unpacks into the phrase 'retroactive need-determination':

> When we experience a need we do not at first know what it is we need. We must search to discover what allays our restlessness or discomfort. This is not found by comparing various objects and activities with some objective, determinate criterion, but through … our sense of gratification. This gratification is experienced as the discovery of what we needed all along, but it is a retroactive understanding and covers up the fact that we were unable to make our need determinate without first receiving that gratification.

Substitute 'discursive resources' for 'gratification', and the parallel with the point we are making here is obvious: when we experience an inchoate unease we need cultural resources to give a form to it (Langer 1953).

In a similar vein, narrative therapists see peoples' lives as storied experiences:

> The structuring of narrative requires recourse to a selective process in which we prune, from our experience, those events that do not fit with the dominant evolving stories that we and others have about us. Thus, over time and of necessity, much of our stock of lived experience goes unstoried and is never told or expressed. It remains amorphous, without organization and without shape
>
> (White and Epston 1990, p.12).

If we put these points about the structuring powers of people using discursive resources and narrative together, then we gain an appreciation that some stories cannot be constructed, some stories cannot be resisted, because there are no resources available for doing this. For example, consider the case of Ian, a 6-year-old who has a nasty temper. This gets him into a lot of conflict with his father, who doesn't believe that boys, especially his, should throw the tantrums that he does: that Ian is a 'spoilt brat'. The conflict is between Ian and his father, and Ian is seen as a problem child. Why does *he* do it? Ian is seen as responsible for his outbursts, and so needs to be held to account over them. He and his father are on opposite sides.

If, however, we linguistically externalize the problem, and talk through with Ian that the problem is not him, or his temper, but 'Mr Angry', who is invisible, and sneaks up on kids because he likes getting them in trouble, then we can start to explore with Ian what makes Mr Angry tick: what is *he* up to; how does he *get* Ian to do these things? Ian, as the insider in all of this, can offer some explanations as to how Mr Angry wants to spoil his relationship with his father, and he finds a way of noticing when and how Mr Angry is able to pick the best times to do that. Ian can begin to fight back at Mr Angry, and not let him get his way. In addition, his father can become his ally in this fight. Ian is no longer a 'spoilt brat', but a brave kid trying to beat Mr Angry with the help of his father. The situation is very different when approached with a different discursive framework.

Discursive therapies

While they have different emphases, the therapeutic perspectives that we are characterizing in this book as 'discursive' share the central points we have introduced above. Discourses construct the objects they talk of, in the sense of pinning down an otherwise inchoate set of human experiences, which could be construed along different dimensions. Discourses are performed, and along with the 'choice of words', the performance of speaking is central to the way conversations proceed. Speaking is not a self-contained activity, but is situated at particular times and places, in particular micro- and macro-contexts. Conversations can be surprising, because their courses cannot be guaranteed by either of the participants at the outset. There's more to talking than meets the ear.

It was Josef Breuer' patient Anna O who coined the phrase 'the talking cure' (Breuer and Freud, 1957/1895), and it became a phrase Freud used to introduce psychoanalysis in his lectures to an American audience at Clark University in 1910 (she also referred to the process she and Breuer were engaged in as 'chimney sweeping', but this description hasn't stuck). Lois Shawver (Chapter 2, this volume) alerts us in her chapter to the changing roles of language in the treatment of people's problems over time. The idea that language might have a central role in sorting through problems is surprisingly recent. As she documents, the role of language in therapeutic work has been, and remains, multifaceted and susceptible to change. In the sense of being multifaceted, language can be used to conceptualize the essence of the problems that can beset people; to describe the various manifestations of these problems; to categorize and diagnose their symptoms; to tell people what to do so as to 'get better'; and so on. It is only late in the day that language has come to be used for the purpose of hearing what sense people themselves make of their problems, and thus the possibility that one goal in therapy might be to assist people in making 'better', or at least a different, sense of these problems, gets opened up.

As family therapist Karl Tomm (1988) suggests, the questions one asks should have something to do with the answers one seeks. This reflexive insight about what therapists can elicit in therapeutic dialogue—via their questions—informs the discursive therapist's efforts to use questions as interventive resources. As Tomm indicates, what matters is what our questions of patients 'bring forth'. When the efforts are to get information alone (symptom accounts, for example) things are back in familiar psychiatric territory. However, when a solution-focused (e.g. deShazer 1985) question gets asked, like 'Suppose your concern resolved itself overnight; what would you be doing differently'—the question itself becomes an invitation to begin to construct a different way of being. Narrative therapists (see Chamberlain, Chapter 6, this volume), in a slightly different manner, invite reflection on linguistically 'externalized' problems, asking questions like 'If anger got the upper hand in your relationship with your kids, where might that take you and your kids?'. These invitations to construct new meanings or deconstruct the taken-for-granted ones in people's lives play a major role in the discursive therapies.

In the next group of chapters in this volume, three of the main contemporary contributors to the general social constructionist (or what we are terming discursive) view consider communication in relation to therapy in various ways. Ken and Mary Gergen (Chapter 4) provide an introduction to the relational view of communication. Their approach has one foot in the tradition begun by Bakhtin, and the other in their relational stance. One of Bakhtin's points (1986, p. 94) was that 'the role of the *others* for whom the utterance is constructed is extremely great . . . From the very beginning, the speaker expects a response from them, an active responsive understanding. The entire utterance is constructed, as it were, in anticipation of encountering this response'. As the Gergens note, saying 'hello' to someone in the street is not just saying something, not a statement, but an act of greeting, which as Bakhtin notes anticipates a response. And as Bakhtin (ibid) again makes clear, many things we might consider as statements have a similar conversational realization:

> The fact is that when the listener perceives and understands the meaning (the language meaning) of speech, he simultaneously takes an active, responsive attitude toward it. He either agrees or disagrees with it (completely or partially), augments it, applies it, prepares for its execution, and so on. And the listener adopts this responsive attitude for the entire duration of the process of listening and understanding.

It is this aspect of speaking with others that gives conversation the constructive nature that the Gergen's accord priority to.

John Shotter's chapter (Chapter 5) takes this constructive concern down to the deep micro-level to focus on the performance of conversations, emphasizing another Bakhtinian point (1986, p. 121) that:

> when one begins to hear voices in language, jargon, and styles, these cease to be potential means of expression and become actual, realised expression; the voice that has mastered them has entered into them. . . . Here one encounters *integral* positions, integral personalities (the personality does not require extensive disclosure—it can be articulated in a single sound, revealed in a single word)

We might revise Shotter's final sentence: 'it is in our *inter*acting that we come to our first understandings, vague though they may be'. But in making this revision, we need to take care to emphasize that we are dealing with embodied interactions that have a spontaneous and expressive character to them. Shotter is moving beyond his nuanced concern with particular examples of therapeutic conversations to sketch a quite radical new stance of performative and ontological constructionism. Rom Harré and Mirjana Dedaić (Chapter 3) provide another micro-level account of language in use, this time through the lens of Harré's 'positioning theory', which provides a framework for considering the way in which rights and duties are actively assigned and contested by the participants in a conversation. After outlining how conversations can be analysed for the ways positions are claimed, contested, and negotiated, they consider two cases of multiple personality from this perspective, and thus directly begin to address the insights their analyses can have in a therapeutic context.

The next section of the book presents overviews of five different schools of therapy that fall under the discursive umbrella. Narrative therapists (see Chamberlain, Chapter 6) take the view that life is best understood and addressed in story-form. In this respect, a personality is a story, as are understandings of relationships, institutions, cultures, and so on. When it comes to concerns presented to therapists, what matters are how these stories' unpreferred plotlines and understandings are sustained, particularly with respect to the identities seemingly assigned. Problems—not people—are the problem is a credo of narrative therapists. Thus, narrative therapists invite patients to reflect on how problem stories acquired their meanings, and how taken for granted understandings and actions might perpetuate them into the future. From such reflection, possibilities to re-author such stories, with more preferred meanings and plotlines, becomes more possible.

Solution-focused brief therapy (SFBT, see Duffy, Chapter 8; and Miller & McKergow, Chapter 9) developed in ways largely associated with Stever de Shazer (e.g. 1985, 1994) and his wife, Insoo Kim Berg (De Jong and Berg, 2007). Influenced by the writings of the Mental Research Institute (Watzlawick et al. 1974), and later by Wittgenstein's view of 'language games', SFBT dialogues focus on client strengths and actionable solutions clients codevelop with therapists. The SFBT therapist's challenge is to plausibly negotiate the client's and conversational focus from 'problem talk', to 'solution talk'. Thus, the therapist's questions and focus become deliberately reflexive with the aim of identifying and mobilizing formerly unheeded resources and competencies.

Collaborative language systems, or as it is currently known, collaborative therapy (see Levin and Bava, Chapter 7) developed from the view that problems coordinate people's understandings and actions, mostly through conversational interaction. In the language of Anderson and Goolishian (1988), 'problem-organizing systems' develop and the therapeutic challenge is to engage in problem-dissolving conversations. Most people have had the experience of having a concern somehow dissolve in good conversation, as new possibilities overtake former seemingly intractable concerns. In Collaborative therapy such conversations do not happen using specific techniques, but are hosted or facilitated according to important discursive principles of practice. Collaborative therapists provide an important postmodern update to the client-focused therapy of Carl Rogers (1961; see Anderson's 2001 update).

Social therapy originated from the group and community work of analytic philosopher Fred Newman and Vygotskian developmental psychologist Lois Holzman (Chapter 10). Their unique hybrid of the ideas of Marx, Vygotsky, and later Wittgenstein (cf., Newman and Holzman, 1997) came to inform an improvisational, 'performative' approach to therapeutic process and change. Social therapists facilitate group and community development processes though the question of 'method' is a central challenge to be addressed by members of each group or community. Social therapists do not provide the methods of change; they invite group and community members to articulate problems, and then improvise ways of getting beyond the meanings and actions that sustained problems as they had been understood. To paraphrase Newman and Holzman, 'we continually become who we are by acting in ways we aren't'. Just therapy (see Maniapoto, Chapter 12; Waldegrave, Chapter 11) developed from a recognition that Euro-American approaches to therapy often run counter to indigenous populations' traditions, and are practised in ways that can obscure or perpetuate social injustices. Just therapists therefore are engaged in welcoming the traditions and ways of knowing patients bring to therapy, while inviting critical reflection upon, and collective action in addressing, forms of social injustice. For this reason, much of their work is focused on community development and in reconnecting patients to the communities and traditions from which they may have become estranged.

In the final section of the book we have included chapters on two issues. The first is whether the approaches that we are introducing here under the term 'the discursive therapies' are effective. On the face of it, this appears a fairly straightforward question with an obvious route to establishing the answer: do people 'get better' after a course of 'treatment'. However, at a practical level, as Ron Chenail and his collaborators point out (Chapter 13), actually pursuing this question is not quite as straightforward as it might first appear. Despite the difficulties that they tease out as endemic to conducting such an endeavour, they do offer us the most comprehensive and synthetic review of the studies relevant to this question.

Robbie Busch (Chapter 14) then sets out a number of challenges for the whole evaluative project. His starting point is that the evaluation of a practice depends on the nature of the evidence available to be judged, and that: (a) evidence is not of itself self-evident; and (b) that it is necessary to be clear when evaluating something that making judgements and making decisions are different activities (a point also developed by Shotter, Chapter 5). The issues here are difficult and challenging, and can be appreciated if we indulge in a thought experiment and some hypothetical questions. Suppose a pharmaceutical cure for schizophrenia was developed, and it was recognized as a cure because former patients no longer heard voices. What would be the effect of this upon someone who had been a long-term sufferer? How would they make sense of their situation? Might the silence drive them mad? If it did, what would the diagnosis be? If the drug treatment had returned them to 'normal' neurological and physiological functioning, then presumably there is 'nothing wrong with them'. Would it be necessary to turn their situation into a new psychiatric condition: 'post-schizophrenic disorder'? Or might we start thinking that what is needed here is to explore how these 'cured' people might be helped to make new understandings and better sense of their situation? And what kind of evidence would we be looking for to decide whether our therapeutic interventions were effective in helping them do this?

The second topic considered in these concluding chapters almost takes us full circle, by returning to the divide that has been present throughout this introductory chapter: the very different ontologies underwriting the medical contextualization of therapy as compared to the discursive conceptualization of therapy. The relation between causes and meanings as forms of explanation has a long and unsettled history. A definitive resolution of this relation is not made any easier once discourse and brains are added to the mix: but attaining such a lofty goal is not our concern here. What is most important in the present context is that a bridge over a long-standing divide might be established.

This divide is rooted in Karl Jaspers early attempts to synthesize an adequate portrayal of psychopathology in his 1913 paper 'Causal and "meaningful" connections between life history and psychosis'. Jaspers arguments were for a hybrid stance towards mental health, disorders, or illnesses. On the one hand, he argued for a biological base to many of these conditions, such that they could be better treated once their underlying causes were appreciated (herein the roots of the modern fascination with diagnosis and pharmacological treatment). On the other hand, he maintained that a practitioner needed to be able 'to "understand" the individual patient's experiences' (Fulford et al. 2006, p. 169). To this end, Jaspers drew heavily on Husserl's conceptualization of phenomenology (e.g. 1912, see also Fulford et al. 2006, pp.160–238). The discursive therapies, drawing from different intellectual bases, set this question of the hybrid nature of practice in a new frame.

We need be wary here, having already raised the topics of 'culture wars' and the different ways that members of the 'opposing sides' would regard the use of language with respect to 'experience' (or reality in general). From a discursive perspective, drawing from both Bakhtin and the deconstructionist strand of continental philosophy, we don't speak language, language speaks through us, and constitutes 'us' on its way through. The notion of selves having 'pure experiences' that 'language' truthfully labels and describes, or of grasping an objective, external reality, is just that in this perspective—a notion. The finding of particular neurological disturbances is one thing: the construction and understanding of them *as they are lived* is not in a one-to-one relation with them (see Duffy, Chapter 15). There is, in this reconceptualization, a fertile ground for progressing towards the hybrid science that Jaspers, and more recently Harré (e.g. 2003; see also Cromby, Chapter 16) have envisioned.

References

American Psychiatric Association (1994). *Diagnostic and Statistical Manual of Mental Disorders*. Washington, DC, APA.

Anderson, H. (2001). Postmodern collaborative and person-centered therapies: what would Carl Rogers say? *Journal of Family Therapy*, **23**, 339–59.

Anderson, H. and Goolishian, H. (1988). Human systems as linguistic systems. *Family Process*, **27**, 371–93.

Bakhtin, M. M. (1984). *Problems of Dostoevsky's poetics* (C. Emerson, Ed. and Trans.). University of Michigan Press, Minneapolis, MN.

Bakhtin, M. M. (1986). *Speech genres and other late essays* (V. W. McGee, Trans.). University of Texas Press, Austin, TX.

Bazeman (1988). Shaping written knowledge: The genre and activity of the experimental article in science, University of Wisconsin Press, Madison, WI. [Quoted by Shotter, 1993, p. 157.]

Behbehani, A. M. (1983). The smallpox story: Life and death of an old disease. *Microbiological Reviews*, **47**, 455–509.

Breuer, J. and Freud, S. (1957/1895). *Studies on hysteria*. (J. Strachey, Ed. and trans.), Basic Books, New York. Originally (1895) *Studien über hysterie*. Franz Deuticke, Leipzig + Wien 1895.

Briggs, L. (2000). The race of hysteria: 'Overcivilization' and the 'savage' woman in late nineteenth-century obsterics and gynecology. *American Quarterly*, **52**(2), 246–73.

British Medical Journal (1976). The search for a psychiatric Esperanto. *British Medical Journal*, **2**, 600–1.

Cameron, D. (2001). *Working with spoken discourse*. Sage, London.

Cooper, R (1999). *Review: Mad Travellers*. Metapsychology on-line reviews. http://metapsychology.mentalhelp.net/poc/view_doc.php?type=book&id=125. (Accessed 22 March 2011.)

Coulehan, J. L. and Block, M. (2005). *The medical interview: Mastering skills for clinical practice* (5th Revised ed). F. A. Davis Company, Philadelphia, PA.

De Cock, K. M. (2001). The eradication of smallpox: Edward Jenner and the first and only eradication of a human infectious disease. *Nature Medicine*, **7**, 15–6.

DeJong, P., & Berg, I.K. (2007). *Interviewing for solutions* (2nd ed.). Brooks Cole, Pacific Grove, CA.

De Shazer, S. (1985). *Keys to solution in brief therapy*. Norton, New York.

De Shazer, S. (1994). *When words were originally magic*. Norton, New York.

Dreyfus, H. (1967). Why computers must have bodies in order to be intelligent. *Revue of Metaphysics*, **21**, 13–32.

Foucault, M. (1972). *The archaeology of knowledge*. Pantheon, New York.

Fulford, K.W.M., Thornton, T., and Graham, G. (2006). *Oxford textbook of philosophy and psychiatry*. Oxford University Press, Oxford.

Gergen, K. J. (1994). *Realities and relationships: Soundings in social construction*. Harvard University Press, Cambridge, MA.

Guillain, G. (1949). *La Semaine des hôpitaux* de Paris, **xxv**(4), 147–60.

Hacking, I. (1998). *Mad travellers: Reflections on the reality of transient mental illness*. Harvard University Press, Cambridge, MA.

Harré, R. (1983). *Personal being*. Blackwell, Oxford.

Higgins, D. (1978). *A dialectic of centuries: Notes towards a theory of the new arts*. Printed Editions, New York.

Howarth, D. (2000). *Discourse*. Open University Press, Buckingham.

Jaspers, K. (1912/1968). The phenomenological approach in psychopathology. *British Journal of Psychology*, **114**, 1313–23.

Jaspers, K. (1913/1974). Causal and 'meaningful' connections between life history and psychosis. In S. R. Hirsch and M. Shepherd (Eds.) *Themes and variations in European psychiatry*, pp. 80–93. Wright, Bristol.

Kirmayer, H. (2001). Cultural variations in the clinical presentation of depression and anxiety: Implications for diagnosis and treatment. *Journal of Clinical Psychiatry*, **62**, 22–30.

Kirmayer, H. (2002). Psychopharmacology in a globalizing world: The use of antidepressants in Japan. *Transcultural Psychiatry*, **39**, 295.

Kirmayer, H. (2005). Culture, context and experience in psychiatric diagnosis. *Psychopathology*, **38**, 192–6.

Kitanaka, J. (2008). Diagnosing suicides of resolve: Psychiatric practice in contemporary Japan. *Culture, Medicine and Psychiatry*, **32**, 152–76.

Koplow, D. A. (2003). *Smallpox: The fight to eradicate a global scourge*. University of California Press, Los Angeles, CA.

Langer, S. K. (1953). *Feeling and form*. New York, Scribner.

Lessa, I. (2006). Discursive struggles within social welfare: Restaging teen motherhood. *British Journal of Social Work*, **36**(2), 283–98.

McHale, B. (1987). *Postmodernist fiction*. Routledge, London.

McHale, B. (1992). *Constructing postmodernism*. Routledge, London.

MacIntyre, A. (1981). *After virtue*. University of Notre Dame Press, South Bend.

Marshall, J.C., Halligan, P.W., Fink, G.R., Wade, D.T., and Frackowiak, R.S.J. (1997). The functional anatomy of a hysterical paralysis. *Cognition*, **64**, B1–B8.

Micale, M.S. (1993). A study in the clinical deconstruction of a diagnosis. *Isis*, **84**, 496–526.

National Alliance on Mental Illness (2011). *Mental illness*. http://www.nami.org/template.cfm?section=about_mental_illness. (Accessed 26 March 2011.)

Newman, F. and Holzman, L. (1997). *The end of knowing*. Routledge, New York.

Riedel, S. (2005). Edward Jenner and the history of smallpox and vaccination. *Baylor University Medical Center Proceedings*, **18**, 21–25.

Rogers, C (1961). *On becoming a person*. Houghton Mifflin, Boston, MA.

Rorty, R. (1980). *Philosophy and the mirror of nature*, Basil Blackwell, Oxford.

Rosenhan, D. (1973). On being sane in insane places. *Science*, **179**, 250–8.

Saussure, F. de. (1916/1977). *Cours de linguistique générale* (C. Bally and A. Sechehaye, Eds. with the collaboration of A. Riedlinger, Lausanne and Paris: Payot; W. Baskin, Trans.) *Course in general linguistics*, Fontana/Collins, Glasgow.

Schwartz, A., Calhoun, A., Eschbich, C., and Seeling, B. J. (2001). Treatment of conversion disorder in an African American Christian woman: cultural and social considerations. *American Journal of Psychiatry*, **158**, 1385–91.

Shorter, E. (1992). *From paralysis to fatigue: A history of psychosomatic illness in the modern era*. Free Press, New York.

Shotter, J. (1993). *Conversational realities: Constructing life through language*. Sage London.

Snow, C. P. (1960). *The two cultures*. Cambridge University Press, Cambridge.

Stephansson, J. G., Messina, J. S., and Meyerowitz, S. (1976). Hysterical neurosis, conversion type: clinical and epidemiological considerations. *Acta Psychiatrica Scandinavica*, **53**, 119–38

Szasz, T. (1960). The myth of mental illness. *American Psychologist*, **15**, 113–18.

Tomm, K. (1988). Interventive interviewing: Part III. Intending to ask lineal, circular, reflexive or strategic questions? *Family Process*, **27**, 1–15.

Tseng, W. (2001). *Handbook of cultural psychiatry*. Academic Press, San Diego, CA.

Voloshinov, V.N. (1973). *Marxism and the philosophy of language* (L. Matejka and I.R. Titunik, Trans.). Harvard University Press, Cambridge, MA.

Voloshinov, V.N. (1976). *Freudianism* (I. R. Titunik, Trans.). Indiana University Press, Bloomington, IN.

Watters, E. (2010). *Crazy like us: The globalization of the American psyche*. Free Press, New York.

Watzlawick, P., Weakland, J., and Fisch, R. (1974). *Change: Principles of problem formation and problem resolution*. Norton, New York.

White, M. and Epston, D. (1990). *Narrative means to therapeutic ends*. WW Norton, New York.

Whorf, B. (1956). *Language, thought, and reality: Selected writings of Benjamin Lee Whorf* (J. B. Carroll Ed.). MIT Press, Cambridge, MA.

World Health Organization (2011) *Smallpox*. http://www.who.int/mediacentre/factsheets/smallpox/en/

Chapter 2

Talking to listen: its pre-history, invention, and future in the field of psychotherapy

Lois Shawver

There is something we therapists do in our offices that is in serious need of a name. Without a name, we can hardly discuss it, write about it, or even search for it on the Internet. For now, I call this something simply 'talking to listen'. Talking to listen in the practice of psychotherapy is the subject of this chapter.

What do we do when we talk to listen? Sometimes we ask questions so as to hear the answers. We might also offer invitations for a client to talk, such as 'Feel free to talk about whatever is on your mind'. We might talk to listen with a command such as 'Tell me what you're thinking', or by wondering out loud as in, 'I wonder how you decided he resented you'. We can talk to listen with a ruse such as, 'I bet you don't know the answer to this'. There are countless ways for creative therapists to talk to listen, even ways that are not yet invented.

I, and some of my friends, believe that how a therapist talks to listen affects the very culture of therapy, gives it a conversational or hierarchical style, fosters intensive engagement or a soothing of emotions. It can speed up the process, or slow it down. It can be appreciated by some clients and not so much by others. There are also special cases that call for better methods of talking and listening. Consider the silent and sullen adolescent, for example.

We would probably all be better therapists if we improved our understanding of the dynamics of talking to listen. But for that to happen, we must notice that we are doing it and that it is part of the therapy that we provide. My own awakening to this concept occurred when I ran across a passage in a philosophy book that mentioned it—although in different words. The author said:

> For us [in western culture], a language is first and foremost someone talking. But there are [forms of language] in which the important thing is to listen, in which the rule deals with audition . . . one speaks only inasmuch as one listens, that is, one speaks as a listener, and not as an author
>
> (Lyotard 1999, pp. 71–2).

I posted this passage in an online community of therapists and, after some discussion, it quickly made sense to some of us. Lynn Hoffman responded with an enthusiasm that further stirred my thinking, as did Tom Strong and many others. And the more we talked about it, the more interested in the new topic I became, and now the concept has slowly begun to appear in the literature.

Tom Strong soon mentioned the concept in an article I liked (Strong 2002). I have mentioned it in a prior chapter (Shawver 2004). I have also noticed that several people have referred to our mention of talking to listen (Bott 2002; Fredman 2004; Haydon 2004; Hoffman 2002, p. 245; Launer 2006; Reynolds 2007; Roth 2004) So it seems that the previously unmentioned concept is gradually coming into view. However, I believe that this is the first article or chapter devoted entirely to the concept of talking to listen.

I should tell you that we therapists who have pioneered the new concept have not always called it talking to listen. Multiple terms for concepts are common and good. The term 'talking' itself has many substitutes (think of 'speaking', 'saying', and 'mentioning' as alternatives for the word 'talking'). We use all these terms in daily speech without misunderstanding. Talking to listen also has alternatives. 'Talking in order to listen', is an example of an alternative, as is 'speaking to listen'. Your ear will likely recognize these phrases as synonyms once you are comfortable with the concept because all these alternatives are based on combinations of words you know and combine in various ways.

Not so with another term we have used for talking to listen. The new term is 'tiotol'. Joe Pfeffer, a colleague and member of our online community, said we should pronounce the term 'tea-yodel', and that has stuck in our minds. 'Tiotol' can serve as a verb (replacing 'talking to listen') but the word also makes a handy noun, as in 'That's an interesting tiotol I hadn't heard before'. Many of the references above refer to the talking to listen concept with the alternative term 'tiotol'. I have come to think of tiotol as a kind of nickname for talking to listen.

This new concept of talking to listen has interested some of us because we are convinced that tiotoling constitutes much of what we therapists do today and, that being the case, it is puzzling that it has not been named and talked about until very recently. To me, it's as odd as if there were a special spice without a name. One sprinkled it liberally, but never mentioned that one did.

Therefore, I have organized my research around the question: Why have we therapists been slow to notice that much of what we do is talking to listen?

My research, I believe, will throw considerable light on this question and yet leave blank spaces that can be filled in by anyone with similar interests. Even more, I hope my findings awaken your eyes, as they did mine, to this rich dimension of therapeutic dialogue.

Before talking to listen began

The historical context: when the humanity of lunatiks was invisible

This tour through history begins at the end of the 1700s when Europe still had one foot firmly planted in the dark superstition of the Middle Ages and one foot planted in cultural reform. It was a time when leprosy had all but disappeared and so it seemed, to this self-transforming culture, that a natural thing to do was to use the buildings that had been built for lepers for another purpose (Foucault 2009, p. 6).

So it was that mad houses began to be common throughout Europe. They were to provide convenient housing for 'lunatiks'. These asylums were used mostly by the well-to-do to house the embarrassing members of their families. While the families paid for this housing, the expense was also shared by the public who paid to gawk at the pathetic people who lived there. Being a 'mad doctor' (as it was called) was a lucrative business (Andrews and Scull 2003). And while there was little reflection on the causes of 'madness' it was typical to presume it was caused by demon possession or other magical forces, such as a full moon.

By our standards, these mad houses were miserable places housing innocent people. The lunatiks were much worse off than the average prisoner today. In the 1700s, the 'mad' were typically kept naked and chained, usually by an ankle to a stake in the floor. They had no toileting facilities, of course, and only scanty food and perhaps a straw bed. When they screamed, or otherwise expressed themselves inconveniently, guards would douse them with cold water, beat them, and further restrain them (Kraepelin 1962, p. 79; Marx 1991/2008). There were no laws restricting what harm the guards could cause (Foucault 2009, p. 49) because, 'It was common currency until the late eighteenth century that the mad could put up indefinitely with the miseries of existence' (Foucault 2009, p. 148).

This very sad phase of the pre-history of talking-to-listen lasted until near the end of the 1700s.

Then came Pinel.

The compassionate moralists: Pinel and Heinroth

At the dawn of the 1800s, several therapists began not only to care about their patients' well-being but also to advocate for them. While it is true that they showed only the flimsiest signs of talking to listen, I believe they had an amazing impact on the emergence and evolution of therapist interest in listening, and thus, eventually, in talking in order to listen to their patients—and so these mad doctors became a key part of my story.

Philippe Pinel (1745–1826)

The idea of using compassion to treat lunatiks began with Philippe Pinel, a French doctor who became famous for freeing many of the lunatiks from their chains and finding that they were not nearly so dangerous as had been imagined. In fact, for the most part, he stopped calling them lunatiks and started calling them 'patients'.

In his celebrated book, *A Treatise on Insanity* (*Traité medico-philosophique*) 1801/1806/1809), Pinel specifically advocated compassionate treatment. He called his methods 'kind treatment' or 'moral treatment' and maintained that such treatment sometimes produced a permanent 'cure'. His moral treatment consisted of teaching patients to be moral, for immorality (indecency), so thought Pinel, was what had most often caused their insanity in the first place. His methods sometimes consisted of playing theatrical tricks on his patients to get them to behave (Goldstein 1987), but tricks were to be played with compassion because of their illness.

Nevertheless, Pinel's compassion had limits. When patients were not cured, Pinel would permit them to be chained or 'intimidated' although, for him, intimidation was only permissible if it was done without violence (Pinel 1806, pp. 63–6).

Is there evidence that Pinel talked to listen? Very little. However he did say he talked with his patients, which was a considerable advance over the traditional practice of doctoring the mad. Once Pinel mentioned that he talked with a particular patient 'in order to console or amuse him' (Pinel 1806, p. 57). Still, he did not mention listening, or describe anything I would call talking to listen to a patient.

In reading him, it is easy to see that Pinel was trying to improve his patients' lives whereas the mad-doctors before him had merely constrained them. In contrast, Pinel's conscience had somehow been awakened. More importantly, Pinel inspired others, awakened their consciences, and thus increased the likelihood that one of his followers would be interested in listening, a definite pre-requisite for having any interest at all in tiotoling patients.

Johann Christian Heinroth (1773–1843)

Among the doctors whom Pinel inspired was Heinroth. Heinroth was a whole generation younger than Pinel and wrote in a different language. However, I imagine him starting the notes for his two-volume set soon after reading Pinel. Pinel's masterpiece was published in 1801 and updated in 1809. Heinroth's important two-volume work (Heinroth, 1818/1975) was published just 9 years after the update. Moreover, Pinel was still a current figure in psychiatry at the time Heinroth started writing his book.

Pinel's ideas echo continuously through Heinroth's work making it clear that he was very influenced by Pinel. He called Pinel 'gallant' and cited him frequently, sometimes argued against him, but never without respect. Clearly Heinroth accepted much of what Pinel taught or mentored: that the inmates should be called patients not lunatiks, that their derangement was caused by immorality, and that they could sometimes be cured. And like Pinel, Heinroth was a moralist who provided 'moral treatment' which instructed the patient as to proper moral behaviour.

Still, there were differences. Whereas both doctors stressed the need for friendly and humane treatment, Heinroth's own theories stressed the need for the doctor to be a conspicuously inspiring character. In fact, Heinroth recommended that doctors develop such an inspiring presence that they could seem to the patient to be a 'visible God' (Heinroth 1975, pp. 337–65). From the position of a 'visible God' the doctor would have enough authority, so he reasoned, to have a positive effect on the patient. To enhance this influence, Heinroth recommended that the doctor put a little condescension in his voice, in order to maximize his power to persuade.

Did Heinroth talk to listen to his patients? He seems to have tried at times, but he felt that 'A man who is out of his senses cannot be interrogated at all, but should be merely observed' (Heinroth 1975, p. 399). Nevertheless, every attempt was made to provide a diagnosis, often on the basis of minute study of files containing information provided by witnesses.

There were many diagnostic categories that he suggested, categories such as 'foolish' or 'apathetic with or without idiocy', and each diagnosis was associated with its own recommended treatment. Sometimes Heinroth offered hope as treatment (Heinroth 1975, p. 367). Other treatment methods included bloodletting, or even 'letting the patient go hungry'. Once Heinroth even listed 'wait and see' as the recommended treatment.

There was only very indirect evidence that Heinroth ever listened to clients as part of his treatment. However, perhaps there was one type of patient he tiotoled, those whom he diagnosed as 'quietly insane'. For such a patient, Heinroth thought the doctor should try to 'penetrate into the innermost soul of the patient and be perfectly familiar with it if he is to be of any use at all' (Heinroth, 1975, pp. 369–370). Although Heinroth did not describe how he managed to 'penetrate the patient's innermost soul' I speculate that this could have involved talking to listen to them—but my evidence is scanty and Heinroth might just have tried to penetrate the patient's soul with his God-like presence rather than a tiotol.

While there was little if any evidence that Pinel and Heinroth (the moralist doctors) talked to listen to their patients as part of their therapy, I do not doubt the importance of their 'compassionate revolution' for the eventual development of different talking to listen styles. The theories of these moralists were carried forwards for a long time. Isaac Ray did much to spread the belief that the insane were morally blind (Ray 1843; Clanon et al. 1982) and thus in need of a treatment based on kindness. A full century after Pinel and Heinroth wrote, the then famous Paul Dubois spoke positively of both of them, saying of Pinel that his work was 'of a man of genius, who gave to the whole science of psychiatry, a new direction, and was a century ahead of his contemporaries' (Dubois 1909, p. 97).

In summary, Pinel and Heinroth brought a dawning of 'compassion' towards mental patients and started the whole process of rethinking how to treat mental patients with understanding and generosity. Also, as the moralist doctors communicated their increasing interest and curiosity about the inner life of mental patients, they no doubt awakened the interest of other doctors in hearing what their patient might have to say.

Quick fix treatments: George Miller Beard, Silas Weir Mitchell, Émile Coué

The year is now about 1879. Queen Victoria will rule England for another 20 or so years, the American Civil War has been over for almost 15 years, and antiseptics are just beginning to be used to prevent surgical infection. Regarding treatment of the mentally ill, the moral treatment that Pinel and Heinroth contributed to is now flourishing. It has become the dominant form of treatment.

However, something quite new was about to splash onto the scene: an entirely new mental illness no one had ever heard of before.

And within a short time there are at least three separate and competing treatments for this new illness, and these treatments, too, had never before been known. All three of these treatments are flashy new remedies, easy to administer, easy to accept, and very stylish—and their popularity just explodes. You can still see traces of these treatments in our own culture today, although the fashion has definitely faded.

George Miller Beard (1839–1883)

George Beard brought a dramatic shift in the public's understanding of mental illness. A prolific and popular medical writer on topics ranging from hay fever to sea sickness, he gained his reputation when he began publishing about a new form of mental illness.

Beard told his readers that this new illness was caused by the times, and he named this new illness 'neurasthenia'. He also called it 'nervousness', and sometimes spoke of it as 'nervous exhaustion' or 'nervous breakdown'.

What was dramatically different about this new mental illness was that it wasn't thought to be caused by moral shame for indecent acts, as the moralists believed. Those suffering from neurasthenia, so Beard explained, had simply exhausted their supply of nerve energy by overworking. This, he said, was the natural result of industrialization. Numerous other authors picked up on these flashy new concepts and the public at large embraced them. It seems that everyone was ready to take the treatments that did not shame them, cutting-edge treatments that promised them brand new tanks of energy.

Moreover, this popular new illness had 'simple fixes'. Beard himself invented the first of these treatments (Beard 1894). You can picture how the treatment worked by looking at the cover of one of his books. There you can find a large line-drawing illustrating the treatment. It involved the patient wearing a skull cap with wires hanging out of it, each connecting to a single large battery. This electrical energy, it seemed to Beard, could flow into the brain where it was to replenish a person's energy supply. Such a treatment was no doubt more credible then than it would be now because the general public, at that time, had little experience with electricity. It would be another year before Edison would produce a practical light bulb and make the use of electricity more evident to everyone (Durgin 1912, p. 120). Fortunately, the electrical current Beard used was quite low.

Did Beard talk to listen to his patients? It is hard for me to imagine him doing so while he was attempting to pass electricity through people's heads. And, not surprisingly, I could find no evidence that he talked to listen to any of his patients.

Silas Weir Mitchell (1829–1914)

A few years later, Silas Mitchell invented another popular treatment for neurasthenia: it consisted of prescribing a short period of rest in a luxurious facility that Mitchell called a 'rest home'. (These rest homes developed a different connotation later in the 20th century.) In Mitchell's time, rest homes were used mostly by the wealthy and they quickly became a symbol of prosperity for the 'wealthy overworked'. Thus, it appears to have become a coveted status symbol. His book explaining the need for such rest homes sold many copies and went through numerous editions (Mitchell and Kimmel 2004).

Whereas moralists like Pinel and Heinroth were compassionate towards mental patients, the mental patients of this new 'quick fix' era were no longer stigmatized as indecent, so they did not need, or particularly want, compassion. The patients who went to rest homes only talked to their doctors to obtain a prescription for a rejuvenating rest. The treatment in the rest homes was performed by attendants, not doctors. The attendants' jobs were to provide as much rest as possible, and not to talk with or otherwise engage the patients.

I suspect rest home patients were sometimes 'cured' by the boredom that soon developed. At any rate, it seems clear that the referring doctors for this quick fix treatment did not bother, or perceive a need to bother, to listen to patients, much less to talk to them to in order to listen more.

Émile Coué (1857–1926)

The third cure, and the most widely practised treatment for neurasthenia, was called 'suggestion'. The notion of suggestion grew out of the concept of 'post-hypnotic suggestion'. (A post-hypnotic suggestion happened, you might recall, when hypnotizers told subjects they would do certain things after awakening from their trance, and then, if the suggestion 'worked', the subjects did as suggested.) Émile Coué's contribution to suggestion theory was the idea that suggestion caused people to change even without actually hypnotizing them. This new kind of suggestion required nothing other than an authority (such as a doctor) to tell the patient that they would get better, or that they would be cured—even if the authority actually believed the patient would die (see Meyer 1980; Walsh 1912, p. 186). In addition, Dr Coué soon claimed that many patients could be taught to cure themselves just by reciting mantras like 'Every day, in every way, I'm getting better and better'.

Both versions of Coué's suggestion technique, the doctor-cure and self-cure variety, became highly popular and spilled over into all walks of life as a method for managing both mental and physical problems (Meyer 1980). Suggestion theory still exists in our thought processes today, but today it is also criticized (e.g. Ehrenreich 2009).

In spite of the fact that suggestion doctors almost certainly did not talk to listen to their patients, I speculate that by removing some of the shame from having a mental problem, they made the public at large more comfortable with the idea of telling their doctors about their personal problems.

Then came Sigmund Freud.

Digging deep with a tiny shovel: Sigmund Freud, Hugo Münsterberg

Now, once again, another important model of mental therapy was emerging: Freudian psychoanalysis. I call Freudian psychoanalysis 'digging deep with a tiny shovel' because Freudians tiotoled just a tiny bit, but they tried to use this tiny tiotol to dig deep into the Unconscious, and thus they became a part of this history of tiotol.

Sigmund Freud (1856–1939)

Freud devised his single standard tiotol that was to take place in the first session. I think of it as a 'domino tiotol'. Just as a row of dominos set on their edge can all fall down by just touching the first one, so Freud's domino tiotol was given to initiate the patient's free flow of voiced thoughts from the beginning of the next session to the end of the last session. The tiotol instruction went like this:

> Your talk with me must differ in one respect from ordinary conversation. Whereas usually you rightly try to keep the threads of your story together here you must proceed differently. You will be tempted to say to yourself: 'This or that has no connection here, or it is quite unimportant, or it is nonsensical, so it cannot be necessary to mention it.' Never give in to these objections. Say whatever goes through your mind. Act as if you were sitting at the window of a railway train and describing the changing views you see outside
> (Freud 1913, 1953, p. 355)

In the next session, the patient took a position on the chaise, and Freud took his position behind the patient. The idea was for him to avoid influencing the flow of the patient's thoughts completely, because, so he thought, the free flow of thoughts in these 'free associations' would enable the analyst to make sense of what the Unconscious needed to say about its desires. That is, Freud's initial tiotol was a technique intended to penetrate the patient's darkest secrets and unmentionable desires—secrets and desires that were almost always sexual and usually indecent, adulterous, or scandalous, and to learn of these desires before the patient knew of them.

Once the psychoanalyst had detected the Unconscious ideas, the job was to 'interpret' them, which meant informing the patient of what indecent acts they unconsciously craved to commit. Such an interpretation was meant to liberate the patient to recognize the truths of his or her unconscious desires. It was not to be stated until the analyst thought the patient was ready to hear it, which sometimes took a very long time.

Notice that there is a similarity between Freud's and Heinroth's ideas. Both of them believed that shameful indecencies were the cause of the mental illness. Heinroth may have thought these indecencies were actual incidents that had happened whereas Freud thought they could be just Unconscious desires to commit 'indecent acts', but they both saw that people in their treatment were fearing and hiding the shame and guilt that was causing their mental illness. For Heinroth, the cure of indecent actions was the Godlike appearance and authority of the therapist. For Freud, it was rather similar. He thought that cure was possible because the patient saw the doctor as a father figure (through transference).

So, in his own subtle way Freud was a 'moralist', a point made earlier by Phillip Rieff (1959/1961). For Freud, like the moralists before him, any curative effect his work provided the patient, was a cure of symptoms caused by unconscious shames and indecent thoughts. Nevertheless, unlike the moralists before him, Freud wanted to listen and though he mostly merely listened, rather than sometimes talking to listen, he has a place in this history. At least, Freud did listen, and he tiotoled each patient at least once.

But why is it that other therapists of this time did not talk to listen?

Hugo Münsterberg (1863–1916)

There is a remarkable clue as to why therapists did not tiotol which is contained in a small passage of a book by Hugo Münsterberg, an American contemporary and an admirer of Freud.

Almost unknown today, Hugo Münsterberg was a well-known figure in his time. He was President of the American Psychological Association in 1898. In 1909, he published a book named *Psychotherapy*. It was an early use of the term 'psychotherapy' and it was a quite complete account of what was counted as psychotherapy at that time.

As a therapist, Münsterberg was apparently eclectic, using moralist persuasion of patients on the one hand, and suggestion therapy on the other in his therapy process. But what made him deserve a place in my history was that he was the only author I found who spent a few sentences explaining (in different terms) why a therapist should not 'talk-to-listen', that while talking to listen was appropriate for a neighbour or a friend, it was inappropriate, he thought, to do with a therapy patient.

Münsterberg (1909, p. 11) explained that in friendly conversation with friends and neighbours he wanted to understand the content of what was being said to see if he agreed with it. In contrast, when he wanted to understand his patients' words, he was looking to understand their 'inner nature', and he was not at all interested in determining if he agreed with what was being said (Münsterberg 1909, pp. 13–15).

This idea of listening to hear the Unconscious was an idea Münsterberg took from Freud. Of course, patients would sometimes talk about the world and practical problems, but Münsterberg, like Freud, took that aspect of the patient's remarks as a kind of noise which a good psychotherapist should ignore in order to discover the hidden problem that was not explicitly stated. It was 40 years later when Theodore Reik (1948) would write a quite readable book saying much the same thing.

Clearly, then, those influenced by the Freudian model tried to avoid talking-to-listen. Talking to listen, they thought, interfered with the patients' free flow of ideas, and distorted the 'true' picture of the patient's Unconscious hidden behind the noise of what the patient actually said.

Nevertheless, three things had happened to prepare a place for psychotherapists to begin to invent talking to listen. All three groups I have reviewed played a role in making talking to listen seem to therapists like a profitable way to go. First, the compassionate moralists (represented here by Pinel and Heinroth) helped make the idea of curing mental patients seem more feasible so doctors stopped treating patients like livestock. Second, the quick-fix doctors (represented here by Beard, Mitchell, and Coué) showed us that we could think of helping people without deliberately shaming them at the same time. Third, those who dug deep into the Unconscious with a tiny shovel (Freud, and Münsterberg in this history) demonstrated that a doctor could listen to patients and learn from them about their troubles.

So, finally, the field was ripe for someone to invent a therapy that involved talking to listen. Of course, there would be those therapists who would not talk to listen, and perhaps most therapists' tiotoled their friends, but now the time was ripe for the idea to occur to therapists that it might sometimes be useful to talk to listen in order to listen in ways that could foster therapeutic goals.

Therapy's invention of talking to listen: the work of Carl Rogers and Harry Stack Sullivan

The cultural context

We have arrived at the 1920s and there is magic in the air. The Great War (World War I) is now old news. Suddenly, women have the right to vote. Young women shocked their Victorian grandparents by cutting off their long skirts to the knees, and dancing the Charleston with their boyfriends to the sound of Big Band music. Hollywood's Golden Age has dawned. Amazing Model T's chug down many city streets. Most people have electric lights. A few have telephones.

Then, in the 1930s, the magic melts. The Great Depression has knocked out life's fresh charm. Long lines of people wait outside soup kitchens while the young boyfriends from the last decade suddenly find themselves selling polished apples on street corners, or hitching rides in box cars to find odd jobs in the next town.

It was at this point in history that I want us to enter the lives of my heroes, the inventors of two different models of therapeutic talking to listen. They were the therapists who thought outside the box of the established practice.

First, I will tell you something about them in a way that I hope will sharpen our comparative study of their different tiotoling techniques.

Rogers (1902–1987) and Sullivan (1892–1949): their careers

During the dark 1930s, there was a time when Rogers and Sullivan each had therapy offices only about six driving miles apart. I picture them at their desks, scribbling notes, as they were prone to do. They had similar looks: both slim and bespectacled with thinning dark hair slicked back with oil. The most striking physical difference between the two, it seems to me, was Sullivan's thin-line moustache. He was also 10 years older than Rogers.

However, there were important differences. First, Rogers was not yet a doctor. He had yet to finish his dissertation, but because of the Great Depression and his having a young family, he was urgently in need of a job. He was relieved to find one at a child guidance centre, but it was a job he would later describe as '… a dead end street professionally' (Rogers 1961, p. 9). Rogers was almost 30 at this time, a young psychologist, just getting started, in bad times—undistinguished except for one thing: his dissertation was published (Rogers 1931), and it sold quite well. It was a test and manual that attempted to measure the attitudes of problem children (Kirschenbaum 1979, pp. 59–60).

On the other hand, at this time, Sullivan had much more name recognition than Rogers. And, while it is true that Sullivan also had financial troubles—he declared bankruptcy in 1930 (Perry 1982)—he did have a good job as a psychiatrist. Moreover, he was already something of a celebrity among the psychiatric elite. People such as Eric Fromm, Karen Horney, Frieda From-Reichman, Edward Sapir, and many others, thought he was brilliant. They marvelled at his success with clients (cf. Perry 1982). He was in demand as a lecturer and he would soon be made head of the Washington School of Psychiatry.

Still in the 1930s an incident occurred that changed the way Rogers thought of doing therapy. The incident began when Rogers told a mother in his office that her son was not progressing in therapy because she was rejecting the boy. So despairing was Rogers that he even told her that it was time for the therapy to stop. It was a waste of time. At that point the mother rose from her chair to leave, but on the way out she stopped at the door and asked Rogers if he ever did therapy with adults. Surprised, Rogers invited her back in, and he listened to her in a way he had not before, and thus he learned the value of non-directive listening (Rogers 1980, p. 36). And, by 1942 he had published his second book, a book seldom noticed today but proving, for those few who were looking, that Carl Rogers was capable of doing quite a lot in his 'dead end' job.

Sullivan, as the 1930s played out, continued to be admired by many people who came to hear his lectures, and his ideas wove into increasingly meaningful patterns, but, still, at the end of the 1930s Sullivan had relatively few published articles and only handwritten notes for a book to be published later.

Then, in the 1940s, a second incident happened that led Rogers to write another book. It happened, so he has told us, on 11 December 1940 (Rogers 1964, p. 17). It was right after listening to a behaviourist criticize Rogers' non-directive ideas. It was on that day that Rogers decided he was saying something new that he wanted to elaborate in another book, a book on non-directive therapy (Kirschenbaum 1995, p. 17). It was to be called *Counseling and Psychotherapy* (1942). In it, he described a completely different kind of therapy than he had been doing before the mother of the troubled boy asked for therapy for herself. After the publication, Rogers' new book quickly became a best seller, perhaps the best selling book ever in the psychotherapy field. And by the end of the 1940s, Rogers had a very good job, a second book and was acquiring considerable name recognition in his chosen field.

Sullivan, on the other hand, published only one book in the 1940s, and that reluctantly. However, he had acquired a growing collection of notes and recordings of lectures and seminars. And he continued to attract enthusiastic followers. Then, in 1949, very suddenly, Sullivan died. Fortunately, he was so popular among a certain set of psychiatrists that over the next half century his followers would manage to pull together his many notes, and turn them into a dozen or so books, articles, and teaching transcripts (cf. Cooper and Guyn 2006).

On the other hand, Rogers lived for another 30 or so years, and during that time, he wrote a dozen more books and many articles and chapters, enjoyed his fame, addressed his critics, served a year as president of the American Psychological Association, and greatly influenced the course of history in the field of therapy (Kirschenbaum and Jourda 2005; Simo 2007).

Those are the two heroes of this chapter, whom I am calling 'the inventors of therapeutic talking to listen'. I call them that, because as far as I can see they were the first therapists to talk to listen.[1] If there were others before them, I believe it was these two therapists who saw that it could be therapeutic to tiotol.

Let's look briefly at their theory of therapy and then study their two styles of talking to listen.

Rogers and Sullivan: explanatory concepts on parallel tracks

Sullivan and Rogers were like two trains going along different but parallel tracks and arriving at similar but importantly different places. In other words, while they seemed

---

[1] There is, however, some evidence that regular interviews of moral treatment patients were beginning to happen by 1887:In my regular morning visits to the various departments of the House, it was my custom to have its immates (sic), who were well enough to leave their rooms, meet me in the parlor attached to their respective halls. Of course private and confidential interviews were frequently required. These every-day family-like gatherings proved far more than formal visits to each room. Such informal meetings, like many of my old-time visits in general practice, were so homelike and natural that their influence readily drew out those genial and social elements of the heart which, in the most extreme developments of insanity, I have rarely, if ever, found beyond our reach. For here was possible "that intangible permeation of a household not too large for the personality at the head of it." The conversations were easy and natural, often bringing out the mental peculiarities of one and another; these in turn leading to timely criticisms, and then to frank and general discussions (Butler 1887, p. 20).

to be going in the same direction, they eventually developed different styles of tiotol. This inconsistency, as I will try to explain, might be useful for the future of therapeutic talking to listen.

Rogers' explanatory concepts

I will show you some segments in their writing that reveal the similarity of their thought. To keep this section brief I am creating a context for each quote with a few words of my own. Do not be bothered by the fact that some of Rogers works were from early writings. I believe the elements mentioned here were ideas he retained through his life.

Rogers and his collaborators felt that people generally came to therapy with concerns that they were unable to talk about and, further, that they generally denied these concerns (as when one denies being angry even to oneself). Then, when in the course of therapy:

> ....these denied elements of experience are brought [by the therapy] into awareness, a process ...of ... reorganization of the self is necessitated [which is therapeutic]
>
> (Rogers 1951, p.77).

And because the self is reorganized when people recall denied experiences, Rogers came to feel that:

> [i]f we [therapists] can create situations in which there is no need of being defensive, unconscious motivations come to the surface [of consciousness] rather easily
>
> (Rogers 1942, p. 361).

Thus, so Rogers explained:

> ...the main aim of the counselor is to assist the client to drop any defensiveness, any feeling that attitudes should not be brought into the open, any concern that the counselor may criticize or suggest or order [the patient to do something]
>
> (Rogers 1942, p. 195).

Talking about such denied experiences made it possible for the client to undergo a helpful reorganization of the self.

> [It] may [be a] most drastic reorganization in which the self and self-in relationship to reality is so altered that few aspects [of the person] remain untouched, [and] the client may go through the most racking torment of pain, and a complete and chaotic confusion
>
> (Rogers 1951, p. 77).

Sullivan's explanatory concepts

Similarly, Sullivan was intent on minimizing the patient's anxiety. That is, he too felt anxiety was what caused 'security operations' or as he sometimes put it 'defensive operations'.

Sullivan said:

> In general, one cannot accomplish good by increasing a patient's anxiety. Any question, and in particular, any explanatory statement—[or] interpretation—that arouses anxiety is apt to prove worse than useless
>
> (Sullivan 1940/1953).

Therefore, much like Rogers, Sullivan felt that:

> The principle problem of the therapeutic interview [a common word used for 'therapy session'] is that of facilitating the accession of awareness of information which will clarify for the patient the more troublesome aspect of his life. This requires that one circumvent the inhibiting processes which, on direct attack, would manifest themselves as severe anxiety, or anger and resentment, with disintegration of the therapeutic situation
>
> (Sullivan 1940/1953).

Can you see the similarity between the way Rogers and Sullivan saw psychological problems and their cure? They both felt, as did Freud, that people who came to therapy had troubles caused by hidden or repressed concerns and needed a therapist to help them disclose in order to talk about what was important to them. To do that, Freud sat and listened quietly, whereas both Rogers and Sullivan talked to listen while trying to avoid making their patients defensive.

However, fortunately I think, they invented two different methods of talking to listen.

Rogers and Sullivan: two different practices of talking to listen

In this section I want to provide some illustrations of their different styles of talking to listen. Unlike the Freudians, neither spent much time listening without comment. Neither did they critique their patients as the moralists did, nor send them to rest homes, nor hypnotize them, nor zap them with electricity. Most of what Rogers and Sullivan did in the therapy office amounted to talking to listen to their patients, although using two distinctively different ways to do so.

A practice of talking to listen: Rogers

If I may summarize him briefly, Rogers (1957) felt that all an effective therapist needed to do was to feel and express a genuine empathy and unconditional positive regard for clients. And, after 1957, at least, he tried to draw attention away from his very distinctive way of talking to listen. He said that he was 'appalled' when he saw imitators mimicking his way of talking to patients because it sounded to him as though they did not have the sincere feelings that made his words work in the session (Rogers et al. 1989, p. 302). He attributed the power of his therapy to help not to his way of phrasing his comments but entirely to his expressed empathy. His evident empathy worked as a kind of 'midwife of change', he thought, to any help he provided (Rogers 1977, p. 21).

Nevertheless, he occasionally explained some of his way of phrasing talking to listen comments (Rogers and Farson 2004). Today his method of speaking to listen is variously called either 'reflective listening' or 'active listening' and is recognized by others as an important component of Rogers' work (Baucum 1999; Blair-Broeker et al. 2003; Prochaska and Norcross 2009.) Ask yourself, as you read the illustration I provide below, if you think it is likely that the way he talked to listen helped Roger's experience of empathy. It might be more difficult to feel empathy, after all, for a client who is not talking. Also, is it that Rogers' empathy was curative? Or is it that the empathy needed to be carried by a wise selection of words, as has been suggested by Wickman and Campbell (2003)?

In the following section I illustrate Rogers' style of tiotol with a composite I have created (from watching films and reading transcripts) in order to contrast and compare Rogers' style of tiotol with that of Sullivan's in a brief and succinct manner. These comparison passages are so brief that they do simplify a bit, but for our purposes that should be helpful.

A Rogerian tiotol:

A woman steps in the door and as she takes her seat she looks over at the therapist, shakes her head and sighs.

1. **Therapist:** (after 15 seconds) I'll be glad to learn what you have on your mind.
2. **Client:** I know, but I'm not sure I want to tell you. (long pause, sigh) It's just hard to know how to explain it to you.
3. **Therapist:** Are you having difficulty putting the problem in words?
4. **Janet:** Not exactly. (long pause) It's just hard to explain without telling you. (laugh) I do this quite a lot, really, struggle over whether to tell people even little things (laughs). (pause) Do you want to know more about how hard it is for me to tell people things? I have lots of stories I could tell, some of them funny.
5. **Therapist:** If that's where you want to go, but I think you were trying to tell me something specific.
6. **Janet:** Yes, that's right. (takes a deep breath) Okay. I want you to know that I had an abortion once. It was a long time ago, but it still bothers me. It has always haunted me. I mean it is really against my religion, although I'm not even very religious.
7. **Therapist:** (nodding) Umhm.
8. **Janet:** Or, maybe what mostly bothers me is that my husband doesn't know about it. I just never could bring myself to tell him.
9. **Therapist:** It's hard to tell him things?
10. **Janet:** Yes, but I've just never told anyone. I guess I'm kind of a private person (sigh). I guess I worry what people would think. (pause) Like I'd like to know what you think.
11. **Therapist:** (nodding and looking sincere) I think telling me you had an abortion was really hard for you, and you're worried I'll think badly of you.
12. **Janet:** You're just repeating me. I want to know what you think.
13. **Therapist:** I'm just very pleased you told me.
14. **Janet:** (laughing) - You're just going to make me worry about what you think. (sighs) I guess I don't so much care what you think. I knew I had to do this if I didn't waste my time, and I'm glad I did it.
15. **Therapist:** I'm glad, too.

The question in line 3 was what Rogers called a 'directive question' which he said encourages the client to answer questions rather than express their flow of concerns through their own evolution.[2]

---

[2] On that page, Rogers analyses the pros and cons of the therapist remarks in a transcript and he says of similar question that a therapist had asked:This one directive question. . .puts the client in the question-answering frame, and hence there comes a pause which the counselor has to break, this time with a less directive question (see Rogers 1942, pp. 268).

Remember I said that Rogers thought that what was important in the session was the therapist's genuine expression of empathy. I tried re-reading the illustration while imaging the therapist speaking mockingly and it seems to me that it clearly would not work with a mechanical or rejecting tone of voice. Still, I suspect that both empathy and supporting words might be required for the most effective form of therapy.

Sullivan's practice of talking to listen

Whereas virtually everything that Rogers did in therapy seemed to involve talking to listen, this was not true for Sullivan. Sullivan tiotoled in a way that brought the patient's stories to life and then he summarized them and advanced tentative hypotheses to help clarify patterns in the patient's social interactions.

The illustrative script that follows was constructed largely from a study of Sullivan's important book *The Psychiatric Interview* (1954). However, I have also relied on Sullivanian illustrations by Chapman (1978) and a book based on recorded transcripts of Sullivan (Kvarnes and Parloff 1976)

To facilitate the comparison, I have composed the following interview so that the patient in the Sullivanian session below is the same patient you have just met in the Rogerian session. Also, at a certain point in this interview, which I will later identify, the therapist tiotol shifts to become more Rogerian:

1. **Therapist:** (after 15 seconds) Maybe at this point we should discuss what we are trying to do in therapy.
2. **Client:** I don't know about you, but I am trying to tell you something—I'm not sure I want to tell you. (long pause, sigh) It's just hard to know how to explain it to you.
3. **Therapist:** Is it important to tell me?
4. **Janet:** Probably. (pause) I just can't tell my husband about the abortion I once had.
5. **Therapist:** Do you think about telling him?
6. **Janet:** All the time. I mean, the subject of abortions comes up now and then, and I think about what it would be like if he learned I had had an abortion.
7. **Therapist:** Give me an example of the subject coming up. When did it happen last?
8. **Janet:** Just a few weeks ago, I guess it was.
9. **Therapist:** Where were the two of you?
10. **Janet:** In a movie.
11. **Therapist:** Where in the movie house?
12. **Janet:** Sitting in a movie house, way in the back. We like to be off to ourselves in movies. The movie hadn't started. We had to wait five or ten minutes.
13. **Therapist:** But the subject came up?
14. **Janet:** Not yet.
15. **Therapist:** Then, what happened?
16. **Janet:** Well, this woman came in we both know. I don't like her. She's a neighbour's daughter. I think her name is Sally. Sally was just walking down the aisle to the front of the theatre. I'm sure she didn't see us. She didn't even look our way.
17. **Therapist:** What happened next?

18. Janet:		Well, nobody could hear us, but I think Jack said something like, 'The last time I saw her she was a lot fatter'. And I said, 'How long ago was that?'. I thought maybe she had lost a lot of weight. Then he said, 'Just a few weeks ago'. It was then that I knew what he was saying, when he said she had lost weight.
19. Therapist:		And what was that?
20. Janet:		He was thinking she might have been pregnant and had an abortion. That's the kind of thing this girl would do, too.
21. Therapist:		And you said this is an example of you thinking of telling him about your abortion?
22. Janet:		What I think of really is his finding out, and then forcing me to tell him. I don't really think of telling him, voluntarily. Not seriously. I just think about what would happen if he ever found out. It kind of scares me.
23. Therapist:		Like you were scared, when you told me about the abortion?
24. Janet:		(looking thoughtful). Maybe… but he's not like you. You accept it. I don't think he would accept it.
25. Therapist:		But you don't know for sure?
26. Janet:		Not for sure, but I don't think I want to take that chance. It's nice to talk to you about it, but I'm not your wife. Still, I think it's good to keep some things private.

The first part of the dialogue is much the same as in the Rogerian illustration.

What made it a distinctively Sullivanian dialogue is illustrated by passage 7 when the therapist asked questions to bring out the story. I believe these two questions would have been unlikely for Rogers, but the facilitation of such stories was central for Sullivan. Sullivan frequently used questions to focus the discussion on significant or thought-provoking events that the patient had experienced.

He explained this practice saying that he wanted to elucidate the patient's characteristic patterns of living (Sullivan 1954, p. 14) and to discover the specifics behind 'obscure difficulties which the patient does not clearly understand' (Sullivan 1954, p. 15).

Sullivan said:

> I want the patient to sketch a little background first [behind the complaint or occasion]. Then I want the point ….at which something relevant to the complaint happened
>
> (Sullivan 1956, p. 278).

> I say to the patient that I want to know what happened, who said what next, and so on and so forth. . .
>
> (Sullivan 1956, p. 275).

In a seminar discussing this point with his followers, Sullivan elaborated:

> Have you gone to town on that topic? Tried to find what he really was talking about? It is a general statement. Has he illustrated at all, told you about attempting to talk with his father and what happened?
>
> (Kvarnes and Parloff 1976, p. 24).

A few of those influenced by Sullivan say much the same thing:

> Of course, as many psychiatrists do, I may also ask for a description of the room or place in which the experience took place
>
> (Fromm-Reichman 1950, p. 78).

What I hope you will see is how tiotols can be similar, but also different. Rogers' tiotols are organized around creating an atmosphere in which the client feels safe to disclose at the deepest level, should he have any impulse to do so. However, as we have seen, Sullivan's tiotol is similarly organized around the goal of making it safe for the client to disclose.

What is different is that Rogers' questions are more open-ended than Sullivan's. Sullivan asks questions to guide the patient into vivid story telling, although what stories are told is largely left to the patient.

This means that it would be possible for a therapist to talk much like Rogers for a while, and then shift to facilitate the patient's story at another time. Both procedures seem to me worthy, although perhaps not for all patients. A client in a Rogerian office, like the one we just studied, might need more support before telling stories. But a therapist who only supports the client's words has fewer resources for helping the patient review incidents and discover new elements in their memories when asked that allow them to reconstruct important events. Yet, because these theorists had a very similar idea of the goals of therapy, one could imagine an eclectic therapist moving back and forth between the Rogerian and Sullivanian model.

Shawver's stupid tiotol

I believe that today there are many kinds of tiotols, and that they can serve different purposes: de Shazer's 'miracle question', is a simple example. Circular Questioning in the Milan Systemic model, is another, and I will give more examples later.

However, as a final example of tiotol, I want to show you one I invented myself. I call it 'The stupid tiotol' because it has felt a little stupid or silly for me to do. But it has, nevertheless, been very useful on the few occasions that I have used it. As you will see, I was talking in order to facilitate my clients' talk, or talking to listen, in situations that seemed to require my assistance.

I give this example of the stupid tiotol as I recall it happening. I will call my patient Cynthia. She was 15 years old. She was brought to therapy by her parents after they found her frequently cutting her wrists, although with very small strokes. Picture me sitting with her for about 5 minutes. I have asked her various questions, but she just sighs, rolls her eyes, chews her gum, and looks away. So far, she hasn't said a word. She looks very glum. Also, picture me in the beginning, talking very slowly, hoping she will interrupt.

Lois:	I can't help wondering what you're thinking (pause) and I find myself guessing what you have on your mind right now. (pause) I'd like to tell you about what I'm imaging you're thinking but I'm afraid I'll look pretty stupid (sigh).
Cynthia:	(looking up at me) Why? Because you think I'm stupid, too?
Lois:	No, it's because I was going to pretend to be you talking to me, telling me what's going on.
Patient:	(She sighed and looked away)
Lois:	I'll be embarrassed but you'll probably think it's pretty funny. Shall I go ahead?
Patient:	She looks at me, rolls her eyes again, and says, 'Whatever'.

I invented a dialogue in which I did all the talking for both of us. I leaned to one side in my chair as I was speaking as myself and to the other side when I spoke as Cynthia.

I will mark the pretend Cynthia by putting her name in italics. If there are no italics, that is the real Cynthia speaking.

> Lois: (leaning to one-side and acting like I am addressing someone on the other side) Cynthia, please tell me what you're thinking.
> *Cynthia:* I don't have to tell you anything. You can't make me.

The real Cynthia laughs then tries to straighten her face. Lois leans to the other side and continues.

> Lois: That's true, but I bet you're not mad at me. I bet you're mad at having to be here, but you're not mad at me.

Now the real Cynthia looks up at me with apparent interest.

> Cynthia: I'm not mad at you, I'm just not going to talk.
> Lois: I think I know what you want to say. You want to be able to talk to me but you don't trust me enough to do that. You don't trust me to keep what you say confidential. After all, you're thinking that because your Mom is paying for this I'm going to tell her what you say.

At this point the real Cynthia interrupted me to say something like, 'That's not how it is. It's that my mom is trying to ruin my life. Everyone else gets to . . .' And thus the conversation started. No need to continue with my 'stupid tiotol'.

I believe other therapists have invented a stupid or perhaps not so stupid tiotol. From listening to therapists, I think such inventions happen even when the inventors themselves do not notice. Therapists sometimes just come up with better ways to invite the next comment, and that is to invent a tiotol. Perhaps this invention is happening today because Rogers and Sullivan, and some less obvious others, have opened the way for therapists to invent new forms of such a practice. Whatever the cause, I am grateful, for it was not that long ago, after all, when the practice of therapy was new, and talking to listen was seldom if ever practised.

Reflections

I have provided you with the findings of my research in this chapter, so I trust that I am not alone in trying to make sense of what I have found. Nevertheless, I have a picture that has emerged from my studies that I am eager to provide.

Remember, my organizing question for this chapter was: why have therapists been slow to notice that much of what we do is talking to listen?

The answer seems be that through the centuries therapists have been highly distracted by a parade of cultural beliefs that made the practice of talking to listen seem irrelevant. There was the belief that listening to mental patients was useless because they were not of their 'right mind' and that nothing they said could be trusted. Then, it seemed to therapists that mental patients were only able to profit from treatment if they were tricked into doing so, perhaps by convincing them the therapist was speaking for God. Next, the belief was that mental patients could be better treated by new, quick and attractive treatments, so listening to patients was irrelevant. And, finally, the psychoanalysts taught us that the only helpful truth patients had to teach us was something they could not tell us directly, something unconscious.

None of these therapy practices used more than the trivial forms of talking to listen, but each shift of framework resulted in a gradually changing attitude towards patients and their therapy in a way that, over the years, made talking to listen seem increasingly relevant. Today, I suspect that the vast majority of therapists of all sorts would see the relevance of at least some degree of therapists talking to listen in the session.

It seems to me that the two men most responsible for drawing to our attention the usefulness of talking to listen were Carl Rogers and Harry Stack Sullivan. Each of these two men invented a style or method of talking to listen, along with a theory of how therapy could be useful. Their theories of what therapy needed to do to be useful were similar, but their methods of tiotoling were distinctive.

Over the next few decades, new ways of talking to listen began popping up like pop corn. The popular question in the 1970s for therapists to ask was, 'What are you feeling?'(McAuliffe and Ericksen 2002, p. 41) and before many years cognitive therapists were asking: 'What's going through your mind?'(Kuehlwein 2000).

More recently we have the Milan Therapy's practice of circular questioning, de Shazer's 'Miracle Question', Michael White's instructions as to how we could look for 'unique outcomes', and the Lacanian method of the analyst speaking as the voice of the Unconscious. You also have my 'stupid tiotol' and no doubt the tiotols of many other therapists who have invented tiotols behind therapy's closed doors.

There is even research on talking to listen questions (cf. Adams 1997; McGee 2005) although do remember that all forms of talking to listen are not questions.

And the future of the practice of tiotoling? I think its future rests with the future of psychotherapy in general, and the future of psychotherapy is currently being written. To see the changes that are happening, glance all the way back to Rogers and notice one of the most pronounced movements in therapy practice over the last 50 years.

In the 1950s, when Rogers wrote, he and every other theorist that I am aware of defined their contributions as part of a school of thought. Rogers wrote, (under the heading 'The Presentation of a "School of Thought"'):

> It is clearly the purpose of these pages to present only one point of view, and to leave to others the development of other orientations
>
> (Rogers 1951, p. 9).

But today, authors who present their ideas as part of a school of therapy are out of touch with dramatic changes that have been happening in our field. Surveys for the last 30 years or so show that therapists are increasingly breaking away from the practice of following the guidelines of specific schools. Instead, more and more, therapists identify themselves as eclectic or integrationist (Garfield and Kurtz 1977; Norcross and Prochaska 2002), and, in addition, when therapists choose a personal therapist for themselves, they prefer a therapist who is not committed to a particular school (Norcross et al. 2009).

Talking to listen has a place in this new eclecticism if we can learn to mix models and, perhaps, add a little salsa of our own. It is not that we must choose which form of talking to listen to practice, but that we need to pick and choose, and also blend and weave, the different models of tiotol more spontaneously. Anything else will tend to sound inauthentic. In fact, I believe it was this kind of parroting that so appalled Carl

Rogers and caused him to draw attention away from the way he spoke and call attention to the emotion he was trying to express.

To ensure this relatively new practice of talking to listen a place in the future, however, we need to adapt it to the other trends happening which make therapy more of a creative art, more like the art of a primary physician, say, than that of a diagnostician following a manual, at least to the extent that a primary physician adapts a personal style to work best with the specific patient in the office and the situation that is happening.

I hope we therapists continue to tiotol. I believe it was a fortunate invention, and I extend this new term talking to listen so we can better collaborate in improving and extending our understanding and the general practice of talking to listen.

References

Adams, J. F. (1997). Questions as interventions in therapeutic conversation. *Journal of Family Therapy*, **8**(2), 17–35.

Andrews, J. and Scull, A. (2003). *Customers and patrons of the mad-trade: The management of lunacy in eighteenth-century.* University of California Press, Berkeley, CA.

Baucum, D. (1999). *Psychology.* Barron Educational Services, Hauppauge, NY.

Beard, G.M. (1894). *A practical treatise on nervous exhaustion (neurasthenia)* (3rd ed.). Lux Tinebra, New York.

Blair-Broeker, C. T., Ernst, R. M. and Meyers, D. G. (2003). *Thinking about psychology: the science of mind and behavior.* Worth Publishers, New York.

Bott, D. (2002). Comment—Carl Rogers and postmodernism: Continuing the conversation. *Journal of Family Therapy*, **24**, 326–9.

Butler, J. S. (1887). *The Curability of Insanity and the Individualized Treatment of the Insane.* Putnam and Sons, New York.

Chapman, A. H. (1978). *The treatment techniques of Harry Stack Sullivan.* Bruner/Mazel, New York.

Clanon, T. L. Shawver, L. and Kurdys, D. (1982). Less insanity in the courts. *American Bar Association Journal,* July, **68**, 824–7.

Cooper, A. B. and Guynn, R. W. (2006). Transcription of fragments of lectures in 1948 by Harry Stack Sullivan. *Psychiatry: Interpersonal and Biological Processes*, **69**, 101–6.

Dubois, P. (1909). *The psychic treatment of nervous disorders: The psychoneuroses and their moral treatment* (9th ed.). Funk & Wagnalls Company, New York.

Durgin, W. A. (1912). *Electricity, its history and development.* A.C. McClurg & Co., Chicago, IL.

Ehrenreich, B. (2009). *Bright-sided: How the relentless promotion of positive thinking has undermined America.* Metropolitan Books, New York.

Foucault, M. (2009). *History of madness.* Routledge, New York.

Fredman, G. (2004). *Transforming emotion: Conversations in counseling and psychotherapy.* Whurr Publishers, Philadelphia, PA.

Freud, S. (1913/1953). Further recommendations in the technique of psychoanalysis: On beginning the treatment. The questions of first communications. The dynamics of cure. In *Sigmund Freud, collected papers*, vol II, pp. 342–65. The Hogarth Press, London.

Fromm-Reichman, F. (1950). *Principles of intensive psychotherapy.* University of Chicago Press, Chicago, IL.

Garfield, S. L. and Kurtz, R. (1977). A study of eclectic views. *Journal of Consulting and Clinical Psychology*, **45**, 78–83.

Goldstein, J. E. (1987). *Console and classify: The French psychiatric profession in the Nineteenth Century*. University of Chicago, Chicago, IL.
Haydon, M. and Elliott, N. (2004). Internal consultancy and the public conversations project: A dialogic consultation. *Journal of Systemic Therapies*, **23**, 91–106.
Heinroth, J. C. (1818/1975). *Textbook of Disturbances of Mental Life, or Disturbances of the Soul and their Treatment* (J. Schmorak, Trans.). Johns Hopkins University Press, BA.
Hoffman, L. (2002). *Family Therapy: An Intimate History*. W. W. Norton, New York.
Kirschenbaum, H. (1979). *On becoming Carl Rogers*. Delacorte Press, New York.
Kirschenbaum, H. (1995). Carl Rogers. In M. M. Suhd (Ed.) *Positive Regard*, pp. 1–90. California: Science and Behavior Books, Palo Alto, CA.
Kirschenbaum, H. and Jourdan, A. (2005). The current status of Carl Rogers and the person-centered approach. *Psychotherapy: Theory, Research, Practice, Training*, **42**, 37–51.
Kraepelin, E. (1962). Cited in Weckowicz, T. E. and Liebel-Weckowicz, H. P. (1990). *A history of great ideas in abnormal Psychology*. Elsevier Science Publishers B. V., North Holland.
Kuehlwein, K. T. (2000). Enhancing creativity in cognitive therapy. *Journal of Cognitive Psychotherapy*, **14**, 175–87.
Kvarnes, R. G. and Parloff, G. H. (Eds.) (1976). *A Harry Stack Sullivan case seminar*, W.W. Norton, New York.
Launer, J. (2006). New stories for old: Narrative-based primary care in Great Britain. *Families, Systems, & Health*, **24**, 336–44.
Lyotard, J. and Thébaud, J. (1999). *Just gaming*. University of Minnesota, Minneapolis, MN.
Marx, O. M. (1991/2008). German Romantic Psychiatry (Part II). In E.R. Wallace IV and J. Gach (Eds.) *History of psychiatry and medical psychology*. Springer, New York.
McAuliffe, G. and Ericksen, K. (2002). *Teaching strategies for constructivist and developmental counselor education*. Bergin & Garvey, Westport, CT.
McGee, D. (2005). An interactional model of questions as therapeutic interventions. *Journal of Marital and Family Therapy*, **31**, 371–84.
Meyer, D. (1980). *The positive thinkers: Religion as pop psychology from Mary Baker Eddy to Oral Roberts*. Pantheon Books, New York.
Mitchell, S. W. and Kimmel, M. S. (2004). *Wear and tear: Or hints for the overworked*. Alta Vira Press, Walnut Creek, CA. [Originally printed as Mental fatigue (1887), Lippincott, Philadelphia, PA.] Available at: http://bit.ly/6iWvL7 [Accessed 25 March 2010.]
Münsterberg, H. (1909). *Psychotherapy*. Moffat, Yard and Company, New York.
Norcross, J. C., Bike, D. H. and Evans, K. L. (2009). The therapist's therapist: A replication and extension 20 years later. *Psychotherapy*, **46**, 32–41.
Norcross, J. C. and Prochaska, J. O. (1988). A study of eclectic (and integrative) views revisited, *Professional Psychology: Research & Practice*, **19**, 170–4.
Perry, H. S. (1982). *Psychiatrist of America: The life of Harry Stack Sullivan*. The Beknap Press, Cambridge.
Pinel, P. (1801). *Traité médico-philosophique*. Richard, Caille et Ravier, an IX, Paris.
Pinel, P. (1806). *Treatise on insanity* (D. D. Davis, Trans.). Messrs Cadell and Davies, London.
Pinel, P. (1809). *Traité médico-philosophique*. J.A. Brosson, Paris.
Prochaska, J. O. and Norcross, J. C. (2002). Stages of change. In J. C. Norcross (Ed.) *Psychotherapy relationships that work: Therapist contributions and responsiveness to patient needs*. Oxford University Press, New York, pp. 303–14.
Prochaska, J. O. and Norcross, J. C. (2009). *Systems of psychotherapy: A transtheoretical Analysis*, Brooks Cole, Belmont, CA.

Reik, T. (1948/1983). *Listening with the third ear: The inner experience of a psychoanalyst*, Farrar, Straus and Giroux, New York.

Ray, I. (1843). *A Treatise on the Medical Jurisprudence of Insanity*. Freeman and Bolles, Boston.

Reynolds, D. (2007). Containment, curiosity and consultation: An exploration of theory and process in individual systemic psychotherapy with an adult survivor of trauma. *Journal of Family Therapy*, **29**, 420–37.

Rieff, P. (1959/1961). *Freud: The mind of a moralist* (3rd ed.). University of Chicago Press, Chicago, IL.

Rogers, C. R. (1931). *Measuring personality adjustment in children nine to thirteen years of age*. AMS Press, Inc., New York.

Rogers, C. R. (1942) *Counseling and psychotherapy*. Houghton Mifflin Company, Boston, MA.

Rogers, C. R. (1951). *Client-centered therapy: Its current practice, implications and theory*. Houghton Mifflin Company, Boston, MA.

Rogers, C. R. (1957). The necessary and sufficient conditions of therapeutic personality change. *Journal of Consulting and Psychology*, **21**, 95–103.

Rogers, C. R. (1961). *On becoming a person*. Houghton Mifflin Co., Boston, MA

Rogers, C.R. (1964). Remarks on the future of client-centered therapy. In *American Psychological Association, symposium on the future of client-centered therapy*. [Cited in Kirchenbaum, H. (1995). Carl Rogers. In: M. M. Suhd (Ed.) *Positive regard: Carl Rogers and other notables he influenced*, Science and Behavior Books, Inc, Palo Alto, CA.]

Rogers, C.R. (1977). *Carl Rogers on Personal Power*. Delacorte Press, New York.

Rogers, C. R. (1980). *A way of being*. Houghton Mifflin Co, New York.

Rogers, C. R. and Farson, F. E. (2004). *Active listening*. In S. Ferguson (Ed.) *Organizational Communication*, pp. 319–334. Transaction Publishers, New Brunswick, NJ.

Rogers, C. R., Kirschenbaum, H. and Henderson, V. L. (1989). *The Carl Rogers reader*. Houghton Mifflin Company, New York.

Roth, K. (2004). Lois Shawver über sprachspiel, paralogie und transvaluation. *Zeitschrift für systemische therapie und beratung*, **22**, 77–98.

Shawver, L. (2004). Therapy theory after the postmodern turn. In D.A. Paré and G. Larner (Eds.) *Collaborative practice in psychology and therapy*, pp. 23–34. Haworth Press, Inc., Binghampton, NY.

Simon, R. (2007). The top 10: The most influential therapists of the past quarter century. *Psychotherapy Networker*, **68**, 24–37.

Strong, T. (2002). Therapy's "Borderzone". *Journal of Constructivist Psychology*, **15**, 245–62.

Sullivan, H.S. (1940/1953). *Therapeutic conceptions of modern society*. W. W. Norton and Co, New York.

Sullivan, H.S.(1954). *The psychiatric interview*. W. W. Norton and Co., New York.

Sullivan, H. S. (1956). *Clinical studies in psychiatry*. Norton, New York.

Walsh, J.J. (1912). *Psychotherapy: including the history of the use of mental influence, directly and indirectly, in healing and the principles for the application of energies derived from the mind to the treatment of disease*. D. Appleton and Company, New York.

Wickman, S. A., and Campbell, C. (2003). An analysis of how Carl Rogers enacted client-centered conversation with Gloria. *Journal of Counseling and Development*, **81**, 178–84.

Chapter 3

Positioning theory, narratology, and pronoun analysis as discursive therapies

Rom Harré and Mirjana Dedaić

Discursive therapy can be none other than an application of the methods of discursive psychology in pursuit of resolutions of personal conflicts and difficulties. Discursive or cultural psychology can be one of the means by which insights into some of the more general features of life among language users can be attained. Furthermore, the insights that have emerged from discursive psychology can shape discursive therapies, in so far as we follow the lead of those who see psychology as a moral science and hence revelatory of local norms. The tensions and strains that arise as people cope with the force and sometimes the oppressive power of local norms in relation to their life projects, can be revealed and their nature at least partially understood by the application of the insights of discursive psychology. Positioning theory is an integral part of the repertoire of methods that constitute the methodology of discursive or cultural psychology. We will illustrate its role in the ground work of discursive therapy. Moreover, the positioning approach is closely allied to two other aspects of discursive psychology, narratology, and pronoun analysis. Each has its own methods and characteristic contribution to make to the repertoire of approaches available to the discursive therapist. In this chapter we illustrate the role that some of the features of discursive psychology might play in enriching the resources of the discursive therapist. The insights of positioning theory are among the products of the development of a range of alternative psychologies, some of which are to be found within the family of discursive or cultural psychologies (Valsiner 2010).

Psychological phenomena are produced as the result of active agents drawing on bodies of knowledge to accomplish intentions and projects. Adherence to this principle in some form identifies discursive psychologists, cultural psychologists, and so on, all of whom reject the simple causal format for expressing knowledge, and particularly those who reject the naive experimental methods of the 'mainstream'. Once again a brilliant expose of the unscientific character of 'scientific psychology' has appeared, this time from Jan Smedslund (2010).

Discursive psychology

The principle upon which the edifice of discursive psychology rests is that people both live and tell narratives. Narratives are shaped by story lines, and story lines are cultural resources.

Understanding an episode in which language is the main medium of the action requires implicit recourse to schemata, a psychologists' word for story lines, though many other terms have been used. For example, Schank and Abelson (1977) used the word 'scripts' to highlight the relation of the technique of discursive analysis with the drama. Algirdas Greimas et al. (1976) described the formal investigation of plots as 'actantial analysis', and Vladimir Propp (1968) called these structures 'plot formats'.

Acting in an intelligible way to accomplish some greater or lesser project during the living out of an intelligible episode requires implicit recourse to such schemata. Only very rarely does one access a discursive representation of a schema and follow its guidance—though this may be typical of the lives of people who are at odds with the social world they find themselves inhabiting.

At another level, episodes that have been lived through become the topics of stories, narratives, and reminiscences in which the schemata are realized in explicit story lines. She said this and I said that and then she said and so on. One might find such a narrative in a courtroom, at a gossip session, in a psychiatrist's sanctum and in many other places as well.

It is an important insight of discursive psychology that any episode, identified by time, place and personnel, may *always* be read as the performing of more than one story. We illustrate this feature of the human life-world later in this chapter. The work of the discursive therapist might well include the extraction of a different story from an episode than the one that is troubling a client.

A person as an actor in an episode sometimes tells a story that is identical to the one that he or she lived in the course of the relevant episode, though not always. Self-presentation is a key intention of many raconteurs. Actors as story-livers and story-tellers are embedded in moral orders—public-collective and private-individual beliefs about the distribution of rights and duties to speak and act in certain ways, the meaning and value of what is said and done and so on.

Every discourse is orderly at some level and that it can be made so is a mark of discursive competence (Greimas 1987, p. 445). Relative disorder is often taken as a sign of pathology of speech and so of thought, that is of discursive incompetence—at least by those who are careless about the danger of slipping into malignant psychology (Kitwood 1988). Orderliness can be expressed or represented by rules—though care must be taken to avoid confusion between rules which are used as regulators of conduct and rules which express tacit norms. The former are instructions, the latter a metaphorical way of giving explicit representation to implicit norms. Some implicit norms exist only in the regularity of certain practices without any implication that they are part of the repertoires for action of individual people.

The role of rules

How is authority constituted and maintained in circumstances in which the usual structures of assigned role and explicit social conventions are weak or in abeyance? This question is complementary to this: how and why do people remain, or even welcome being trapped in webs of rules onto which responsibility for action is loaded? An important role for discursive therapy is to relieve people of the burden of rules which seem to enclose them in a web of necessities. One way of looking at such matters is in terms of the beliefs people have about their rights and duties as social actors, even as private thinkers, and their beliefs about the rights and duties of others. Rules and the imperatives they seem to impose are human constructions and often times their oppressive force can be lifted. 'Rule-anxiety' is a condition susceptible to discursive therapy in the light of the place it may have in discursive psychology.

Let us start with *cultural dopes*, those for whom the positions they have been assigned or taken on or inherited are apparently final. Here are some anecdotes to illustrate the puzzling character of 'resort to rules'. Many years ago one of the authors was living in Wisconsin, USA, from which train services had long since been withdrawn. To catch a train to Chicago one had to take a cross country bus ride to the nearest 'depot' on the main line. As the bus ambled through a forest we came across an abandoned line, with small trees growing up between the rusty rails. Just before the crossing the driver stopped, opened the bus door with one of those scissor like devices, moved the bus across the derelict line, stopped and closed the door. I was intrigued—'Why did you do that?' I asked him. 'It's the rules' he said. 'We have to do that'. 'But' I said, 'the line is derelict'. 'Doesn't matter', he said. 'It's the rules!'

Here is another story. A long line had formed at the interval of Nabucco at the bar of the Lyric Opera House in Baltimore. The one young lady behind the bar was taking forever to serve the patrons because she was slowly pouring out each can of soda into a glass. When it came to the turn of one of the authors he said 'I'll do that, so you can serve the next person'. 'Oh no', she exclaimed horrified. 'We are not allowed to let a customer handle a can.'

And another. Recently at the Concert Hall at the John F Kennedy Center in Washington DC an even more startling example occurred. A lady sitting in the middle of a row began to cough very badly and struggled to get over the legs of the others in the row to make her way outside. There was a long pause between the items in the first half of the concert and it was clear that the last block of seats, over 60 in all, were empty. When the unfortunate woman came back someone suggested to her that she should move to one of the block of empty seats at the back of the hall, near the door. She tried to do so but one of the ushers rushed up saying that she cannot be allowed to sit there—someone might come in—what about the other 59 seats? The senior usher than chipped in that no one was allowed to occupy another seat because it might have been assigned to someone else. Disconcerted, the anxious patron came back to the row, but everyone moved along one place so she could sit on the aisle in case she was overtaken by another attack. At the end of the concert the 60 empty seats at the back of the hall were still empty.

Of course, all this is the consequence of a social order in which personal responsibility is so heavy a burden that most people try (successfully) to unload the authority on to rules. Here too is a place for the discursive therapist! How can you help an anxious cultural dope?

Among the many useful ways of looking at incidents like those described is to relate what happened to the local moral order—the distribution of rights and duties in the local social group. The bus driver was surely a duty-dope, and perhaps it never occurred to him that he was adult enough to take upon himself the right to abrogate an empty custom. The young lady in the opera house is different. As a very junior employee she knows she has no rights. Like the bus driver, her life is all duty.

The Kennedy Center episode is different again. It displayed a clash of two systems of duties. The ushers had imbibed the American respect for rules, rules which according to Piaget only infants cannot query. The demeanour of the senior usher was not the frightened agitation of the middle-aged lady who showed people their seats. He was obviously torn between his duty to the rules, however stupid, and his duty to the welfare of the patrons. Unfortunately, and as so often happens, adherence to the lesser duty overcame loyalty to the greater.

In each episode the distribution of rights and duties is the salient feature of the unfolding the events described. The study of the way that rights and duties are distributed, and the methods by which they are created and maintained *in the absence of a formal code of instructions,* is the topic of positioning theory.

Positioning theory

Positioning theory addresses the question complementary to that raised by the predicament of anxious rule-dopes. In a situation in which the distribution of rights and duties is not determined by the local moral order, how is an assignment of these important moral stances achieved and anarchy kept at bay? In the several examples we have cited above there was a 'positioning discourse', since it challenged the existing distributions of rights and duties, but to no avail. The most interesting cases for the social psychologist are those in which there is a prior discussion in which positions are assigned or a discussion in which existing distributions are challenged successfully and a new local moral order comes into being. Here we come across *cultural refuseniks*.

Positioning theory came into being as a fusion between two more basic concepts of personal positions. One sense of 'position' was used to describe how an individual person was related to others with respect to assessments of personal qualities, real or imagined or even stereotypical. In another sense a person's position was his or her beliefs about the cluster of rights and duties that that person was thought to have in a certain situation with respect to the rights and duties of others. Research into the way the latter sense of position worked in real life episodes soon disclosed that the position beliefs that people had were often derived, directly or indirectly, from assessments of person qualities, significant biographical incidents relative to the matter in hand, and so on. The important discursive practices of assignments and challenges to positions often turned on such beliefs. The assignment of a certain duty to someone might be rescinded on the disclosure of an inability to carry out an essential part of the task, witnessed to by some prior incident. To keep track of these variants we have come to call assessments of skills, capacities and biographical incidents acts of 'pre-positioning', leaving 'positioning' for the discursive processes by which rights and duties are ascribed, taken on, rejected, refused, contested and so on. 'You have no right to do that because . . .' is the sort of discursive act that relates positions to pre-positioning claims. It is important to bear in mind that the source from which larger scale positioning discourses are derived, even to the positioning of nations, are small-scale personal encounters—the Alzheimer sufferer and the care-giver, the IT manager and the staff member, the mother and her child, the Prime Minister and the members of the cabinet, the bus driver and the passengers, and so on endlessly through the fabric of everyday life.

The method for research in discursive/cultural psychology is simple to state:

1) Work toward the discovery and classification of working bodies of knowledge, meaning, and the schemata with which they are shaped into the forms of thought and action with which we are familiar.
2) Given that people, even cultural dopes, are agents, at least in principle, research must include the monitoring and analysis of the methods people use for their management of actions of all kinds so that all, *ceteris paribus*, shall conform to local standards of correctness and propriety. The meanings of their actions, speeches, environmental situations, happenings, and so on, are assigned according to local bodies of knowledge.

Life goes on fairly smoothly. What is the status of the products of positioning theory research? We list situations, pre-positioning acts, positioning beliefs, and so on. However, people rarely attend to such items in living through an episode in which positioning was at issue. Like all cognitive psychology, positioning analysis offers a representation of the tacit knowledge and beliefs of the actors that could be a model of fictional cognitive processes that would account for the way episodes unfold.

How do we investigate the way that unequal access to resources, and unequal rights to exercise skills a person of a certain category (child, woman, medical doctor), come into being, are sustained, and could be challenged? How can we analyse the situation that then obtains, and how can we explore the discursive means by which a certain distribution of rights and duties was established? Positioning theory has grown up as an answer to these kinds of questions. It is part of the burgeoning growth of 'psychology as a moral science', the idea that psychologists are as much concerned with ideals as they are with how those ideals are or are not realized in practice (Brinkmann 2010).

The basis of positioning studies is to be found in a grouping of four components into a positioning cluster. There are *positions* (beliefs about rights and duties which are ascribed in any episode to the actors). There are the *repertoires of acts* available to a person positioned in a certain way in a group. There are the *story lines* that are lived out in everyday encounters. Finally there are the '*selves*' which are produced in the course of an unfolding episode. Methods of analysis are part of the repertoire of discursive psychology, concerned with the ethnomethods (cf. Garfinkel 1967) for distributing and contesting the distribution of positions among people, locally and ephemerally. Positioning theory is one way that the overall approach of cultural psychology is idealized. As Valsiner (2010) argues, culture is mediated to the psychologies of people through sign systems, of which the vernacular, wherever you may be, is the prime vehicle. Positioning is a discursive practice: that is, it expresses a moral order mediated by speech act types and pronoun choices.

Features of positioning clusters

Rights and duties

A position is a set of beliefs held by actors as to their own rights and duties and those of others engaged in an encounter or a longer strip of life, unique or part of a series of similar encounters. These beliefs are grounded in characterological and other attributions to the actors in the current scene.

The sources of beliefs about duties and rights stem ultimately from certain necessary empirical conditions realized among the actors; their vulnerabilities and 'matching' powers. There are many cases in everyday life where the vulnerabilities of one person can be matched to the powers of another. However, that fact alone does not determine whether the latter person will help the former or even have slightest inclination to do so. The tall fellow looks on with amusement while the little chap jumps up and down in a rage as he tries to reach the high shelf.

Interpreted through the lens of a moral theory, asymmetries of powers and vulnerabilities yield distributions of duties and rights, in which duties often routinely accrue to the powerful and rights to the vulnerable. There are several moral principles that might be invoked in a formal analysis of this thought—for example the Golden Rule—use my powers to assist the vulnerable in the hope that someone from among the one time vulnerable will have the power to help me deal with one of my vulnerabilities. Locating vulnerabilities and powers in Kant's Kingdom of Ends might suggest that treating everyone as an end rather than wholly as a means might effect a moral connection between someone's plight and someone else's help. Jesus' use of this situation was more as a way of highlighting a moral principle than as a substantial argument for it.

Note that there can be viable social systems that recognize only duties. In the European Middle Ages some of the societies of knights, such as the original Knights Templar, or the feudal hierarchy of duties ratified by King John in Magna Carta, delineated duties in much greater detail and with much greater significance than it did rights. Fealty was the most prized mediaeval virtue. But as the fiction of the Arthurian legend suggests fealty sometimes falls victim to desire. *Tristan and Isolde* covers much the same moral ground. Later stages of the originally fealty based Samurai system with the code of bushido tied honour to fealty in the way the code was interpreted morally. It is a moot point whether there could be social systems which recognized only rights. There have been warnings, for example, Jack Kennedy's famous exhortation that the American people should not ask what society can do for them but what they can do for society. When Western society is in its 'client' mode, there are almost endless demands that people make on each other and the institutions of the state. In this instance, it has come close to being a society with a deformed positioning basis, in which only rights are recognized and exercised. Again, sometimes we must attend to supererogatory duties from which formally recognized duties can crystallize. For example, many people took on themselves duties to protect the environment, as a matter of personal choice outside the domain of the officially designated duties of the citizen. Now such duties are formally recognized in law and there are penalties for their neglect.

Speech-acts and other social meanings

We owe to John L. Austin (1959) a new way of looking at the meanings of utterances germane to the application of positioning theory. Austin began the study of speech acts, that is, utterances which are intended to have social effects and are understood as such by the interlocutors. However, the social force of an utterance is not a simple consequence of grammatical form or choice of vocabulary. What a certain sentence means as uttered depends on the positions that have been established in the conversation so far. 'Do you want any help?' could be a genuine offer of assistance or in certain circumstances a snide remark.

The basis of Austin's analysis is a distinction between the locutionary force of an utterance, what it means in a decontextualized dictionary sense, the illocutionary force, what it means as an embedded social act, and the perlocutionary force, what effect it has on the world around. Austin's criterion for distinguishing illocutionary force from perlocutionary force was to ask what am I doing *in saying* 'p' and what am I doing *by saying* 'p'. In saying 'You idiot' I am reprimanding you, while by saying 'You idiot' I might be reminding you of the right way to do something. These distinctions can be extended quite naturally to para-linguistic and other symbolic actions where they play a role as the bearers of psychologically and socially significant acts.

Story lines

We have noted that a basic principle of positioning analysis is that strips of life unfold according to narrative conventions. There are implicit generic scripts such as 'doctor/patient', 'confessor/sinner', 'mother/child', 'commander/vassal' and so on. Moreover, we also find implicit and explicit specific scripts, such as interrogation of suspects, shopping, obtaining a meal in a restaurant, and so on. These story lines have been analyzed by several relevant *methods,* such as Greimas' search for actants, Burke's (1945) dramaturgical analysis, positioning theory, and so on

The presentation of selves

'Self' is such a weasel word and yet so deeply embedded in the literature that there is no alternative but to use it. However, in positioning theory the meaning of 'self' is clear—the attributes of a person—including their bare presence as an identifiable location in space and time (nowadays perhaps an identifiable location in cyberspace and cybertime). The self is not a person—it is not a unitas multiplex. It is not a being at all, but a labile group of collocated cognitive and affective attributes, including those sometimes reified as personality and character.

From the beginning positioning theorists have been interested in the way acts of positioning impact on selves, that is, on the beliefs a person has about him or herself and the beliefs that others have of the attributes and history of someone. A feminist slant on this was a feature of Davies and Harré (1990), while Sabat and Harré (1994) demonstrated its importance in the lives of Alzheimer sufferers.

'Positioning' example in discursive therapeutic practices A striking example of the way that using positioning analysis can illuminate a problematic situation is to be seen in a study by Stephen Sabat (1994). Mr and Mrs R present a complex pattern of positioning, only revealed when two story lines are brought into juxtaposition. In the day care centre Mrs R was reported to be able to manage tableware and the business of eating quite well. However, according to Mr R, he essentially had to feed her. Though Mr R admitted his wife could pick out her clothes, he would do so when he deemed the situation important, such as her birthday. She wanted to wear an outfit she had worn recently, and he thought that this was because she thought that her birthday had already been celebrated—though according to a third party this was not so.

Similar narrative disparities reappeared in reports about her using make-up, about following instructions and her willingness to help in the house—in the day care centre story line she figured as a busy and thoughtful helper of those less able than herself.

One can look at this narrative in terms of positioning—Mr R pre-positions Mrs R as helpless, thus defining a range of duties for himself, while denying certain rights to self-grooming and so on to Mrs R. But another narrative emerges as we incorporate the day care centre story. Mrs R can be seen as pre-positioning herself as competent in the day care centre, where she thus accrues certain duties and rights, while at home she pre-positions herself as helpless, thereby positioning her husband as having certain duties. In the extended day care centre story, Mrs R is the active person who claims the right to position her husband.

With the help of this analysis the discursive therapist comes to understand that the situation is as good as it could be—each of the couple has created a story line that makes the life of the Alzheimer sufferer tolerable and the caretaker.

Narratology Episodes of our lives are rarely chaotic. Careful study of the records of what people think, feel, do and perceive reveals the presence of schemata in the background of what has been said and done. How such schemata exist, how welcome it is to have them, and how they play a role in thought and action, is a central concern of theoreticians of the discursive turn. For the purposes of this chapter we need only acknowledge their role and the forms they take when presented explicitly.

In introducing the idea of the role of schemata in the orderliness of everyday life we can turn to the management of ceremonies as a model. Ceremonies are routines which initiate or change social realities: for example, swearing in a President; sentencing someone to a term in prison; graduating from university, and so on. For the most part, a ceremony is a fixed sequence of action/acts usually explicitly defined in a set of rules in a manual or order of service. Importantly, ceremonies may initiate, maintain or relieve conflicts. War can be declared, actions can be brought in court, a truce may be brokered and formally ratified. The short-term outcomes of ceremonies are certain, if the speech act conditions of sincerity and legitimacy are fulfilled. Games, too, are usually played within a framework of rules that are taken by all concerned to be proper and legitimate for the occasion. There is often an authority that is given the task of maintaining, and sometimes revising, the rules. However, though bound by explicit rules, games are set up so that the outcome of an encounter is uncertain. If Manchester United always won their matches there would be little point in the UEFA cup.

These are formal episodes and the story lines are determined by agreement to accept a formal code. However, most talk and writing occurs in, and also can be about, informal episodes; that is, those without explicit governing rule systems. These can be analysed to reveal two different ways in which the discourse is ordered in relation to the event recorded. There are 'chronicles', stories in which the episodes are ordered by their temporal relations, usually in the West, past, present, and sometimes future. The ordering principle of a chronicle is a 'proairetic code', for example by centuries, by days of the week, by the death of kings and so on. However, for the purposes of the application of discursive psychology and positioning theory to the analysis of interpersonal encounters, the problem for the analyst is to disentangle the narrative, and here we make use of hermeneutic codes. In narratological analysis we can ask, 'What is the significance of the offer to make tea?' and the answer will depend on the catalogue of meanings appropriate to this analysis, the people who offer to go to the kitchen, the situation and the milieu in which the incident is taking place.

There are several useful formal schemes available in extracting a relevant story line. There are Vladimir Propp's 31 categories of episodes within a complete story (Propp 1968). This scheme has been used in the analysis of environmentalist discourse (Harré et al. 1998). Algirdas Greimas's concept of 'actants' (1987) is another useful scheme which focuses analytical attention on the dynamics of a storied episode. Finally, important because it was a major influence on the narratological analyses developed by Erving Goffman in such works as *Frame Analysis* (1974), there is the dramaturgical analysis of Kenneth Burke (1945) with its five narratological categories of Scene, Actor, Agent, Agency, Purpose-Motive.

Narratology in discursive therapy

Lived narratives manifest three stages of positioning: (a) pre-positioning, (b) positioning, and (c) holding (reaffirming, reinforcing) one's subject position. Pre-positioning relies on the actors' familiarity with the script within which they take, negotiate, or accept a subject position (Davies and Harré 1990). Since actors are committed to the pre-existing idea of selves, their selves are embedded in certain narrative worlds that delimit ideas, notion, actions, stories, and discourses that are allowable in such worlds. This delimitation can be understood through the conceptualization similar to that of Goffman's framing (1974).

In the case of a non-pre-existent narrative world that is acquired in the process of socialization, the idea of pre-positioning acquires a new meaning. In an emergent stepfamily, there are no pre-given social frames that delimit allowable discourses and that give them meaning, except for those appearing in folk and fairy tales, or obtuse movies aimed at either raw emotional or sexual arousal. The pre-positioning has to be accomplished by settling for a new script based on metaphorical mappings from similar non-step-family frames. In other words, the new set of rules and regulations needs to be constructed within the interactional immediacy.

The 'repertoires of acts' for positioning in a stepfamily are scarcely populated, and tainted by the skewed examples given in the childhood narratives and popular culture which, both implicitly and explicitly, attaches negative meanings to the rights and duties of the step-familial members: stepmother is *not* 'a real mother' (and she is also not an aunt, or a friend, etc.); stepdaughter is *not* 'a real daughter'; stepfamily is *not* 'a real family', etc. A stepfamily is, to this day, stigmatized and commonly understood as an artificial construct that has no biological basis necessary for the familial attribution.[1]

In a narrative episode discussed below, four actors position themselves and others in an effort to create a story that they believe to be an ideal one. To achieve this, each actor seems to occasionally wrestle for their position, negotiate both self- and the

---

[1] This holds true despite the impressive statistics: up to a third of 74 million American children live in a stepfamily household (Forum on Child and Family Statistics, accessed on 8 May 2010 from http://www.childstats.gov/AMERICASCHILDREN/index.asp).

other-positioning and accept/reject a proposed position. Their narrative story lines reveal their agenda. However, we can see that each family member struggles to advance several competing narratives. We follow these multiple narratives in a single transcript; therapeutically one can say that there are always alternative narratives that can be displayed for the understanding of the persons involved. Or another way of making this point—there is nothing absolute about the narrative or story line that has been taken to be unfolding—another is always possible.

The stepfamily

In the family dynamics represented by the conversation below among three members of a new emerging stepfamily—father (F), stepmother Anamaria (SM), daughter/stepdaughter Renee (D), and a house guest, stepmother's female friend visiting from Europe (G), the actors do not produce a stable square with an equal chance of engagement. The conversation consists of four integral stories, which we identify as 'The Apron Story' (lines 1–23) 'The Cookbook Story' (lines 24–31 and 87–93), 'The Refrigerator Story' (lines 32–42 and 52–56) and 'The Young Vegetarian' (lines 43–51 and 55–86). Clearly, the *fil rouge* of this conversation is the food that the family consumes together, the centre of their daily family routine.

The rights and duties in a traditional family are established within the moral order of the given society. These conventions do not apply to some non-traditional family formations, especially one in which the central family actor—mother—has been replaced by another person. In addition, the family whose conversations provide the material for this illustration has a teenage daughter who lived for a while alone with her father, thus assuming some of the identity of the household female proprietor. This position is manifested in the excerpt below as she continues to maintain her position in the foundational establishment of the family structure. However, as positions are momentary and ephemeral and can be challenged (Harré et al. 2009, p. 10), the actors negotiate a new family script that would be more adequate to accommodate their emerging relationships. However, as we shall see, the conversation affords more than one reading.

We drop in on a dinner table conversation as SM had offered more food, but everybody had enough to eat.[2]

```
1  D:   Did you hear what I said
2       to you before dad
3       I said
4       Anamaria needs-
5       we need to get her an apron
6       that says 'laud the chef'
7  F:   Yeah.
8  SM:  A lo- what?
9  D:   Laud the chef
```

---

[2] Transcription conventions: /xxxxxxx/ marks undecipherable speech; @ marks a second of laughter; [transcriber's comments are placed in brackets].

10	F:	Laud. Mean-
11		meaning bow before it
12		and give-
13		SM:Oh:.
14	D:	/xxxxxxxxxxxx/
15	SM:	@@@@@@
16	G:	@@@@@@
17	D:	/xx/ have it just written@@
18	SM:	No, no. I-
19		I don't think I'm that bad.
20	F:	[CLEARS THROAT]
21	SM:	But I certainly enjoy
22		when people eat.
23		With pleasure.
24	F:	Well, y'know, when Anamaria
25		united with our little family
26		I mean it was the case that
27		y'know mainly-
28		mainly what she cooked was
29		was things with meat of course.
30	G:	@Hmh.
31	F:	So, one of the first things that I got-
32	D:	I remember seeing it-
33		dad, remember she had like
34		big chunks of meat
35		in the refrigerator
36	F:	Yeah.
37	D:	and stuff when we
38		visited her apartment and-
39		w- dad and I were just like
40		Blaah! [MAKES REVULSION SOUND]
41	F:	Blaah! [MAKES REVULSION SOUND]
42	D:	@@@@@@@
43	G:	You were-
44		you were vegetarian
45		when you met already?
46	F:	Yeah.
47	D:	@@@@@@
48	SM:	Yeah.
49	D:	@@@@
50		Yeah.
51	G:	And Renee too?
52	D:	It was so funny.
53		Because we came to visit her
54		when she lived
55	SM:	Oh, she would sin sometimes
56	D:	in that apartment.
57	SM:	in McDonald's.

58 G: Oh, really?
59 D: What?
60 SM: You would sin sometimes
61   at that time still
62 D: I would s- what?
63 SM: Sin.
64 D: Oh, I would sin-
65   I thought you said sing
66   and I was like 'what'?
67 G: @@@@@
68 D: No, but-
69   not when I met you though
70 SM: Not anymore?
71 D: I was phasing it out then but-
72 SM: Oh,
73   phasing it out.
74 F: Phasing it out.
75   Phasing out sin.
76 D: It was just chicken.
77 SM: @@Chicken.
78 D: I got rid of red meat
79   that was the first thing
80   I got rid of.
81   And then
82   I was still eating chicken and turkey
83   but then eventually
84   that—I was rid of that too.
85 SM: Mh-mh.
86 G: @@@
87 F: But one of the first things
88   I did buy for Anamaria
89   was *The Ultimate Vegetarian Cookbook.*
90   Which is-
91   Was it *New York Times*?
92 D: For Christmas.
93 SM: Mh-mh.

In a previous analysis of this narrative (Dedaić 2001), the focus was on the ways the stepmother was self- and other-positioned within the emergent family confines. Here, we expand the analysis by looking at it from the perspective of narratology as to ascertain the immanent positions that each actor takes in order to participate in the positioning negotiation that evolves in the narrative.

First reading: power struggle

Each of the family members acts within a specific set of moral obligations and rights, their joint work producing the first frame: the power struggle in which the stepmother and the daughter are fighting to set up the new family according to their specifications, while the male figure attempts a reconciliation.

The power struggle is engendered by the opposing projects recognized in the daughter's and stepmother's (SM) story lines. Daughter (D) positions all participants according to her project—to exclude the SM from the family core. D takes up the leading role in the conversation and pre-positions her stepmother as (a) not knowing the language properly, (b) having been a carnivore who kept big chunks of meat in her refrigerator, (c) being 'tamed' by the family (and should be lauded for that). D also draws her father into the display of disgust (40–41).

Speech acts issued by D go through F, or by invitation to him to join in. They involve reminders and remembrances ('did you hear what I said to you before, dad'), suggestions for joint actions ('we need to give her an apron') or confirmation of joint actions (giving a cookbook 'for Christmas'). D's direct speech acts position SM as lacking the pre-family rights, that is she is 'out of the loop', as she explains to SM the meaning of words or corrects SM's statement that D was still eating meat at the time of the family's initiation. Note, also, that the pronominal use indicates that D casts herself as an agent while SM is objectivized: 'when I met you' (69).

D's pronouns confirm the centrality of her self-positioning. The communal pronoun '*we*' in D's discourse excludes the SM. The position of 'us as the core' and 'you as the periphery' is attained by the steady use of the 'dad, you and I' formula (1–2, 42–43, 49) which invites F to join the story line, and foregrounds the former 'dad and I' unit.

F's project is to incorporate Anamaria into the family core while simultaneously maintaining solidarity with D (c. f. echoing the disgust performance, 40–41). His discursive work is much more transparent in terms of pre-positioning his wife as a member of the family and hence having all the rights and duties that accrue to her as such. He mentions a deliberate act of incorporation—symbolic gift of a vegetarian cookbook as means of entering core family practices, and joins SM in teasing D for her delusive story line (74–75).

SM's project is to objectify or counter how D positions her in order to neutralize them. When praised in a circumlocutory manner (an apron with the words 'laud the chef'), SM takes it as a backhand compliment and refutes the positioning by saying 'no, I don't think I am that bad'. It could be that she finds the D/F united front exclusive enough so that the symbolic gift of a praising apron becomes less appealing.

SM is seemingly a topic of the whole segment, and therefore the other-positioning is taken upon by other participants towards her. The ratified listener, in Goffman's terms, is G, while SM was pushed into a position of a forced eavesdropper. However, she takes the positioning helm over while repudiating D's claim on early vegetarianism (55–57). The exposure of D's hypocrisy is done in a teasing manner, which swells as F collaborates and G laughs when D clumsily attempts to reposition herself as 'phasing out' her secret carnivorous habits (71–86).

Pre-positioned into an uncertain role that draws upon a number of potential ones—a mother, a friend, a wicked witch, or aunt-like female relative—SM does not respond very strongly to the carnivorous exaggerations in stepdaughter's second order positioning (Harré et al. 2009, p. 12). D's positioning of SM exudes power as she is able to position her stepmother as a 'lower-level member', the one who hasn't yet achieved the status of vegetarian nobility like her father and herself. Her participation in converting her stepmother into a better human being, that is a vegetarian, is then made into a story line that maintains the positioning imbalance while simultaneously working towards the familial balance. The new position within the family gives stepmother an opportunity to reposition herself towards the moral ideal.

Second-order positioning can be implicit or explicit. Story lines reveal the implicit beliefs of members, but they are reinterpreted explicitly. With SM's objection to the stepdaughter's positioning of her, she, SM, repositions herself while simultaneously casting her stepdaughter as a hypocrite, effectively re-positioning her too. D thereby loses her upper hand at the other-positioning.

SM also attends the story line established with her friend G. Serving as a corrector of story lines offered by F and (most often) D, SM positions herself in the construction of the narrative presented to the person who has the longest historical knowledge of her. Pre-positioned as a friend and an equal, she attempts to maintain that subject position as her narrative acquired a new context within her new family.

Second reading: united front

While the first reading highlights the management of the new social formation around the core family of father and daughter with the arrival of the stepmother, a second reading makes salient the fact that her friend (G) is the ratified listener to the family stories already known to the other listeners. The individual projects find a shared goal in looking for a successful way of affirming all family memberships and creating a family unit. All three family members participate in erecting a family front, collaborating in explaining to G their uniqueness, affirming their superior moral status as vegetarians, *including SM*! The *key events* in this story are: (1) the plan to present the apron, honouring the quality of the veggie cooking, (2) the presentation of the Veggie cook book at Christmas, confirming conversion, and (3) the explanation that D too had gone through the conversion at essentially the same time. The salient story line is the gradual transformation of the family, *including SM and D*, via temptations overcome to the pure state of being vegetarians.

It is up to the therapist to recognize the braided story lines and to sort out the one deemed most beneficial to the client. In the first utterances by D (1–6), we can recognize two stories. The first one is the making of two fronts—the father/daughter opposite to the stepmother. This reading clearly comes from the pronominal use ('*we* need to give *her* an apron'). However, giving such a gift can also mean a token of acceptance of the stepmother as the family cook, not intrusive but rather a desired member of the family. Both readings are 'correct' since the text is susceptible of the either without strain or implausibility.

However, there is also a third reading, which might be less usable in the therapeutic sense. However, we want to mention it in order to shed light from another possible angle because we talk to position ourselves, but also to ascertain and construct positions for the interactant(s). Thus, a narrative micro-system (Ricoeur 1989, p. 583) incorporates the relationship of a family to their guests as a general rule, and is epitomized in their approach to their guest G. Pleasing a family guest might be seen as a duty of a family. In reverse, the family gains rights as it confirms itself as a family by fulfilling that duty.

Third reading: pleasing and educating the guest

For G, vegetarianism is an unfamiliar practice. Having come from a culture which appreciates meat dishes, she sounds surprised that everybody is vegetarian and enquires about the ways and times of the members becoming vegetarian. Her positioning efforts are minimal; she mainly accepts family members' positions but expresses disbelief in D's story (51) and directs to the 'adults' a question about her explicitly. On this and several other occasions, the directions of her questions and laughter indicate her alignment with SM. Despite her minimal active involvement as a speaker, G's active listening attention moves the story forward. After all, for whom is this elaborate charade performed?

G's project is to learn about a new family and the place her friend SM takes in it. G senses a struggle, and takes sides, albeit ever so slightly. After all, she is a guest, a pre-position that culturally assigns her a duty of respect to the household that hosts her. In addition, she modifies her own pre-existing subject position of SM whose pre-positioning has radically changed from a single woman to a wife and a mother.

Upshot

The ideal outcome of the stepfamily narrative would be a united front, in which all actors are interested in advancing the same goal—to position each person within an idealized structure in which everybody finds a happy place. However, as the normative step-frame suffers from deficient description and even more deficient practice, the actors are left to construct not only their selves, but also the context for the embedding of those selves.

In a stepfamily, the pre-positioning is the most interesting part because there is no given story line to follow; every stepfamily has to construct their own anew. The saliency of story lines is determined locally, but the cluster of rights and duties distributed among actors is global. In a stepfamily, those rights and duties need to be constructed locally, at the conversation site, and distributed according to the interlocutors' epistemic relevancies to the perceived duties and rights of the participants.

It is worth remembering that ascriptions of rights and of duties are often symmetrical in the sense that for every right someone or some institution has a duty to satisfy it. This derives from the basic principle that rights are reflections of the vulnerabilities of a person or class of persons, while duties are reflections of the powers of correlative persons and classes of persons.

Pronoun grammars as psychologically relevant schemata

Among English speakers the lost distinction between thee/thou and you/ye leaves relative social status unmarked grammatically. However, almost all Indo-European languages have a T-V (named after the French 'Tu' and 'Vous') second person grammatical resource open to them—while the available pronouns in some oriental languages offer even greater resources for marking relative social status grammatically. Thus in Spanish native speakers have 'tu' and 'Usted' available. Brown and Gilman (1960, p. 257) express this resource in a pair of Cartesian axes, the formal/informal axis and the 'solidarity' or intimate/distant axis. Further research has yielded some refinements, but T-V has stood the test of time as the most revealing analytical scheme.

To express social intimacy one can use the reciprocal T-T form in address and response and social distance can be expressed by the reciprocal V-V usage. To express respect a social inferior addresses his or her social superior with the V form while the high status interlocutor uses the T form in response. One perhaps should say 'used to use' since this degree of marking of social superiority and inferiority is fading fast in Europe, and even in Japan.

The principle of indexicality

Whatever may be the fate of the T-V grammar in any particular social setting the distinction between 'I', 'we' and 'you' as indexicals, and all third person pronouns as serving an anaphoric function, is of crucial importance, as we shall see when we turn to pathologies of personal discourse.

The first person singular indexes the speech act it introduces with some relevant attribute of the speaker. For example, if someone says what they can see or feel or hear, the hearer understands that the point of vantage is where the speaker happens to be at the moment of utterance. The grid of places is implicit in the discourse. Tenses are more complex, but still require that the speaker uses the first person to index what is said with the time it is spoken—'now' is implicit in every act of speaking. To complete the meaning of a first or second person statement the hearer must know something about the speaker that is extrinsic to the conversation. However, the anaphoric pronouns 'he', 'she', and 'they' get their meaning from within the discourse from reference back to a name or definite description. Thus in the statement 'Barack Obama said that he would regulate the banks' the 'he' gets its meaning from the occurrence of the prior proper name.

Moreover, the use of the first person has a further indexical force—to use 'I' is to commit oneself to the content of the speech-act—for example a promise. This indexing is also tied to knowledge of something outside the discourse, namely the moral standing of the speaker. To understand the utterance properly, for example whether or not to rely on it, one needs knowledge of the moral standing of the speaker, a feature which is not available in the discourse itself.

Pronoun analysis in discursive therapy: intrapersonal positioning

In the case now to be discussed the person displaying multiple personality syndrome (MPS) offers two story lines to the therapist (Beran and Unoca 2004, pp. 151–61). There is the story of herself as Elsa and the story of herself as Marian. These story lines are tied in with primary acts of character pre-positioning that support claims of positioning each persona as having rights to be heard as authentic independent voices. The psychiatrist attempts to meld the two story lines into one as a single autobiography. In so doing, a single personality is restored or recreated. In the classical study of MPS, Morton Prince's (1905) record of the discourses in which Christine and

Sally Beauchamp appeared, an important aspect of the therapy was 'grammatical'. Prince insisted that Miss Beauchamp refrained from talking of her life events in terms of three pronouns, 'I', 'you', and 'she', thus recreating a single autobiographical story line, with the suppression of one the original protagonists, Sally.

Autobiography can be viewed as a device for positioning *oneself* in the act of presenting a self-narrative. An autobiography is not a chronicle because it is not only a history but also a manifestation of personhood, and ordered in accordance with the meanings that an event may have in the autobiography then being presented rather than any other that might have been. Every normal human being has a repertoire of autobiographies each freely accessible from every other. This is not the case with the story telling of someone presenting MPS.

A narratological analysis of MPS can be set out in formal schema as an analytical tool for the study of the problems of a patient, P:

1) P tells two distinct autobiographies, A1 and A2 which are not freely accessible one from the other.
2) Each autobiography displays a distinctive set of personal qualities, including knowledge of past events.
3) When living out A1, events relevant to A2 are apparently not accessible to memory (or at least as tellable as recollections), and when living out A2, events relevant to A1 are not accessible to memory (or at least tellable as recollections).
4) Each A1, A2, etc. establishes a position as someone, a distinct voice, having the right to speak and the right to be heard—even also the duty to reprimand other claimants to those rights, even if embodied in the same material being.

Morton Prince and the discursive therapy of Miss Beauchamp

In this classic case, Christine Beauchamp is referred to Morton Prince by her family, worried by her seemingly erratic behaviour. Prince records conversations with her in which she produces a variety of narratives, indexed via the personal pronouns of English to various voices/speakers/actors. These are not the voices of Joan of Arc but speaking positions functioning indexically. Some of these narratives are reminiscences, some about life events and some meta-reminiscences about her sense of herself. Using hypnosis as an auxiliary technique Prince collects a corpus of material in which he discerns three major voices. The patterns of cross reference between these voices are complex, as we shall see.

In the first part of his report Morton Prince describes the way that his patient, Miss Christine Beauchamp, displayed distinct personalities in the character traits that were evident in the content of what she said and in the pronouns she used to refer from one personality 'stance' to that of another. Prince elicited these 'personality stances' by the use of hypnosis, though later they appeared spontaneously when Christine Beauchamp was awake.

Prince labelled Miss Christine Beauchamp, identified by displays of normal personality traits, BI. BII appeared first as a hypnotic 'artefact'. BIII was a coherent personality with distinctive memories and, after some time, an independent proper name,

'Sally'—introduced by Miss Beauchamp herself. Eventually both Christine and Sally referred to another way Christine Beauchamp could be, that is BIV to Dr Prince but as 'the Idiot' in Christine's and Sally's talk.

At a certain point in Prince's therapeutic dialogue with his patient the question of pronouns comes up. As BII, she referred to herself as BI by the third person 'she' (Prince 1905, p. 55). He tries unsuccessfully to persuade her to use 'I', which she steadfastly refuses—'I' is the pronoun with which one takes responsibility for what is said. She declares that she is justified in staying with 'she', 'Because "she" does not know the same things that I do'.

We use indexicals to claim memories as our own—and on p. 33 Morton Prince lays out the relation between claims of personal knowledge in a table—BIII knows what BI and BII know, though BI does not know all that BIII knows. BII knows what BI knows but not all that BIII knows.

Still later in the story BIII addresses BI as 'you'—still further sharpening the divide between herself as Christine Beauchamp, the hard working neurotic student, and BIII, the fun loving, mischievous young woman. After a complicated pattern of hypnotic trances and invitations to be herself, the real Miss Beauchamp, Morton Prince reports the following dialogue in which a stable synthesis is presented *pronominally*. 'Who are you?' the doctor asks. 'I am myself' answers Miss Beauchamp. 'Where is BI?' asks the doctor. 'I am BI' she declares. 'Where is BIV?' he asks. 'I am BIV. We are all the same person, only now I am myself' she replies. 'Sally' is never evoked and the 'real' Miss Beauchamp knows nothing of her (Prince 1905, p. 533). Perhaps, at the end of this long series of conversations Morton Prince managed to persuade Miss Beauchamp to adopt a consistently singular indexical grammar. We do not know.

E. Beran and Z. Unoca and the discursive eherapy of Elsa/Marian

Beran and Unoca (2004), like Morton Prince, use pronouns as persona and position indicators. Their analysis displays two persona positions presented sequentially and tied in with proper names in the same manner as the referential system revealed in Miss Beauchamp's case. The story lines are tied discursively to distinct voices in the following manner, first with proper names and then with pronouns, one indexical and one anaphoric:

Elsa: she positions herself as an authoritative witness of the past having the right to be heard and believed. Her narrative's original past tense changes to present tense, as she retells the story of the trial of the man who raped her.
Marian: she is evoked by Elsa when she, Elsa, is asked to tell the story again, as one who is trying to stop her (Elsa) telling the tale. This is a positioning move since Marian is resisting Elsa's self-positioning as one who has a right to tell the story and to be believed.

The therapist induces Elsa to talk as Marian to explain why the story should not be told. In this telling Elsa is referred to in the third person and Marian adopts the first person, positioning herself as authoritative, that is, as having the right to be believed. Then the therapist induces Elsa to tell the story as Elsa in the first person. In this way the therapist makes both stories available, the telling of the original story and the telling of the story of the resistance to the telling. In the new situation Elsa is able to explicate the significance of the second voice. Marian is the name of her husband's mistress with whom she had a quarrel. The implication is that through this process of discursive readjustment of indexicalities and rights to speak of certain events, at least one of the disturbances with which Elsa has been troubled will or has already been dissolved. The storied life of Elsa has moved forward into what we may hope are calmer waters.

Conclusions

We have set out several aspects of discursive psychology, each of which can find a place as a source of techniques and inspiration to those who use discursive therapies.

1) Much of social life is ordered by implicit schemata, the content of which we can express as rules—with various levels of coercive force. Sometimes the schemata are offered as explicit instructions. However, whatever their status, rules are human constructions. What can be constructed can be deconstructed. No one ever need be a cultural dope, a rule-slave. The most important cases for discursive therapy must surely be those where someone mistakes the force of the rule, taking advice for coercion, for example.

2) Life is lived as, and in the framework of, narratives. There are story lines that are so firmly embedded in a culture, and which endlessly repeat themselves to us, that we cease to notice, if we ever did, that there is nothing inexorable about them. A new story line could always be lived and told. From the nursery through the folk tale to the popular soap, these tales seem to have a kind of necessity about them, but we must remind ourselves, they are just stories. However, they can be fateful.

3) What one does is shaped by the interplay between what one is capable of and what is acceptable in the local moral order. Locality may be ethnicity, it may be social class, it may be profession or job, it may be age group or religious affiliation. The study of this interplay reveals positions, clusters of rights and duties, within which people are trapped. Change the story line and the trap is sprung open. Positioning theory also tracks the many ways that positioning is refused, accepted and, in Sabat's fascinating case, subverted. The story of the stepmother's *rite de passage* illustrates the enormously important point that many different story lines with associated positionings can be underway at any time and within the very same conversation. Clearly, an important part of the work of the discursive therapist is to help to highlight the most constructive and life-enhancing reading that can be made available to the participants.

4) Finally, there are those little words that are scarcely attended to but which are hugely important as the language of life unfolds in everyday conversations. Multiple personality syndrome can come to be seen as a matter of the uses of pronoun grammar. Furthermore, one can hardly be unaware of the fatefulness of the use of pronouns, the most socially loaded of all the parts of speech.

5) Discursive psychology has much to offer the discursive therapist.

References

Austin, J. L. (1959). *How to do things with words: The William James Lectures delivered at Harvard University in 1955* (J. O. Urmson, Ed.). Clarendon Press, Oxford.

Beran, E. and Unoca, Z. (2004). Construction of self-narrative in a psychotherapeutic setting. In U. M. Quasthoff and T. Becker (Eds.) *Narrative Interaction*, pp. 151–64. Benjamins, Amsterdam.

Brinkmann, S. (2010). *Psychology as a Moral Science*. Routledge, London.

Brown, R. and Gilman, A. (1960). The pronouns of power and solidarity. In T. A. Sebeok (Ed.) *Style in Language*, pp. 253–76. MIT Press, Cambridge, MA.

Burke, K. (1945). *A grammar of motives*. Prentice Hall, Englewood Cliffs, NJ.

Davies, B. and Harré, R. (1990). Positioning theory. *Journal for the Theory of Social Behaviour*, **20**, 43–63.

Dedaić, M. N. (2001). Stepmother as electron: Positioning the stepmother in a family dinner conversation. *Journal of Sociolinguistics*, **5**, 372–400.

Garfinkel, H. (1967). *Studies in the ethnomethodology*. Prentice Hall, Englewood Cliffs, NJ.

Goffman, E. (1974). *Frame analysis*. Harvard University Press, Cambridge, MA.

Greimas, A. J. (1987). *On meaning*. Minnesota University Press, Minneapolis, MN.

Greimas, A. J. Courtès, J., and Rengstorf, M. (1976). The cognitive dimension of narrative discourse. *New Literary History*, **7**, 563–79.

Harré, R., Brockmeier, J., and Muhlhausler, P. (1998). *Greenspeak*. Sage, London.

Harré, R., Moghaddam, F. M., Pilkerton Cairnie, T., Rothbart, D., and Sabat, S. R. (2009). Recent advances in Positioning Theory. *Theory and Psychology*, **19**, 5–31.

Kitwood, T. (1988). The technical, the personal, and the framing of dementia. *Social Behavior*, **3**, 161–80.

Prince, M. (1905). *The dissociation of a personality*. Longmans, Green and Co, London.

Propp, V. (1968). *The morphology of the folk tale* (L. Scott, Trans.). University of Texas Press, Austin, TX.

Ricoeur, P. (1989). Greimas's narrative grammar (F. Collins and P. Perron, Trans.). *New Literary History*, **20**, 581–608.

Sabat, S. (1994). Excess disability and malignant social psychology: a case study of Alzheimer's disease. *Journal of Community & Applied Social Psychology*, **4**, 157–66.

Sabat, S. and Harré, R. (1994). The Alzheimer disease sufferer as a semiotic subject. *Philosophy, Psychiatry and Psychology*, **1**, 145–60.

Schank, R. C. and Abelson, R. P. (1977). *Scripts, plans, goals, and understanding: An enquiry into human knowledge structures*. Erlbaum, Hillsdale, NJ.

Smedslund, J. (2010). The mismatch between current research methods and the nature of psychological phenomena: what researchers must learn from practitioners. *Theory and Psychology*, **19**, 778–94.

Valsiner, J. (2010). *Culture in minds and societies*. Sage, Los Angeles, CA.

Chapter 4

Therapeutic communication from a constructionist standpoint

Kenneth J. Gergen and Mary Gergen

Many therapists are familiar with the landscape of social constructionist thought. Indeed, many of those represented in the present volume have contributed significantly to its development. However, for those presently joining these explorations, some preliminary remarks may be helpful. Specifically, our attempt in this chapter is first to sketch out several major assumptions shared by those engaged in constructionist endeavours. After describing some of these central ideas, we will take up the challenge of therapeutic communication. Here we will move beyond existing accounts to demonstrate what might be called a *radical relationalism* that constructionism invites. Finally, we shall explore significant implications of this account for therapeutic practice.

The social construction of the real and the good

There are many ways to tell the story of social constructionism. Each account would construct constructionism in a different way; each would be useful in a different context. In what follows we shall briefly describe three of the most widely shared narratives circulating today. These accounts are elaborated more fully elsewhere.[1] We have selected these particular stories because they are simultaneously among the most unsettling and profoundly liberating. They also relate most clearly to the discursive theme that links together the chapters of the present book.

The social lodgment of knowledge

Perhaps the most generative idea emerging from the constructionist dialogues is that what we take to be knowledge finds its origins in human relationships. What we believe to be true as opposed to false, objective as opposed to subjective, scientific as opposed to mythological, rational as opposed to irrational, moral as opposed to immoral is brought into being by historically and culturally situated groups of people. This view stands in dramatic contrast to two of the most important intellectual and cultural traditions of the West: the individualist and the communal. On the one hand is the tradition of the individual knower—the rational, self-directing, morally centred,

---

[1] See, for example, Gergen (2009a), and Gergen and Gergen (2004).

and knowledgeable agent of action. In effect, the constructionist dialogues challenge the longstanding individualist tradition and invite an appreciation of relationship as central to human well-being. It is not the individual mind in which knowledge, reason, emotion, and morality reside, but in relationships.[2]

The second view of knowledge, that is the communal view, is also challenged. The possibility that the accounts of scientists, or any other group, reveal or approach the objective truth about what is the case is cast into doubt. In effect, propose the constructionists, no one arrangement of words, mathematical formulae, or symbolic system is necessarily more objective or accurate in its depiction of reality than any other. To be sure, accuracy may be achieved within a given community or tradition—according to its rules and practices. Physics and chemistry generate useful truths from within their communal traditions, just as psychologists, sociologists, novelists, and priests do from within theirs. But from these often competing traditions we cannot locate a transcendent truth, a 'truly true'. Any attempt to determine the superior account would itself be the outcome of a given community of agreement. All claims to Truth must be viewed from some perspective, and beyond any perspective, one has no resources for speaking at all.

Unsurprisingly, these arguments have provoked strong and sometimes angry reactions among scientific communities in particular. Let's say you have devoted a lifetime to pursuing what you believe to be objective knowledge, and you despair of the unverifiable myths, credos, and folk beliefs by which common people lead their lives. Under these conditions it is difficult to be told that science is itself a social construction and not intrinsically superior to other traditions. Yet, it is our view that such anguish is based on a misreading of the constructionist message. Western medical science, for example, does indeed offer useful truths; most of us would scarcely wish to abandon them. However, these truths are based on an enormous array of culturally and historically specific constructions, for example, about what constitutes an impairment, health and illness, life and death, the boundaries of the body, the nature of pain, and so on. When these assumptions are treated as universal—true for all cultures and times—alternative conceptions are undermined and destroyed. To understand death, for example, as merely the termination of biological functioning would be an enormous impoverishment of human existence. The point is not to abandon medical science, but to understand it as a cultural tradition—one among many.

Thus, social constructionism first serves an enormous liberating function. It removes the rhetorical power of anyone or any group claiming truth, wisdom, or ethics of universal scope—necessary for all. In this sense, social constructionist ideas tend to support those who would speak out against the dominant discourse. All voices may justifiably contribute to the dialogues on which our futures depend. It is also important to understand that although knowledge claims are socially constructed, this does not render them insignificant. Again, it is to recognize that each tradition, while limited, may offer us options for living together. In this way constructionism invites a posture of infinite curiosity, where every tradition may offer us riches, and new amalgams

---

[2] For a more extended account of both the critique of individualism, and its relational replacement, see Gergen (2009b).

stand ever open to development. At the same time, because all traditions will tend so suppress, all should be open to critical reflection. Every voice has the potential for both good and evil from some perspective. The future of the planet depends importantly on how disparate or conflicting discourses may be reconciled, amalgamated, or transformed.

The centrality of discourse

Many scholars believe that Ludwig Wittgenstein was the most significant philosopher of the 20th century. After reading his later work, most especially *Philosophical Investigations* (1953), one can never see the aim of philosophy in the same way again. In large measure this is because Wittgenstein's work challenged the capacity of philosophy to yield true understanding of knowledge, rationality, ethics, the self, and all the other subjects of longstanding concern to philosophers. As Wittgenstein proposed, our descriptions and explanations of the world are formed within language, or what he calls 'language games'. Games of language are essentially conducted in a rule-like fashion; to make sense at all requires that one play by the rules. The rules of grammar present the most obvious case; but there are also myriad other rules. For example, it is not acceptable for me to say that 'my love is oblong'. The utterance is grammatically correct, and it cannot be falsified with empirical data. Rather, our ways of talking about love in the 21st century do not happen to include the adjective 'oblong'. Expanding on this point, we can describe the major questions asked by philosophers as language games. For example, the longstanding question of whether the mind truly has access to the external world—the 'problem of epistemology' as it is called—is a problem only within a given game of language. To play the game we must agree that there is a 'mental world' on the one hand and a 'material world' on the other (an 'in here' and an 'out there'), and that the former may possibly reflect the latter. If you do not agree to play by these rules, there is no 'problem of individual knowledge'. It is dissolved.

Yet, to view language as simply a game is limited. As Wittgenstein proposed, language use is lodged within broader 'forms of life', as he called them. Consider the form of life we call a 'soccer match'. To be sure, there are traditional ways of talking about soccer—about teams, scores, penalty kicks, and so on. But these forms of talk are embedded within forms of action and material. One cannot simply yell out 'Score!' on a busy street corner, without arousing suspicion. There are only specific conditions in which such a cry makes sense, and this depends on a specific array of objects (such as the playing field and the ball) and people (such as the players and referees).

Wittgenstein's ideas are highly congenial with the view of knowledge as social in origin. As people coordinate their actions, a major outcome is often a system of signals or words. The words often serve to name the world for the participants. This is 'a goal', you have the 'flu', that is 'a stolen car', and so on. These words are enormously important to sustaining our daily relationships. Not only do they represent the agreements regarding what exists for the participants, but they essentially constitute the glue by which their very forms of life—or traditions—are held together. What sense is there in a jury trial without a language of guilt and innocence; what would the profession of psychology be without a language of the mind; and what would become of religion if we abandoned the language of the spirit?

Objectivity as ideology

Social constructionism shares much with a pragmatic view of knowledge claims. That is, traditional issues of truth and objectivity are replaced with concerns with practical outcomes. It is not whether an account is true from a god's eye view that matters; rather we ask what will happen if we take any truth claim seriously. There can be many truths, depending on community traditions, but as the constructionist asks, what happens to us—for good or ill—if we accept one as opposed to another account? There are no meaningful words without consequence. In this sense, the increased awareness of the communal construction of the real and the good does far more than unsettle our traditional beliefs in truth, objectivity, and knowledge—beyond history and culture. Placed in question is also the right of any particular group—scientific or otherwise—to claim ultimate authority of knowledge. And with such questioning, we are also invited into deliberation on what we judge to be worthwhile, good, or desirable

Such a conclusion has had enormous repercussions in the academic community and beyond. This is so especially for scholars and practitioners concerned with social injustice, oppression, and the marginalization of minority groups in society. If communities create realities (facts and good reasons) congenial to their own traditions, and these realities are established as true and good for all, then alternative traditions may be obliterated. Regardless of whether we are speaking of scientific fact, canons of logic, foundations of law, or spiritual truths, as we formulate the world we implicitly favour certain ways of life over others. Thus, for example, the scientist may use the most rigorous methods of testing intelligence, and amass tomes of data that indicate racial differences in intelligence. However, to presume that there is something called 'human intelligence,' that people differ in their possession of this capacity, that there is something called 'race', that race can be clearly determined, and that a series of question and answer games can reveal one's intelligence or race, is all specific to a given tradition or paradigm. Such concepts and measures are not required by 'the way the world is'. Most importantly, merely entering the paradigm and moving within the tradition is deeply injurious to those people classified as inferior by its standards. Or to put it another way, the longstanding distinction between *facts* and *values*—objective reflections of the world, and subjective desires or feelings of 'ought'—cannot be sustained. Rather, values are intrinsic to facts.

As we see, sensitivity to the politics of the real and the good invites a broad critical posture. The interested reader may wish to explore such critiques and their rejoinders.[3] Unfortunately, however, many of those drawn into a critical posture simply remain there. The gadfly rarely becomes a butterfly. To understand the politics of knowledge also opens the door to appreciation. It is not simply 'what we lose' within any tradition of knowledge that is important, but what we gain as well. We may ask of all claims to knowledge, wisdom, insight, and the like, 'what follows', 'who benefits', and 'who is silenced?'. All constructions will place limits upon our lives; but without construction there is nothing worthy of any pursuit. From these new amalgams we may move towards richer and more inclusive forms of life.

---

[3] See for example, Parker (1998) and Nightingale and Cromby (1999).

These three themes—centring on the social construction of the real and the good, the pivotal function of language in creating intelligible worlds, and the political and pragmatic nature of discourse—have rippled across the academic disciplines and throughout many domains of human practice. To be sure, all such developments are controversial. However, such ideas also possess enormous potential. Such is the case in therapy as it is in the global context. The therapeutic community has long participated in the constructionist dialogues and richly extended their potential. The present volume, for example, brings into common dialogue the voices of narrative, collaborative, and brief therapists—among others—and suggests a broad sea-change in thought and practice. However, the full implications of a constructionist orientation remain unclear. It is within this context, that we now explore the topic of therapeutic communication. The process is of singular significance, not only to the outcomes of therapy, but to the very idea of a constructed world. This discussion will also help to clarify differences between constructionism and contrasting traditions, and to appreciate its radically relational character. After treating some of the rudiments of the communication process we turn to therapeutic implications.

Therapeutic communication in question

The question of what it is in the therapeutic encounter that brings about change has been central to the endeavour since its very inception. Perhaps the central candidate for answering this question is therapeutic communication. There is something about the nature of communicative interchange that seems pivotal to the change process. Yet, such an answer is scarcely sufficient. How are we to understand the process of communication? What precisely is it about communication that brings about transformation? What forms of communication are invited; how might we be more effective? There are significant differences among schools of therapy in their approach to communication, and they are highly consequential. Consider the client who complains of his lack of sexual desire. If one is a marital counsellor, these words may be treated as an accurate representation of reality, and the basis of a programme of support. In contrast, if one is a psychoanalyst, the content of the client's account might be disregarded, and his words examined for messages from the domain of the unconscious. For the cognitive-behavioural therapist, however, the same words are neither descriptions of the real world nor manifestations of repressed desires, but indicators of the world from the client's perspective. The therapist might thus launch inquiry into the logic of this perspective, and its possible distortions. And, for the structuralist family therapist, the client's words may be understood in none of these ways, but as indications of the configuration of family relations. In this case the therapist might address the ways this expressed lack of desire is related to the actions of other family members. Each presumption about the nature of language and the process of communication yields a different therapeutic posture.

In what follows we first consider several major assumptions that underlie most therapeutic practices developed to date. Although there is much to be said on behalf of these assumptions, in each case we shall single out major shortcomings. While our conceptual heritage is rich, traditional assumptions about therapeutic communication erect barriers beyond which our practices cannot proceed. We shall then sketch out the rudiments of a constructionist theory of communication. In this account we find a dramatic disjunction with the past and a shift to a radical relationalism. We then present significant implications for therapeutic practice. Consider, then, several traditional assumptions and the critical problems they create:

The realist assumption

One of the most broadly shared views of language is based on the assumption that words are (or can be) reflectors of the real. That is, language can (and should) function so as to provide accurate accounts of what is the case. This is the view inherited by most of the sciences, as they set out to replace misleading, fallacious, or superstitious beliefs with true and accurate accounts of the world. For many therapists it is also essential to distinguish between client accounts that are accurate, realistic, and truthful, versus those that are distorted, fanciful, or duplicitous. The realist assumption is also central to those attempting to develop diagnostic categories and measures of pathology. In daily life it is a view that lends support to the distinction between objective facts and subjective opinions, and moral weight to demands that people 'tell the truth'.

There is much to be said about the importance of this tradition both to scientific and cultural life. However, as the preceding discussion makes clear, the realist assumption is deeply flawed. There is no privileged relationship between a given language and the state of things; there is no particular arrangement of words and phrases that is uniquely tailored to the 'world as it is'. Rather, as we have seen, declarations of the real and the true are always located within relationships—friendships, families, communities, and traditions. Within these relationships there can be undisputed realities— 'myocardial infarction' in medicine, a 'three-point shot' in basketball, and so on. In this sense, to tell a lie is not to misrepresent the world, but to violate a communal tradition.

The subjectivist assumption

Often coupled with the realist assumption is a second view of longstanding. As it is typically said, we each exist in our own private worlds of experience, a mind set apart from, and reflecting upon nature—a state of subjectivity that variously grapples with understanding the conditions of the objective world. On this account, the words we speak are held to be outer expressions of the inner world, the subjective mind made manifest. This view has played a major role in science, as we count the scientist's words as representing his or her experience of the world, and demand that observations be shared to insure agreement among subjectivities ('objectivity' as shared 'subjectivity'). The assumption is critical to most schools of therapy in the past century. In almost all cases we listen to a client's language as an outer expression of private experience (or, as in the Freudian case, that which lies beneath conscious experience to give it shape). And, the assumption is a common feature in daily relations, as we speak of the difficulties in knowing what others mean by their words, or how they 'really feel'. Intimacy, we believe, is a reflection of the closeness of two otherwise independent subjectivities.

Here we touch briefly on only two problems of subjectivity, the first conceptual and the second ideological. On the conceptual level, it is important to realize that no one has yet been able to give a defensible account of how a person's words give us access to his or her inner world. Given another's utterances, we have no way of knowing what they say about the speaker's subjective state. Hermeneutic theorists, concerned with how it is we can accurately understand the intentions behind the words of the Bible or holy writs, have worried about the problem of 'inner access' for over three centuries now. A satisfactory answer to this question has never been forthcoming. In Hans Georg Gadamer's (1975) pivotal work, *Truth and Method*, the major emphasis shifts to the 'horizon of understanding' that the reader inevitably brings to the text. As Gadamer reasoned, all readings must necessarily draw from this forestructure of understanding—what it is the reader presumes about the world, the writing, the author, and so on. And reading must inevitably take place from this horizon. Much the same conclusion is reached by a host of 'reader response' theorists in literary studies. As Stanley Fish (1980) has put the case, every reader is a member of some interpretive community, a network of people who understand the world in certain ways. And whatever interpretation of the text is made will inevitably rely on these understandings. In effect, the reader never makes authentic connection with the subjectivity of the writer; there is no escape from the standpoint one brings to the interpretation.

The dismal conclusion of this line of criticism is that we never gain access to the other's subjectivity; we never understand each other! We shall revisit this problem shortly. However, there is a second line of attack on the subjectivity assumption, one that resonates with our earlier discussion of the politics of knowledge. Here it is variously proposed that by placing such importance on individual subjectivity we give further support to an individualist ideology, an ideology detrimental to our cultural future. To reiterate some of the earlier critiques, when we hold individual subjectivity as the essential ingredient of the person, we simultaneously construct a world of fundamentally isolated individuals, each locked within their own private world. All we have to count on, ultimately, is ourselves. Others are by nature alien and because self-seeking is the obvious choice under such conditions, others may indeed be seen as potential enemies. When the quality of individual subjectivity is paramount, all forms of relationship—marriage, friendship, family, and community—are necessarily artificial and secondary. If this form of ideology retains its pervasive grip on cultural life, the future seems grim. In effect, the subjectivist assumption is socially corrosive.

The strategic assumption

There is a third problematic assumption regarding communication, one often made by therapists in particular. It is frequently held that communication operates as the major means by which individuals influence each other's actions. More specifically, it is reasoned, each of us uses language to achieve our goals, satisfy our desires, etc. Because of the complexities of daily life, we must rationally consider what we can say, when, where and to whom. Language typically functions, then, as a strategic implement through which we achieve their goals. It is in this sense, as well, that the therapist may select his/her words carefully, insert them into the conversation at the proper juncture in order to change to client or the pattern of family relations.

In light of the preceding discussion, the problems of the strategic assumption require but brief attention. For one, the position borrows heavily from the subjectivist tradition—'I desire and plan, and therefore I speak'. In this sense, the strategic assumption suffers from the same conceptual enigmas and the ideological shortcomings just discussed. Private goals are pre-eminent; others become secondary, mere utilities in the service of self. When we play out the implications of the strategic assumption the critique is intensified. When we understand communication as primarily serving private ends, human relations become a sea of manipulation. When we view communication in this way, acts of trust seem naïve, commitment a sign of weakness, and the pursuit of human rights little more than a political ploy. Even the therapist undermines his/her credibility, as the motive behind his or her communication to the client becomes suspect The therapist may be viewed as a master manipulator, and clients may come to see themselves as mere pawns. A strategic orientation can be fractionating.

Communication as collaborative action

The question we now address is whether an alternative conception of human communication can be developed. And, can such a conception avoid repeating the problems inherent in the earlier traditions? In our view, an alternative view of human communication can indeed be drawn from the constructionist dialogues, not only as they are taking place within therapeutic circles, but as they have developed in the neighbouring domains of ethnomethodology, the history of science, the sociology of knowledge, and literary theory.[4] In each of these cases there is a strong tendency to place the locus of meaning within the process of interaction itself. That is, the individual agent is de-emphasized as the source of meaning; attention moves from the *within* to the *between*. Yet, how are we to understand such a move, and what are the action implications? For purposes of furthering the dialogue, in what follows we make a preliminary incursion into these domains. We offer here a series of rudimentary propositions that place meaning squarely within the relational matrix:

Individual utterances possess no meaning

We pass each other on the street. I smile and say, 'Hello, Anna'. You walk past without hearing. Under such conditions, what have I said? To be sure, I have uttered two words. However for all the difference it makes I might have chosen two nonsense syllables. You pass and I say 'Umtot gigen...' You hear nothing. When you fail to acknowledge me in any way, all words become equivalent. In an important sense, nothing has been said at all. I cannot possess meaning alone.[5]

---

[4] See, for example, Garfinkel (1967); Kuhn (1970); Latour (1987); Edwards and Potter (1994); Fish (1980); and Shotter, (1993).

[5] One may object: 'well, even if not acknowledged, what I say might mean something to me personally', and that may be. But the question then becomes, how did your utterances come to have personal meaning? We take up this issue shortly.

Meaning is realized through supplementary action

Lone utterances begin to acquire meaning when another (or others) coordinate themselves to the utterance, that is, when they add some form of supplementary action (whether linguistic or otherwise). Effectively, I have greeted Anna only by virtue of her response. 'Oh, hi, good morning…' brings me to life as one who has greeted. Supplements may be very simple, as simple as a nod of affirmation that indeed you have said something meaningful. It may take the form of an action, e.g. shifting the line of gaze upon hearing the word, 'look!'. Or it may extend the utterance in some way, as in 'Yes, but I also think that…'. We thus find that to communicate at all is to be granted by others a privilege of meaning. If others do not treat one's utterances as communication, if they fail to coordinate themselves around the offering, one is reduced to nonsense.

To combine these first two proposals, we see that meaning does not reside within either individual, but within the relationship. Both act and supplement must be coordinated in order for meaning to occur. Like a handshake, a kiss, or a tango, the individual's actions alone are insufficient. Communication is inherently collaborative. In this way we see that none of the words that comprise our vocabulary have meaning in themselves. They are granted the capacity to mean by virtue of the way they are coordinated with other words and actions. Indeed, our entire vocabulary of the individual—who thinks, feels, wants, hopes, and so on—is granted meaning only by virtue of coordinated activities among people. The birth of 'myself' lies within relationship.

Supplementary action is itself a candidate for meaning

Any supplement functions twice, first in granting significance to what has preceded and second as an action that also requires supplementation. In effect, the meaning it grants remains suspended until it too is supplemented. Consider a client who speaks of her deep depression; she finds herself unable to cope with an aggressive husband and an intolerable job situation. The therapist can grant this report meaning as an expression of depression, by responding, 'Yes, I can see why you might feel this way; tell me more about your relationship with your husband'. However, this supplement, too, stands idle of meaning until the client provides the supplement. If the client ignored the statement, for example, going on to talk about her success as a mother, the therapist's words would be denied significance. More broadly, we may say that in daily life there are no *acts in themselves*, that is, actions that are not simultaneously supplements to what has preceded. Whatever we do or say takes place within a temporal context that gives meaning to what has preceded, while simultaneously forming an invitation to further supplementation.

Acts create the possibility for meaning but simultaneously constrain its potential

If one gives a lecture on narrative therapy, this lecture is meaningless without an audience that listens, deliberates, affirms, or questions what one has said. In this sense, every speaker owes to his or her audience a debt of gratitude; without their engagement the speaker ceases to exist. At the same time, the lecture creates the very possibility for the audience to grant meaning. While the audience creates the speaker as a meaningful agent, the speaker simultaneously grants to them the capacity to create. They are without existence until there is an action that invites them into being.

Yet, it is also important to realize that in practice, actions also set constraints upon supplementation. If one speaks on narrative therapy, audience members cannot supplement in any way they wish. They may ask a question about object relations theory, but not astrophysics; comment on the concept of externalization but not on the taste of radishes. Such constraints exist because the lecture is already embedded within a *tradition of act and supplement*. It has been granted meaning as a 'lecture on narrative therapy,' by virtue of previous generations of meaning makers. In this sense, actions embedded within relationships have *prefigurative* potential. The history of usage enables them to invite or suggest certain supplements as opposed to others—because only these supplements are considered sensible or meaningful within the tradition. Thus, as we speak with each other, we also begin to set limits on each other's being; to remain in the conversation is not only to respect a tradition, but to accede to being one kind of person as opposed to another.

Traditions of coordination furnish the major potentials for meaning

To amplify a preceding line of reasoning, it is important to recognize that the words and actions upon which we rely to generate meaning together are largely byproducts of the past. If another approached you and began to utter a string of vowels, 'ahhh, ehhhh, ooooo, uuuu…'. you would surely be puzzled; perhaps you would make for an exit, as this individual might well be dangerous. This is so because this utterance is nonsense, or to put it another way, not recognizable as a candidate for meaning within Western traditions of coordination. Similarly, if you began to dance with someone, and he or she suddenly crouched and gazed at the floor, you would scarcely continue dancing. Such actions are not part of any coordinated sequences with which you are familiar. Our capacity to make meaning together today thus relies on a history, often a history of centuries' duration. We owe to traditions of coordination our capacities for being in love, demonstrating for a just cause, or taking pleasure in our children's development.

Most often, our traditions of coordination are not recognized as traditions by the actors. They simply become a 'natural' way of life. This is so even with patterns that are detrimental to most relationships, such as relational patterns involving anger, blame, criticism, disinterest, jealousy, contempt, and so on. This is scarcely to say that there is no room for novel words and actions. Indeed, in the past century we have witnessed an explosion in new vocabulary terms, sporting activities, dance steps, and so on. Because we are not determined by the past, we are free to play, to violate expectations, and to explore the outrageous. This is indeed a major challenge for the therapeutic profession: collaborating in the generation of new and more viable forms of action.

Meanings are subject to continuous reinterpretation

In light of the above, we find that what an utterance means is inherently undecidable. No amount of discussion, discourse analysis, conversation analysis, or other attempt to determine what has been said, can be conclusive. The meaning of any utterance is a temporary achievement, born of the collaborative moment. Further, as relations continue over time, what is meant stands subject to continuous alteration through an expanding arena of action/supplements. Sarah and Robert may find themselves frequently laughing together—affirming each other as humorous persons—until Robert announces that Sarah's laughter is 'unnatural and forced', just her attempt to present herself as an 'easy going person' (in which case the definition of the previous actions would be altered). Or Sarah could announce, 'This is all very pleasant, Robert, but really you are so superficial; we really don't communicate at all' (thus reducing Robert's humour to banality). At the same time, these latter moves within the ongoing sequence are subject to further reconstitution. (In reply to Robert's accusation of being unnatural, Sarah replies, 'Robert, are you worried about your job again? What's bothering you?'. Or, Robert replies to Sarah's ascription superficiality with, 'Now I see... You are only saying that, Sarah, because you find Bill so attractive'.) Such instances of alteration may also be far removed from the interchange itself (e.g. consider a divorcing pair who retrospectively redefine their entire marital trajectory), and are subject to continuous change through interaction with and among others (e.g. friends, relatives, therapists, the media, etc.).

In summary, we find the exclusive focus on the face-to-face relationship is far too narrow. For whether one 'makes sense' is not under one's control; nor is it determined by others, or fixed by the collaborative process in which meaning struggles towards realization. At the outset, we largely derive our potential for coordination from our previous immersion in a range of other relationships. We arrive in the relationship as extensions of the past. And, as the current relationship unfolds, it serves to reform the meaning of the past. These interchanges may be supplemented and transformed by still others in the future. In effect, meaningful communication in any given relationship ultimately depends on an extended array of relationships, not only 'right here, right now,' but how it is that you and I are related to a variety of other persons, and they to still others—and ultimately, one may say, to the relational conditions of society as a whole. We are all in this way interdependently interlinked—without the capacity to mean anything, to possess an 'I'—except for the existence of an extended world of relationship.

Therapy as collaborative action

Developed here is a particular way of understanding the process of communication from which meaning emerges, is sustained and transformed. This account avoids certain pitfalls of most traditional accounts, and simultaneously realizes some of the potentials of constructionist reasoning. It is important to point out that we are not saying that we have explicated 'the true nature of communication'. Rather, this view is offered in the spirit of constructionism itself; it is simply an alternative way of making communication intelligible. The question is not whether it reveals the 'reality of communication,' but what follows from such an exposition? In what way would such an understanding alter any of our practices, and would such alterations be useful for the therapeutic venture? To be sure, such questions cannot be answered all at once.

There are many implications, both great and small, and further dialogue is needed to glimpse the potentials and problems. Some of the implications of this collaborative account are already well integrated into practice; other implications may prove too radical for contemporary application. However, to open discussion on therapeutic communication as collaborative action, we offer the following points:

There is no mental illness in itself

Because no human expression comes into meaning save through others' supplements, there is no suffering and no mental illness prior to collaboration. To be sure, one may 'feel depressed,' or encounter an 'obvious schizophrenic'. But the fact that one 'feels depressed' is already prepared by a previous immersion in a culture of circulating meaning. (Prior to the 20th century I could not 'feel depressed,' because the very intelligibility of depression only emerged within this century.) In the same way we 'see schizophrenics,' because there are already participants in a culture that collaborates to create the meaning of 'mental disease'. Here it is important to lay stress on the responsibilities of the therapist in creating and/or sustaining the life of anguish and illness within the therapeutic relationship. The therapist functions as a major collaborator in the generation of meaning; whether the client is anguished or ill, resourceful or resilient, is importantly dependent on the continuing collaborative process. It is in this light that deliberation is imperative on the movement towards increasing diagnosis, neurological explanation, and pharmacological 'cures'. Such constructions represent both an extension of a singular, medical model of human problems, and a Western ideology of individualism. Together they function to limit—in many unfortunate ways—conversations about human maladjustments and misery.[6]

There is no therapeutic treatment in itself

Although the therapist bears some responsibility for how clients come to understand themselves, their feelings, their relationships and so on, they are not omnipotent. Their supplements to clients' statements do not acquire meaning until supplemented by the client in turn. To put it more broadly, there is no 'therapeutic treatment' in itself; the actions that we might normally describe as 'therapeutic' do not become so until clients supplement the actions of the therapist in this regard. Custodians in mental hospitals know this very well. Often their honest attempts to help patients produce angry and resentful responses. Good treatment from the custodian's perspective may be regarded as manipulation and control by the patient. We must ask, then, whether we should reconsider what we, as professionals, call 'good treatment'. If the concept of 'good treatment' is not collaboratively generated, then 'therapeutic help' becomes unlikely.

Understanding a client is a form of collaborative action

We inherit a psychological view of interpersonal understanding. As we say, understanding occurs when subjectivities are linked or reflect each other accurately.

---

[6] For further discussion of these issues, see Gergen (2006).

Earlier we located important flaws in this view. As argued, if understanding were a matter of intersubjective synchrony, we would never understand each other. Yet, we do believe that understanding occurs, and we are certain when another misunderstands us. How can we account for understanding from the collaborative view? Here it is useful to view understanding not as a mental activity, but as a particular form of supplementation. To be 'understanding' is to coordinate one's actions to those of another; it is to be a certain kind of person in relation to the other. If another speaks of their anguish, a listener 'understands' when he or she responds in a particular way, with certain words, tones of voice, and gestures as opposed to others. If the listener simply gazed out the window during the tale of sadness, the speaker might justifiably say, 'You just don't understand, do you?'. There is no peering into the mind of the other here; there is only coordinated action within a tradition.

The effective therapist is a skilled coordinator

What is actually changed through therapy? Consistent with its individualist base, this question is typically answered in terms of the individual psyche. It is through the removal of repression, a process of catharsis, a gain in insight, the enhancement of self-esteem, or the alteration in cognitive schemas, as it is variously reasoned, that long-term change is effected. From the present perspective the landscape is dramatically altered. The psychological condition is not the centre of concern; it is relational existence. The individual arrives in therapy as a participant in a relational network, a network that extends outward from intimates to the culture at large, and backward in time to pre-existing relationships and traditions. It is this matrix of relationship out of which 'the problem' is created and designated as a problem. The therapeutic relationship represents the establishment of a new coordination, a coordination that will develop from the resources that both the therapist and client bring to the relationship. The major challenge confronting the therapeutic relationship is whether the collaborative trajectory of client/therapist can unsettle or transform the generative matrix in such a way that the problem is resolved, dissolved, or reconstructed.

In this sense we see that the therapist's most valuable resources are conversational actions. In the same way that skilled basketball players possess a rich vocabulary of actions enabling them to score, so are skilled therapists those who are able to coordinate effectively with the client in such a way that agreeable outcomes may be achieved within the extended matrix. It is not the storehouse of facts, concepts, distinctions and so on that the therapist has at his or her disposal that counts, but the capacity for flexibility in relationship. 'Knowing how' as opposed to 'knowing that'. This relational capacity will surely be verbal. Required are capacities to move in narrative, metaphor, exploration, irony, humour, pathos, curiosity, imagination, and much more. Yet, it is not simply the language content that is important. Posture, gaze, tone of voice, facial expression, gait, and so on all contribute to the form and ramifications of relationship. All may be used to unsettle or transform the matrix. All may provide the client with models for action outside the therapeutic relationship.

Because therapy is inherently a coordination, and no two clients will enter from the same relational matrix, there should be no hard and fast rules for the therapeutic encounter. Specific techniques or canons of therapeutic practice will only narrow the capacities for coordination. If the client recognizes the therapist's utterances as 'technique', they may indeed be disregarded or resented. If the therapist must ask questions according to some manual of prescribed practice, only dis-ease will follow. Thus, there is no unequivocal answer to a therapist's question of 'how should I proceed?'. The same words and phrases, useful in one context, may be crippling in another. Again the basketball analogy is useful; with experience the skilled player develops a repertoire of usable actions. There are no rules for which action is most effective; the conditions of play are complex and rapidly changing. The skilled player is one who can rapidly draw from the repertoire as the 'conversation of the court' unfolds. A skilled player can 'unsettle' the opponent's 'traditions of action'. At the same time the opponents will also model these skills and become more proficient. The patterns of play continue to unfold. The therapeutic encounter shares the same potential for innovative activity. In the case of therapy, however, there are no opponents; there is only the collective construction of well-being at stake.

A major challenge is to enter conversations already solidified

When working with a concept of meaning as relational coordination there is a strong tendency to stress the here and now—'us talking together at this moment'. It is in the present moment that meaning is under construction, and thus the future in the balance. Yet, this focus often obscures the ways in which the resources imported into the therapeutic session are anchored in relational history. This history can stand as a major impediment to change. On the simplest level, people develop modes of talking and acting that are comfortable and reliable. In an important sense, they are skilled in these forms of action. Thus, depressive, angry, or self-critical styles of being may seem dysfunctional from the therapist's standpoint. However just such modes of action may serve as reliable, 'natural,' and finely honed skills for the client. 'I know so well how to attack others for their shortcomings,' a client may say. 'Even if others avoid me for this reason, this is what I know how to do'. Without new skills or performance capacities in hand, a client may scarcely relinquish the old.

On a more subtle level, all of us carry with us residues of past relational patterns. As proposed earlier, it is the private recirculation of these residues that we speak of as 'thought' or 'emotion'. Such forms of recirculation may establish themselves as recurring scenarios. There is the voice, for example, that says, 'You are no good', and a following one that gives you a lift, 'Yes you are, you are great!'. You perform with the latter voice at hand and things go well. The cycle repeats, and you develop what might be called a private 'coping scenario'. Such privately re-circulated scenarios may not always be so functional, as in 'You are no good… I will hurt you for saying that… but everybody agrees that you're no good… I will fight them all…'. Performances derived from such a scenario may be suspicious and hostile. These privately re-circulated and well-worn scenarios may be the most difficult to interrupt. Anyone who has worked with what we commonly label as 'eating disorders' has encountered the strangulating grip of the private conversation. In our view, one of the most challenging problems confronting contemporary therapy is that of linking the face-to-face conversation with the client to the off-stage scenarios.

Meaning is subject to continuous transformation

From the collaborative perspective, each move within a conversation grants meaning to what has preceded. The meaning of all our words and actions is importantly dependent on those who respond to them. And their responses are denied significance until they too are supplemented. In effect, meaning is always in process, never complete, forever open to the next move in the conversation. This is to say that any attempt to specify the meaning of a past action—'what I intended...', 'what I was trying to say...', 'what you did to me...', 'what this meant to me...'—is itself a supplement that transforms the past. Such attempts give the past shape and consequence that could not be acquired save through the attempt itself. And these attempts as well stand mute until supplemented. There is no final moment of illumination, a moment at which meaning becomes indelible and undeniable.

The therapeutic implications of this reasoning are many. First, and to underscore an earlier argument, any therapeutic interpretation of a client's words or actions create the meaning of those words and actions. Any attempts by the therapist to point out continuities or discontinuities within the client's life, are themselves creations of continuity and discontinuity. Further, any attempt by the client to speak about the past, to reveal its secrets, to render it meaningful is itself a transformation of the past. Amplifying Donald Spence's (1982) arguments, this is to make prominent the significance of narrative as opposed to historical truth. Accounts of the past are created within the conversational space of the present.

Returning to an earlier issue, it also follows that all attempts at psychodiagnostic testing and therapeutic outcome assessment are essentially transformations of meaning. In both cases, whatever has occurred, whatever has been said or done, is granted a certain meaning that it did not itself possess. There is no pathology until the testing instrument has transformed the individual's words and actions into pathology. There is no positive or negative outcome of therapy until the assessment device renders certain patterns meaningful as outcomes. Important questions must thus be addressed: for whom is this pathology, what makes this diagnostic category more useful than another; are illness categories useful for clients; who is deciding on what constitutes a 'good outcome', what clients and therapists are benefited (or marginalized) by a given conception of outcome; whose voices are allowed into the conversation; and when does the conversation terminate? Again, from the view of communication as coordination, the practices of diagnosis and outcome assessment should be opened to full re-examination.

A major challenge is bridging the gap between meaning-making within the therapeutic relationship and the worlds outside

If we follow the collaborative logic, therapy represents a conversation in which participants borrow heavily from their relations outside, but in which they simultaneously create the grounds for a new and unique reality (discourse patterns shared by them alone.) Under these conditions it might be possible for therapist and client to locate a wonderfully agreeable mode of relating—a shared sense of harmony and fulfilment within the encounter. However, this same reality may also be wholly contained within the relationship. That is, it may have little or no 'street value', little transportability into other relations. Given the collaborative view, the major question is whether the conversational resources generated within the therapeutic relationship can be transported outside of this context. Can the metaphors, narratives, deconstructions, re-framings, multiple selves, expressive skills, and so on developed within the therapeutic encounter be carried into other relations in such a way that these relations are usefully transformed?

At one level, it is easy enough to conclude that such reverberations do occur. However, more effective demonstrations of the ways in which therapeutic conversations actually insinuate themselves into the life worlds of clients would be very useful. Further, more concerted attention is needed to how the contexts of therapy and other life worlds can be made to converge. The most obvious means, and one very congenial to the family therapy movement, is to work with relationships rather than single individuals. In this way new discursive forms and practices are set directly in motion. However, this does not fully solve the problem, as the group reality of the therapeutic hour may not be transportable; family members are also embedded in multiple relationships outside the family circle. The family in the therapy room is not the same family at the dinner table.

In order to remain effective, therapeutic practices must be continuously transformed

For over a century now, therapists have searched for 'the cure' to the problems confronted by their clients. It is thus that we have witnessed a parade of therapeutic schools, each eager to champion their particular form of treatment, and typically dismissing the remaining field of contenders. In the USA, there are longstanding attempts to assess the comparative efficacy of various practices, thus to winnow out the 'mere pretenders'. In other nations, the laws only recognize a narrow range of schools as worthy of health insurance coverage; the remaining are left to perish.

When we understand meaning as collaboration, we open a new vista of discussion. Every therapeutic school contributes to the discursive resources of the culture. Their distinct moves in the collaborative process of meaning-making offer possible departures from convention. In this sense, the plethora of therapeutic schools is not an embarrassment—somehow an indication of the pre-scientific status of the field. With the immense variations in cultural history from which clients emerge, we must cease to think in terms of a 'master conversation', useful to all. Rather, we have here a case in which multiple realities are to be valued.

To extend the argument, we must also recognize that therapeutic schools are themselves self-sustaining traditions. Typically they tend to reaffirm a particular vocabulary and honour certain moves in conversation over others. In this sense schools of therapy become culture-conserving. Yet, while the internal discourses of a school remain stable, the meaning-making process within the culture continues to evolve. New forms of coordination (and dis-coordination) are everywhere in motion. Today's profundity becomes tomorrow's platitude. Passions are cooled and values forgotten in the continuously unfolding illuminations generated by active and creative innovation.

In this way we see that every school of therapy that sustains the dogmas of their founders and resists cultural changes is in danger of becoming irrelevant. Rather, the continuous evolution of therapeutic language and practice is necessary to sustain its relational efficacy. It is when therapeutic conversations are continuous with those of the culture that they will most effectively 'make sense'. It is when the client can coordinate the discourse of therapy with his or her life outside that therapy is most likely to succeed. As a result, new schools of therapy should not only be anticipated, but welcomed.

In conclusion, the present chapter has sketched the contours of what many see as major transformations in our understanding of truth, objectivity, rationality, morality, and progress. These transformations can conveniently be understood in terms of treatises on the social construction of the real and good. As these traditional assumptions are challenged, so can we move into new forms of understanding and practice. Here we have outlined a radically relational view of communication and understanding. Moving away from the traditional view of communication as intersubjective connection, we find meaning created within the spaces of coordination among persons. Thus, meaning is in continuous motion, over which no one has ultimate control. In this light, we took up a range of central issues in therapy. Issues of defining 'mental illness' and 'cure', client/therapist negotiation, the flow of meaning into and out of the therapeutic relationship, and the need for continuous transformation of the therapeutic process all demanded attention. In our view, these are scarcely the 'last words' on social construction and therapy. Rather, our hope is that they sustain what is now a global dialogue on discursive issues in therapy.

References

Edwards, D. and Potter, J. (1992). *Discursive Psychology*. Sage, London.
Fish, S. (1980). *Is There a Text in this Class? The Authority of Interpretive Communities*. Harvard University Press, Cambridge, MA.
Gadamer, H. G. (1975). *Truth and Method*. The Seabury Press, New York.
Garfinkel, H. (1967). *Studies in ethnomethodology*. Prentice Hall, Englewood Cliffs, NJ.
Gergen, K. J. (2006). *Therapeutic realities, collaboration, oppression and relational flow*. Taos Institute Publications, Chagrin Falls, OH.
Gergen, K. J. (2009a). *An invitation to social construction* (2nd ed.). Sage, London.
Gergen, K. J. (2009b). *Relational being, Beyond self and community*. Oxford University Press, New York.
Gergen, K. J. and Gergen, M. (2004). *Social Construction, Entering the Dialogue*. Taos Institute Publications, Cleveland, OH.
Kuhn T. S. (1970). *The Structure of Scientific Revolutions*. Chicago University Press, Chicago, IL.
Latour, B. (1987). *Science in action*. Harvard University Press, Cambridge, MA.
Nightingale, D. J. and Cromby, J. (Eds.) (1999). *Social constructionist psychology: A critical analysis of theory and practice*. Open University Press, Buckingham.
Parker, I. (Ed.) (1998). *Social constructionism, discourse, and realism*. Sage, London.
Shotter, J. (1993). *Cultural Politics of Everyday Life: Social Constructionism, Rhetoric, and Knowing of the Third Kind*. Open University Press, Milton Keynes.

Spence, D. P. (1982). *Narrative truth and historical truth, Meaning and interpretation in psychoanalysis.* Norton, New York.

Wittgenstein, L. (1953). *Philosophical Investigations* (G. E. M. Anscombe, Trans.). The MacMillan Company, New York.

Chapter 5

Ontological social constructionism in the context of a social ecology: the importance of our living bodies

John Shotter

I see life as the moving of myself and my surroundings and the surroundings of those surroundings towards the future. The shifts of life around me come by themselves, not by me. The only thing I can do is to take part in them

(Andersen 1992, p. 54).

To get clear about philosophical problems, it is useful to become conscious of the apparently unimportant details of the particular situation in which we are inclined to make a certain metaphysical assertion. Thus we may be tempted to say 'Only this is really seen' when we stare at unchanging surroundings, whereas we may not at all be tempted to say this when we look about us while walking

(Wittgenstein 1965, p. 66).

– and by reality here I mean reality where things *happen*, all temporal reality without exception. I myself find no good warrant for even suspecting the existence of any reality of a higher denomination than that distributed and strung-along and flowing sort of reality which we finite beings swim in

(James 1996, p. 213).

A central question I want to explore in this chapter is: do all our understandings consist in our using *concepts* to think about things, or is there another much less cognitive, more embodied, non-conceptual way in which we experience and orient ourselves towards the world in which we have our being and in which we must act? Or, to put it another way: when we confront a confusing event or situation, do we try to understand it by finding recognizable features within it, thus to assimilate it to a category of events or situations already well-known to us, or can we, by actively living and moving around within it, come to an understanding of it as the qualitatively *unique* situation it *is*? I think we can. Indeed, not only do I think of this second option as merely being a possibility for us, but that we are in fact always and very basically relating ourselves to our surroundings in this fashion—in which we eventually *come to* an understanding of a situation as a result of our particular *bodily* activities within it—without our being aware of our actually having arrived at it in this way (for we tell of our experiences in terms merely of their namable 'contents', not in terms of the unnamable dynamic *relations* emerging between our outgoing bodily activities and their incoming results).[1]

Indeed, as I see it, rather than being the predominant agencies in the construction of our own destinies, as living organisms who are *spontaneously responsive* to events occurring around us, we are merely participant parts within a much larger network of still dynamically evolving relationships. And as we come to embody (some of) the consequences of our living involvements in this *social ecology*—within the different regions and moments of activity such an ecology *affords* us (Gibson 1979)—we can come to develop into different kinds of people, with different kinds of 'ontological skills' (Shotter 1984)[2] at *being* such different kinds of people.

There is, then, it seems to me, another, more embodied, more situation-specific way of understanding which just 'happens' or 'emerges' between us and within us in the course of our active, living involvements with the others and othernesess in our surroundings, than those forms of understanding which we actively 'construct' as a result of our more rationally planned and deliberately conducted inquiries. And that it is as a result of these more spontaneously occurring forms of involvement with our surroundings that we learn how *to be* a competent, morally autonomous, and responsible members of our cultural community. We do not, like logicians, have to 'to work out' how to act in each situation we encounter by a self-conscious observance of rules or principles. As we grow into the everyday lives of those around us, we come to embody *ways* of spontaneously responding to occurrences both in our surroundings (and with ourselves). As we develop such ways or styles of acting—what we often call our 'second nature' (Corcoran 2009)—we become capable of being able to relate ourselves to others around us, *and* also to ourselves, with many different sensitivities *at the ready*, so to speak, thus to be selectively *attentive* and *responsive* to what they, and we ourselves, do and say.

Thus below, I want to explore the very basic role played in our interactions with the others and othernesses around us by the spontaneous responsiveness of our living bodies, and how it is that in the course of such unplanned, spontaneous activities—of which we are very largely unaware—we can develop the skills and capacities *to be* this, or that, or some other kind of person. But I also want to explore the relations between this embodied, non-conceptual realm and the much more salient conceptual realm of our mature thought as adults. For, as Vygotsky (1978, 1986, 1987) makes very clear to us, what we at first we do spontaneously, often all unawares, we can come later to do deliberately by being able to direct or instruct ourselves through our use of words—words often given to us at first by others.[3] Further, in giving prominence to phenomena

---

[1] See William James' (1890) comments, quoted later, about the anticipatory 'feelings of tendency, often so vague that we are unable to name them at all' (p. 254), but of which we nonetheless can have an 'acutely discriminative sense' (p. 253). Such feelings, although not easily identifiable, can of course still be very precise guides to action.

[2] For an account of 'ontological skills' see Shotter (1984, pp. 71–2, pp. 86–7, and pp. 122–3).

[3] The general law of development says that awareness and deliberate control appear only during a very advanced stage in the development of a mental function, after it has been used and practiced unconsciously and spontaneously. 'In order to subject a function to intellectual and volitional control, we must first possess it' (Vygotsky 1986, p. 168, my emphasis). And a main

that our ordinary forms of thought and talk easily make us overlook, a number of other rather unfamiliar themes will come to light below: 1) Besides the multi-dimensional nature of dialogical forms of talk currently coming to prominence with the study of Bakhtin's (1981, 1984, 1986, 1993) work; 2) I will discuss Wittgenstein's (1980) distinction between difficulties of the intellect (problem-solving) and difficulties of orientation (to do with coming to know one's 'way about' within a practical situation); I will also 3) discuss what is involved in coming to a *judgement* (Nussbaum 2001) as distinct from making a decision.

On relating and re-relating ourselves to ourselves: inside the unfolding dynamics of our 'inner dialogues'

I want to begin with two episodes in which a person's relation to themselves—and as a result, their relations to those around them—is changed by the use of what I will call *deconstructive* moves, i.e. actions and utterances by therapists which disturb clients' expectations, and which cause them to re-orient, i.e. to 'turn in another direction' towards a just recounted event. Both were conveyed to me in personal communications: The first was reported to me by Jaakko Seikkula (but see Seikkula 2009). S is a woman who came into therapy after a prolonged upset over her relations with her other family members, T1 is Seikkula:[4]

> S: I have not been recognized.
> T1: You have not been recognized?
> S: Throughout my life I've been excluded from the family. At last I want to get rid of this symbiotic mess.
> T1: You said that 'Throughout my life I've been excluded from the family'. Then you said that 'At last I want to get rid of this symbiotic mess'.
> It sounds like you are saying two things at the same time?
> S: (10) . . . yes... that's what I said . . . But so far I cannot say anything more about it.
> T1: (7) . . . yeah.

---

theme in Vygotsky's whole approach is that these spontaneously acquired understandings, which are at first only spontaneously expressed in relation to events actually occurring in our surroundings, can come to be expressed by us under our own control, in accord with our own verbal formulations—as he puts it: 'Learning to direct one's own mental processes with the aid of words or signs is an integral part of the process of concept formation' (Vygotsky 1986, p. 108). What Vygotsky outlines here, however, as applying mainly to childrens' development also applies, I want to suggest, to our own further development in adulthood, in acquiring what we speak of as new knowledge: if it is not just to consist in empty verbal formulae, it must also be 'rooted' in our previous practical involvements in our surroundings.

[4] It will be a help in thinking with the episode—to get a sense of it—if readers try to read it out loud to themselves, along with all the pausing and pacing, intonations and other seemingly expressive features (facial expressions and bodily movements and postures) that seem appropriate (as if, say, reading a play script at an initial rehearsal of it).

Seikkula is responsible for these two long pauses, one of 10 seconds, the other of 7 seconds. After having commented to her (S) that it sounds as if she is saying two different things, while Seikkula might have felt the urge to clarify when she doesn't reply, he doesn't. He lets his comment 'hang', unresponded to, for quite a long time. And even then, when S does reply, he lets her reply again go unresponded to for some time. Why? What is the function of these silences, this lack of response?

What is the function of these peculiar silences, are they therapeutic, or was it just that Seikkula couldn't think of anything useful to say in those moments? No, not at all. What Seikkula does here, by pausing after having confronted his client with what, logically stated, appears to her (and to us) to be a paradox, is to give her (S) a distinct *point of entry* (as I will call it) into the complex, multi-voiced and multi-dimensional, dynamically intertwined, non-conceptualized, experiential reality of her family relations. And it is to this stable point of entry, to what conceptually is a paradox, that she can return to time and again, and in relation to which she can begin to *organize* and to put into some intelligible *order* her own actual lived (re)experiences as she herself explores in detail the living actuality of her own bewildering family relationships.

Her task, then, is to find a resolution of this seeming dilemma, to find an intricate way forward within her relations to her family members that allows her to, at least partially, resolve the tensions she feels—a task that involves, as we shall see, a certain kind of *imaginative work* that she must conduct for herself in her own inner dialogues. And this, eventually, is what she did. And what Seikkula did in pausing for 10 whole seconds,[5] was to resist the temptation (as a knowledgeable expert) to do this work for her. Instead, after having confronted her with the apparent paradox expressed in her statements, he stepped back to allow her the time to do that work for herself, in her own terms—although this, in fact, took her quite a while.[6]

In moving from the non-conceptual into the conceptual realm, from an embodied, experiential to an intellectual, conceptual understanding of things, we move from being spontaneously responsive to events occurring around us, to being able to exert our own agency in relation to them—thus to be able to pick out aspects from them that we *will* respond to, and others that we *won't*; and in this activity, the way our utterances can work in directing or guiding our attention towards *this* rather than *that* aspect of a complex circumstance is crucial.[7] This is the power of our being able to

---

[5] 10 seconds is a very long time, as one will discover if one attempts the play-script style of reading suggested above. Indeed, we might surmise that a less experienced therapist than Seikkula would have found it difficult to cope with the tension/anxiety occasioned by such a long silence.

[6] I first heard Seikkula recount this incident (that happened in February 2009) in August 2009. And now as I write, in March 2010, he reported to me (in an e-mail) that, as the account outlined above suggests, that that was 'actually the precise experiences that she (the client) told afterwards as being her aim. Actually that has happened now about 10 months after that saying [after her stating her seemingly paradoxical desires]: They [the family] spent Christmas together the first time for 20 years, in the last meetings they have started to ask of each other and showing caring emotions to each other. I am always moved while meeting these clients every 3–4th months' (Seikkula pers. com.).

[7] Vygotsky (1986) describes how we can use our own wordings in 'instructing' ourselves how to act in a particular situation under our own control, i.e. wilfully, thus: 'Our experimental

come to an *intellectual* 'grasp' of a circumstance; we can exert our own agency in changing our own ways of being in a spontaneously responsive contact with our surroundings by changing our orientation towards them, and in so doing, we can change the conditions determining our embodied ways of being in the world.

And this, I think, is precisely what Seikkula succeeded in doing in confronting S with the seemingly paradoxical nature of her expressions. By making this deconstructive move, he not only occasioned within her a deeply felt tension of a unique and qualitatively distinct kind to which she had to seek satisfaction, but he also turned what was, for her, a continuous flow of only diffusely connected experiences into a verbally expressed seeming contradiction. In doing this, he provided her with what I will call a conceptualized 'point of entry' into her diffuse feelings of disquiet, a point of entry which, as Wittgenstein (1969) puts it, 'stood fast' for her,[8] in the sense that she could return to it time and again as a stable starting point for her inner, exploratory movements involved in the imaginative work she carried out in gradually *differentiating* her diffuse feelings into an articulated and articulable structure.

The second episode I want to discuss arose in an earlier draft version of Andersen (2008) that Tom Andersen sent to me. As in the episode recounted above, the therapist aids the client in gaining an articulable and thus voluntary grasp of an otherwise spontaneous, impulsive, un-self-controlled and inappropriate response to a situation, but in this instance, much more within the immediate moment. Andersen wrote of talking with a father who got easily irritated, and, in such situations, often hit his son. He asked the father the following rather strange question: '*When your hand is on its way to hit, if that hand could stop and talk, what would the words be?*' As Tom goes on to say: "He did not understand the question and it had to be repeated several times until he finally said: "*Stop what you are doing because that is not what you shall do*". And, how would you say it?'. He needed much time and this question was repeated even more until he said: '*I will say it clearly . . . calmly . . . with conviction*'. During this talk where the father was brought back to the hitting moments, it was extremely important to go slow and all the time see if he followed the movements of the talk or stopped. At the same time, when he was back in the hitting moment, he could take part in investigating other expressions than hitting' (Andersen, pers. comm.).

---

study proved that it is the functional use of the word, or any other sign, as means of focusing one's attention, selecting distinctive features and analyzing and synthesizing them, that plays a central role in concept formation ... Words and other signs are those means that direct our mental operations, control their courser, and channel them toward the solution of the problem confronting us' (pp. 106–7). And elsewhere (Vygotsky, 1966) he describes the process thus: 'We could not describe this new significance of the whole operation otherwise than by saying that it is mastery of one's own process of behaviour. It is surprising to us that traditional psychology has completely failed to notice this phenomenon which we can call mastering one's own reactions' (p. 33).

[8] As Wittgenstein (1969) remarks: 'I do not explicitly learn the propositions that stand fast for me. I can discover them subsequently like the axis around which a body rotates. This axis is not fixed in the sense that anything holds it fast, but the movement around it determines its immobility' (no. 152).

Again, we can see Andersen here as also, like Seikkula, making a couple of deconstructive moves, moves which in ordinary conversation would be treated as strange, and which would—and in this instance, at first did—bewilder one's recipient. Thus each strange question Andersen asked of the father had to be repeated a number of times. But as Andersen himself remarks, their purpose was to ask the father to take himself back 'into' the hitting moments, to re-live them again and again as if in 'slow-motion', so to speak, to imagine his hand 'on its way' to hitting. Unfolding the hitting event step-by-step, slowly in time, gave the father the *possible* opportunity to move from the impulse within him that drove its outgoing expression to consider the incoming responses to it from his son (and wife and son's mother)—the 'relational meaning' of his impulsive expression—a possibility that, with Andersen's persistent prompting, he took up. But why did Andersen go further and ask the father about his tone of voice? Because, as we will see, it was a way of inviting the father to explore the *relational* meaning of his actions even further—to explore what Bateson (1973) called metacommunication, and Bakhtin (1986) a speaker's 'evaluative attitude' (p. 85) toward the subject of his or her speech.

The diffuse, multi-dimensional nature of the dialogical: 'losing the phenomena'

Taking these therapeutic episodes in turn, then, as they are set out, the first seems to depict a woman, S, as facing the seemingly impossible resolution of a logical paradox, while the second portrays a father as also facing an impossible task, that of giving a hitting hand a voice. But is this really the case? Is this really how it is for them, S and the father, when they are actually involved in living out the activities in question? Or is this how it seems to us when we view their activities retrospectively, when they can be viewed logically as representing a static, already completed, spatially arrayed state of affairs? Perhaps if we were to view them *dialogically*, their uses would be very different? For then their *uses*—their meaning(s)—would emerge over or through time within the unfolding dynamic flow of the continuously intermingling living and non-living activities all occurring together within the exchanges depicted.

As Bakhtin (1984) points out, if we consider the two separate judgements: 'Life is good', and 'Life is not good', there exists between them 'a specific logical relation: one is the negation of the other' (p. 183),[9] and as such, they would seem to cancel each other out. But once they become embodied utterances, voiced by living beings *in response to* specific circumstances at different moments in time, then things become very different. *Dialogic* relations may 'arise between them and toward them' (p. 183) and their relations to each other cease to be of a logically contradictory kind. They become *related* to each other in a very different way. What is missing in the merely logical relations between them when presented as referential statements representing

---

[9] This example of Bakhtin's is reminiscent of Dickens' opening line in his The Tale of Two Cities: 'It was the best of times, it was the worst of times …'—a line which straightaway, of course, expresses the confusing complexity of the situation within which the rest of the tale is to unfold.

a static state of affairs, but is present in the *dialogical relations* between them when expressed as living *utterances*, is not only both their responsiveness to their context within a specific, unfolding *flow* of events, but also their orientation towards the future within that flow: for the utterance of the first arouses (both in listeners and the speaker alike) a felt *anticipation* as to what might occur next within the flow of activity between them, while the second differentiates or articulates these shared momentary anticipations yet further:

> 'The word in living conversation,' says Baktin (1981), 'is directly, blatantly, oriented toward a future answer-word; it provokes an answer, anticipates it and structures itself in the answer's direction. Forming itself in an atmosphere of the already spoken, the word is at the same time determined by *that which has not yet been said but which is needed and in fact anticipated by the answering word*. Such is the situation of any living dialogue' (p. 280, my emphasis).

But even more than this, as we move from the more traditional, referential-representational to a relationally-responsive understanding of language use (see Shotter 2008), we must note the intrinsic responsiveness of our utterances to the surroundings within which they are uttered. Thus, as I intimated above, we express our *relations* to the others and othernesses in our surroundings in the compositional structure *and* the intonation, and other expressive features of our utterances. Again, as Bakhtin (1986) puts it:

> The speaker's evaluative attitude toward the subject of his speech (regardless of what it may be) also determines the choice of lexical, grammatical, and compositional means of the utterance ... [And] one of the means of expressing the speaker's emotionally evaluative attitude toward the subject of his speech is expressive intonation, which resounds clearly in oral speech (p. 85).

In other words, our talk always points beyond itself to a not-yet-determined-something, to a 'world', to the emerging unity of the event encompassing us, within which our talk *will* have its meaning. And if we orient towards people's words as merely already completed patterns of word shapes or forms (as we do in a transcript or recording, say)—instead of towards the expressive movement of their words in their speaking of them—then we will, in Vygotsky's (1987)[10] and Garfinkel's (2002) terms, 'lose the phenomena' (pp. 264–7). That is, what will be crucially lost are the guiding anticipations aroused by each unfolding event within such a process, the felt anticipations aroused in those who might *respond* to that event in ways intelligibly related to it—and it is these particular understandings and anticipations which function as the 'glue'

---

[10] Vygotsky's (1987) draws a distinction between the analysis of a whole into its separate elements and what he calls 'unit analysis'. In making this most important distinction he notes: 'The first of these forms of analysis begins with the decomposition of the complex mental whole into its elements... The essential feature of this form of analysis is that its products are of a different nature than the whole from which they are derived... Since it results in products that have lost the characteristics of the whole, this process is not a form of analysis in the true sense of the word. At any rate, it is not "analysis" vis a vis the problem to which it was meant to be applied' (p. 45, my emphasis).

holding the sequences of separate utterances in a dialogue together into a unitary whole, the feelings or sensings that at each moment in an unfolding process *relates* it to the rest of what is happening in the process.[11]

If we now return to examine the qualitative nature of S's experience of her complex family life, such that it afforded her expressions of it in two seemingly contradictory utterances without, at first, arousing in her any feelings of contradiction, I want to suggest that we can see its complex, non-conceptual nature as being dialogically-structured in Bakhtin's sense—that is, in being multi-dimensional and only diffusely structured it is *capable of being organized into an orderly structure* in a large number of different ways (Shotter 1993, 2008). What seems to me to have been crucial in Seikkula repeating her utterances to her—along with the comment (with a questioning intonation) that it 'sounds like you are saying two things at the same time?'—is that it not only focused her on her *relations* to her family members, but also (by calling them contradictory) motivated her to seek to put them into an *orderly* structure, i.e. to conceptualize them. This, I suggest, is why his comments worked to occasion within her the kind of imaginative work on herself that was therapeutic.

From the diffusely dialogical to a conceptual orderliness: becoming intellectual—some advantages

But why is gaining a *conceptual* 'grasp' on what, qualitatively, is essentially a continuously flowing, dialogically-structured process, unfolding in time, so important to us? Why do we so often feel driven to seek such a grasp? In coming to an understanding of this *urge*, we will find the last writings of William James to be of direct relevance (although we could also have drawn here on Bergson's (1896/1911) account which was a powerful influence on James).

In his lectures at Manchester College, Oxford, in the spring of 1908, published under the title of *A Pluralistic Universe*, he discussed his concern with the fact that our concepts seem to break up 'our world of objects . . . quite as much as our world of subjects' into 'discontinuous pieces' (James 1996, p. 206). And he went on to say that, in his heart of hearts, he knew that this 'situation was absurd and only provisional . . . [and] that secret of a continuous life which the universe knows by heart and acts on every instant cannot be a contradiction incarnate' (p. 207). So why do we ignore what it is that makes for the *continuity* in a flow of events, and divide continuous time into a series of static instants, and try to think of movement as made up of sequence of 'conceived positions' which, as James (1996) puts it, 'however numerously multiplied, contain no element of movement' (p. 234)?

Because, as James (1996) sees it (clearly drawing on Bergson here), 'we of course need a stable scheme of concepts, stably related with one another, *to lay hold of* our experiences and to co-ordinate them withal' (p. 235, my emphasis). In other words, only if we can do this—that is, to abstract out *aspects* of experiences that just seem 'to happen' to us, outside of our agency to control, in such a way as to gain a 'grasp' of them—can we begin to exert our own agency in trying to modify what we might call

---

[11] See Shotter (2005) and also endnote 1, on William James' 'feelings of tendency'.

the 'determining conditions or surroundings' (Shotter 2009) of our lives. Thus, in moving into the conceptual realm we move from being spontaneously responsive to events occurring around us, to beginning to exert our own agency in relation to them—we begin to pick out aspects from them that we *will* respond to, and others that we *won't*, and in doing this, the way in which our utterance of words can work to direct our attention towards *this* rather than *that* is crucial.[12]

And this, I think, is precisely what Seikkula succeeded in doing in confronting his client with the seemingly paradoxical nature of her expressions, and Andersen did in having the father 'go back into' his hitting movements. By their deconstructive moves, they did two things: 1) they occasioned within their clients deeply felt tensions of a *unique and qualitatively distinct kind* to which they needed to seek satisfaction, but they also provided them with distinct points of entry into these tensions, stable starting points to which they could continually return in making the exploratory moves needed in carrying out the imaginative work involved in gradually *differentiating* a flow of diffuse feelings into an articulated and articulable structure.

This, as I see it, is the power of our being able to come to an *intellectual* 'grasp' of a circumstance: we can exert our own agency, not so much in changing it, as in changing *our own ways of being in a spontaneously responsive contact with our surroundings by changing our orientation towards them*, and in so doing, we can change the conditions determining our embodied ways of being in the world. This, I need to point out, is to turn our intellectual powers in a rather unusual, ontological rather than an epistemological direction—to see our working to influence ourselves and how to get ourselves 'ready', so to speak, to go out to meet the events confronting us, rather than as our working out how, instrumentally, to influence those events themselves.

Being intellectual—some disadvantages

The idea of working on ourselves, and on how we *relate* ourselves to what occurs around us, is still a rather unusual idea at the moment. Much more usual is the idea that, as we have seen, when we take an *intellectual* attitude towards the continuous flow of events occurring around us, 'what does not of itself stand out, we learn to *cut out*' (James 1996, p. 235). We abstract salient features from that flow which we then treat as *things* that we can 'grasp' and thus move around to 'engineer', piece-by-piece, new forms and entities into existence. And each new reality that we encounter can, of course, give rise to a new concept constructed in this manner. But once we have done that, we then feel obliged to seek the rules, laws, or principles in terms of which they can all be joined together as fixed *partes extra partes*, i.e. as externally related parts, in constituted a state of affairs out in the world—when in fact, if they are aspects of a living process, they only initially occurred as internally related parts of a still unfolding

---

[12] Vygotsky (1966) describes how we can use our own wordings in 'instructing' ourselves how to act in a particular situation under our own control, i.e. wilfully, thus: 'We could not describe this new significance of the whole operation otherwise than by saying that it is mastery of one's own process of behaviour. It is surprising to us that traditional psychology has completely failed to notice this phenomenon which we can call mastering one's own reactions' (p. 33).

unitary whole. It is 'the immutability of such an abstract system' that is, of course, 'its great practical merit,' says James, for 'the same identical terms and relations in it can always be recovered and referred to' (p. 235).

This, of course, is a major advantage. For all our deliberate actions and planned achievements, all our designs on paper, all our scheming and conniving, depends on our being able to construct in a conceptual realm what we will try later to construct in fact.

But this is only an advantage, we must add, in *some* spheres of our activities. In others, things are different. Indeed, as James himself adds to the comment above, a major disadvantage is that 'change itself is just such an unalterable concept' (p. 235) like all the others—which (mis)leads us, of course, into thinking that when living change is in question, that it too can be brought about in this same fashion, i.e. 'engineered' into existence according to a pre-designed plan or strategy. However, when it come to living change, says James, 'all these abstract concepts are but as flowers gathered, they are only moments dipped out from the stream of time, snap-shots taken, as by a kinetoscopic camera, at a life that in its original coming is continuous' (p. 235)—and if they were gathered flowers, it would mean that the soil in which they grew, the seeds from which they grew, the whole ecological cycle of dynamic inter-dependencies upon which they depended for their growth, all this and more, would be ignored.

In other words, how our experiences 'grow' or 'emerge' both from 'seeds' within previous experiences, and in responsive relation to our immediate surroundings, is unrepresented in such a sequence of 'snap-shots'. While we might be able to construct automobiles piece-by-piece in this decontextualized manner, to try to construct something like a living flower in this manner (notwithstanding the many stunningly authentic artificial flowers now available) would be crazy. In other words, our intellectualist methods cast no light at all on the emergent processes within which our experiences in fact *get made*. For, to repeat, we cannot depict the way events within a continuously unfolding process reach out towards the future within a sequence of self-contained, objective discontinuities—yet that is what our concepts, by their very discontinuous nature, force upon us.

Intellectually, then, when we 'stop to think', this is the attitude we adopt. We take on the role of rational beings, thinking in terms of the logic of concepts—a tendency, as John Austin (1962) once put it, to think *with* the idea of 'moderate-sized specimens of dry goods' (p. 8) in mind as paradigms of what a concept was a concept of.[13] And it is this style of thought that makes us try, *per impossible*, 'to represent as some single *kind of things* the things which the ordinary man says he "perceives",' said Austin (p. 8), whether they are tables or chairs; cats, plants, trees, and rocks; people or poems; rainbows; or what someone failed to say—they all come to be treated in the same way, as existing in terms of explicit and finished products, as spatial shapes or *forms* of a 'finalized' kind (Bakhtin 1986, p.139).

---

[13] Like Wittgenstein (1953), Austin is here pointing out that without our realizing it, various 'pictures' are implicitly already at work in our philosophical concepts; thus, from the very beginning of our philosophical discussions, say, of the idea of a sense-datum, 'the expression "material object" is functioning already... simply as a foil for "sense-datum"' (p. 8).

Our intellectualism, then, leads us to try to think *with* a sequence of disconnected, static moments in mind to guide us when orienting ourselves to reflect on and to attend to the living processes that concern us. And this (mis)leads us, once again, into conceptualizing them in yet another discontinuous manner, and into failing to notice features of them that work to arouse distinct anticipations within us as to what might come next. Consequently, if the logic of concepts seems to drive us to such conclusions, then so much the worse for logic, says James: a logic that works in terms of static, incomplete abstractions, must yield to reality, not reality to logic. Thus, if we want to go on living in a way well adjusted to the world around us, 'our intelligence cannot wall itself up alive, like a pupa in a chrysalis. It must at any cost keep itself on speaking terms with the universe that has engendered it' (James 1996, p. 207). 'The whole process of life is due to life's violation of our logical axioms' (James 1996, p. 257).

But since Descartes (and, indeed, since Socrates before him) we have made a very good attempt at not doing so—for in seeking to experience ourselves as merely *observers* and *exploiters* of the world around us, we have sought to separate ourselves from it; to separate ourselves as subjectivities (minds) from our merely objective, mechanical bodies; to separate *thought* and *theory* from our spontaneously responsive *doings* in the unique situations of our everyday practical activities. But the *knowledge* we acquire in this fashion is, as James (1996) puts it, only 'knowledge *about* things, as distinguished from living or sympathetic acquaintance with them, [it] touches only the outer surface of reality . . . That inner dimension of reality [which] is occupied by the *activities* that keep it going, . . . the intellect, speaking through Hume, Kant & Co., finds itself obliged to deny . . . . What exists for *thought*, we are told, is at most the results that we illusorily ascribe to such activities . . . . Thought deals thus solely with surfaces. It can name the thickness of reality, but it cannot fathom it' (p. 250).

If James (1996) is correct in thinking that 'what really *exists* is not things made but things in the making' (p. 263)—and I think he is—it means that we do in fact live in a reality that is in continuous flux, that is still evolving and developing—and we have totally deceived ourselves into thinking the opposite. We spend our efforts in seeking the fixed and unchanging entities we think of as constituting the basic materials of the world, and the laws of nature we think of as governing their motions. But if James is correct, rather than fixity and finality being basic and change being problematic, things are the other way around for us: achieving stability and constancy is what is difficult for us, not change. And indeed, our concerns with and efforts at the enforcement of laws, rules, principles, protocols, and the suchlike are a testament to this. What bothers us, of course, is that rather than being *subject* to changes that just happen to us, we want to steer such changes in ways according to our own desires, to exert our own agency in shaping our own lives.

However, as we have seen, so predominant is this impulse, that every time we experience a difficulty, a bewilderment or a confusion, we feel 'called by the circumstance' to adopt an intellectual attitude towards it, and begin the first steps of an *analysis*—the breaking of it up into a sequence of discontinuous parts, named in terms of various specific abstractions. Yet, as we have seen, the very fact that we can do this means that what we are drawing from must itself be qualitatively specific—it cannot be like an amorphous, homogeneous fog. Indeed, as I indicated above, the specific character of an experience becomes apparent to us *in our efforts*—and if it was an amorphous fog, no effort would be needed, for we could just say what we liked—to give aspects of it expression.

But this move, this shift in focus of our attention—from already made things to things in the making—is not easy to make. James (1996), along with Bergson (1911), talks of it as 'put[ting] yourself *in the making* by a stroke of intuitive sympathy with the thing', and that when you do this, a 'whole range of possible decompositions' comes into view, and as result, 'you are no longer troubled with the question as to which of them is the more absolutely true' (pp. 263–4).

What is involved in executing *a stroke of intuitive sympathy with the thing* is, however, somewhat vague. If we can make use of Polanyi's (1958, 1967) distinction between our ability to integrate and to 'disattend from' a set of particulars of which we are only *subsidiarily aware*, to 'attend to' their integration as something of which we can become *focally aware*, then we could say that as living embodied beings, the move we need to make is to learn to attend to, i.e. to notice within ourselves, what we have previously learnt to *disattend from*, i.e. the unique particulars from which we abstract aspects in order to place them in one or another general category. If we can do this, it becomes apparent that we have two fundamentally different ways in which we can make sense of ourselves and of the world around us, not just one. For although the particulars we *attend from* lie in the background to what we are focally aware of, that doesn't mean to say that we are wholly unaware of them—as we have seen, we become aware of their nature whenever we try to express to someone the nature of our own unique experiences.

Indeed, as I see it, this is the nature of Wittgenstein's (1953) discovery of what he calls the 'logical grammar' at work in influencing our *use* of words in this, that, or some other particular situation. And our task in trying to bring to light the usually unnoticed *background* influences at work in shaping our behaviour, then, is not a task of an intellectual kind, but is, as he put it, 'more a working on oneself... On one's *way of seeing* things. (And what one expects of them)' (Wittgenstein 1980, p. 16, my emphasis). But what, exactly, is at issue here in talking of a 'way' of seeing, hearing, etc., and in what kind of vocabulary of terms can it be done? How is seeing and hearing as such done?

Difficulties of the intellect and difficulties of the will

Ryle (1949) distinguishes between what he calls 'achievement verbs' and 'task verbs', words describing activities in which something is 'got' or 'brought of', and the activities which when appropriately sequenced or organized can be aimed at 'getting' something or at 'accomplishing' something. 'Verbs like "spell", "catch", "solve", "find", . . . and countless others, signify not merely that some performance has been gone through, but also that something has been brought off by the agent going through it' (p. 143), he notes. But then goes on to complain that: 'The differences, for example, between . . . . hunting and finding, . . . listening and hearing, looking and seeing, . . . have been construed, if they have been noticed at all, as differences between coordinate species of activity or process, when in fact the differences are of quite another kind' (p. 143). For, to find something (achievement) one has to hunt for it (task); to see, to look; to hear, to listen, and so on—where the tasks of 'hunting', 'looking', 'listening' have all to be conducted in a particular *way*—in a sequentially organized and integrated fashion—if one's conduct of them is to bring off the sought for achievement. In other words, our setting out to *do* something is not quite as straight forward as it might at first appear, because what we call our initial *approach* or *orientation* to the situation in question is of crucial importance.

With his sensitivity to qualitative issues of this kind, Wittgenstein (1980) notes that there are *two* very different kinds of difficulties we can face in our lives: difficulties of the *intellect*, and difficulties of the *will*. He introduced these two kinds of difficulty thus: 'What makes a subject hard to understand . . . is not that before you can understand it you need to be trained in abstruse matters, but the contrast between understanding the subject and what most people *want* to see . . . What has to be overcome is a difficulty having to do with the will, rather than with the intellect' (p. 17).[14] Difficulties of the intellect arise for us when we take an intellectual attitude to the circumstance before us and formulate the difficulty we face in dealing with it as a *problem*, as something which, with the aid of clever theories, we can solve by the use of reasoning. Difficulties of the will, however, are of quite a different kind. For they are to do with how we *orient* ourselves bodily towards events occurring around us, how we *relate* ourselves to them, the *ways* in which we ready ourselves for seeing, for hearing, for experiencing and valuing what we encounter as we move forward with our lives—for these are the *ways* that will organize our lookings and listenings, our sense-makings and judgements of value, and thus ultimately, determine the lines of action we *resolve* on carrying out further.

But unlike the static contemplative thinker, we must do all this while we are already in action, while in motion, *from within* our engaged, spontaneously responsive activity with the others and othernesses, either actual or imagined, we encounter within the situation of our activities. For as soon as we stop moving in relation to one or another practical purpose in our surroundings, our relations to our surroundings cease to be structured by the aims and goals implicit in our movements, and become structured by one or another of our ways of thinking—thus to substitute a very different system of organizational valences.

This distinction between difficulties of the intellect and of the will is not easy to grasp, for the difference between them cannot be captured formally, i.e. they cannot be named and described in terms of objectively observable features, for an orientation to a situation, a way of relating ourselves to it, is something that emerges, that is arrived at only slowly as we explore the 'terrain' of possibilities around us for a satisfactory way forward. Indeed, very generally, it can be likened to the task we continuously face in understanding the speech of a unique speaker, with something unique to say to us. Merleau-Ponty (1962) describes it thus:

> Here there is nothing comparable to the solution of a problem, where we discover an unknown quantity through its relationship with known ones. For the problem can be

---

[14] As I see it, what Vygotsky (1966) calls 'mastering one's own reactions' (p. 33), is what concerns Wittgenstein (1960) in our overcoming what we 'want to see' (p. 16). Both are concerned with resolving difficulties of the will.

solved only if it is determinate, that is, if the cross-checking of the data provides the unknown quantity with one or more definite values. In understanding others, the problem is always indeterminate because only the solution will bring the data retrospectively to light as convergent, only the central theme of a philosophy, once understood, endows the philosopher's writings with the value of adequate signs (pp. 178–9).

The criteria we use, then, in assessing the progress of our 'journey' towards assuaging our disquiet, towards relieving the qualitatively distinct tension motivating it, cannot be formal, namable criteria. They can only be 'practical criteria' of a qualitatively distinct kind; they arise and have their being only within the situation as we 'journey' through it, as the initial tension we felt at its beginning is laid to rest in the course of the line of action we resolve on taking within it. So, although they can be justified retrospectively (if necessary), they cannot be identified ahead of time. Because of this, the qualitative uniqueness, the *singularity* of the difficulties we face in life, individually and/or collectively, has long been ignored—for a science of singularities would seem to be a contradiction in terms.

So although our difficulties in life can be generalized and placed into categories for *some* purposes, to do it for *all* the difficulties that we each individually face as the unique individuals we are, is seriously to mislead ourselves: To tell ourselves we are 'bipolar', or that we have a 'personality disorder', or are simply suffering from 'anxiety', is to ignore (no matter how 'medical' the disease may seem from which we are suffering) the guidance we can receive from the feelings of restlessness, of things not being quite right with us, that can guide us into (perhaps) bettering our circumstances. Rather than as pathological symptoms of something being 'wrong' with us needing a cure, on some occasions at least, we need to treat our disquiets as uniquely important spontaneous responses to our surroundings that can, perhaps, as we move around within them, guide us towards the satisfaction of still as yet unrecognized needs.

The emergence of new ways of acting

In this respect, the account given by Tom Andersen,[15] of the importance of what he called 'crossroads' or 'road-forks' in his working life—when he took a new direction and changed his orientation towards what he attended to in his therapeutic practice—is instructive. In an interview with Per Jensen (Andersen and Jenson 2007), he talked of being strongly affected in his meetings with people and of the worries and disquiets they could arouse in him—Per: '*How would you say such meetings have affected you? Your own practice, own thinking?*' Tom: 'I don't really know, myself. I certainly get very moved by people. Go along thinking a great deal about it and get filled with a restlessness in my body that won't leave me alone. So I have to often formulate something and formulate something that can be taken into other contexts' (p. 171). Per: '*It was the choice of a new direction?*' Tom: 'A crossroads, I call it—because I am very uncertain of to what extent it was a choice. It was more having to give something up, really give it up . . .' (p. 159)—and strangely, what he found was that as he and his team turned away from their old way, away from a reliance on what he felt uncomfortable

---

[15] Tragically, Tom Andersen died on 15 May 2007 from the injuries he received when he fell on the rocky Norwegian coast. He was a close and dear friend and I miss him greatly.

with—when 'we stopped saying what people should do and think—then alternatives popped up almost by themselves' (p. 159).[16] 'It was a big transition—from "either-or" to "this *and* this". Without realizing it then, I would say now that "either-or" belongs in the world one can describe as immovable and to what one can also call "the non-living". So that is to say we worked with living people as though they belonged to "the non-living". It felt uncomfortable, and it was a relief to move over to the "this *and* that" perspective' (p. 159). Indeed, Tom Andersen articulates throughout the whole of this interview how a non-intellectual, felt restlessness in his body that will not leave him alone, functioned as an ethical 'loadstone' in guiding him towards a practice he felt less and less uncomfortable with, a practice which, as Per Jensen put it, resulted in 'speaking less and listening [becoming] an important crossroad in his practice' (p. 158).

It is an important fact, I think, that Tom Andersen's new practice was not something chosen, but emerged, and was only appreciated later as the 'big transition' it was.[17] And to grasp a bit more clearly what is involved in such a process, I want to examine here the sequence of steps involved in both the processes of problem-solving and of re-orienting, a little more closely: (1) first, *problem-solving*: approaching a newness or strangeness as a problem to be solved requires us to first analyse it into a set of identifiable elements; we must then find a pattern or order amongst them; and then *hypothesize* a hidden agency responsible for the order (call it, the working of certain rules, principles, or laws, or the working of a story or narrative). We then seek further evidence for the influence of this supposed agency, thus to enshrine it in a theory or theoretical system. We go on to make use of such theories in giving shape to our actions. In other words, we manipulate the strangeness (now known in terms of the theory) to produce an advantageous outcome which we call 'the solution' to our problem, and we then turn 'to apply' the theory elsewhere.

Importantly, we as investigators remain bodily unchanged in this process; we remain *outside* and *separate* from the others or othernesses we are investigating. Thus, rather than being engaged or involved with them, we set ourselves 'over against' them as if viewing them from afar. The extra knowledge we acquire *about* them—in the form of new facts or information—is in fact aimed at seeking *mastery* or *control* over them, to change *their* behaviour by *our* 'interventions' within it.

(2) Alternatively, in *resolving* on a line of action: Instead of immediately trying to analyse the situation we face into its elements, we can treat it as a being a 'something' that is still radically unknown to us, and, by 'opening' ourselves to being spontaneously

---

[16] Instead of saying to people 'we think you should think this way', he and his team began to say, for example: 'In addition to how you are thinking, we have thought ...' or: 'In addition to doing what you've been doing you could also consider this ...' (Andersen 2007, p. 159).

[17] Senge et al. (2006) also note that choice among alternatives is not always involved in the occurrence of changes in one's ways of acting: While 'standard theories of change revolve around making decisions, determining "the vision"', they suggest many changes are much more to do with, 'reaching a state of clarity about and connection to what is emerging, [coming] to an "inner knowing" where, in a sense, there is no decision making. What to do just becomes obvious',and what is achieved 'depends on where you're coming from and who you are as a person' (p. 89).

'moved' by it, we can 'enter into' a living, dialogically-structured relationship with it. As James (1996) puts it: 'The only way to apprehend reality's thickness is either to experience it directly by being a part of reality oneself, or to evoke it in imagination by sympathetically divining [its] inner life' (pp. 250–1). In other words, if we can become involved or engaged in an active, back and forth relationship with the others or othernesses in our surroundings and can develop relationships with them within which—if we go slowly, and allow time for the *imaginative work* that each response can occasion within us to take place—we can gain a sense of the 'inner landscape of possibilities' available to us for making a next move in relation to them. If, that is, we can gain an initial point of entry into it

To exhibit what I mean here, it would be useful if the following sequence of statements is read quite slowly, in fact, almost sub-vocally uttered while reading them, with a pause at the end of each one to take 'time out' to imagine oneself in the situation depicted:

- We enter a new situation; (pause ... what situation?).
- We are confused, bewildered, we don't know our way about; (pause ... how does it feel?).
- However, as we 'dwell in' it, as we 'move around' within the confusion, and apply one or another descriptive concept to a crucial aspect of it as a 'point of entry', a 'something', then an 'it' begins to emerge; (pause ... what do we begin to notice?).
- It emerges in the 'time contours' or 'time shapes' that become apparent and pertinent in the dynamic relations we can sense between our outgoing activities and their incoming results; (pause ... what kind of unique, qualitative 'feel' does it have?).
- An image comes to us, we find that we can express this 'something' in terms of an image; (pause ... what image?).
- But not so fast, for as we find different aspects to which we can apply different descriptive concepts, we can find another, and another image, and another— Wittgenstein uses a city, a toolbox, the controls in the driving cab of a train, and many different types of games, all as metaphors for different aspects of our experiences of the use of language (pause ... what is 'motivating' all these image?).

Having found a number of points of entry and gone through a number of different images, we can come to a sense of the actual landscape of possibilities giving rise to them all. Indeed, we can gain a sense of familiarity with such landscapes, such that we can come to feel confident of knowing our way around within them, and of being able to *resolve* on a way or ways of *going on* within them. I want to suggest that the imaginative work done by Seikkula's client was along similar such lines. By turning a moment that was for her, at the time, a continuous flow of diffuse but connected experiences into a seeming contradiction, Seikkula turned an aspect of her confused feelings of turmoil over her family relations into a distinct 'something' that she could work with and on, into a something that she could, in William James' words, get on 'speaking terms' with.

This process, then, of *coming to a judgement and resolving on a line of action* is not at all like carrying out a calculation, or of *making a decision or choice* among a set of already clear alternatives. It involves moving around within a landscape of possibilities, and in so doing, being *spontaneously responsive* to the consequences of each move, and *judging* which one (or combination of moves) seems best in resolving the initial tension aroused in one's initial confusion—*judgement* is involved because, to repeat, we are operating here only in the realm of possibilities, not actualities that can be named and formalized (Shotter 2010).

As investigators, we ourselves are changed in such encounters. For, in becoming involved with, immersed in, the 'inner life' of the others or othernesses around us, everything we do can be partly shaped by being in response to what *they might do*. Thus, rather than an objective *knowledge* of their nature, we gain—and come to embody—an *orientation* toward them. We grasp how to 'go on' with them in terms of the *possible* ways they might respond to us. And although at first we can be wholly 'bewitched' (Wittgenstein 1953, no. 109) by their 'voice', as our familiarity with them grows, their voice can become just one voice among the many other voices within us, and we can even become 'disenchanted' with what they 'call' upon us to do. However, we can never gain complete mastery over them—they can always surprise us, no matter how familiar to us they have become. Our constant vigilance is required; the precise words we use are important—for their *grammar* commits us *now* to what is expected of us in the future.

Conclusions: from decontextualized knowledge to contextualized knowing-from-within

> For more clearly *(but not differently)* in my experience of others than in my experience of speech or the perceived world, I inevitably grasp my body as a *spontaneity which teaches me what I could not know in any other way except through it*
>
> (Merleau-Ponty 1964, p. 93).

What I have been exploring above, then, is that fact that, as living bodies, we are inevitably spontaneously responsive in some way or ways *related to* events occurring within our surroundings, or to aspects of them that we attend to. In other words, we only exist as participant parts within a larger ecology, of which our social ecology is also only a participant part, a system of inter-dependencies within systems of other such systems which we all rely on for being sustained in our existence.[18] Further, I have been emphasizing that, as we move around within our surroundings—due to our spontaneous living responsiveness to them—it is hardly at all the carry over from our past experiences that 'shapes' our conduct within them at the present moment; it is what we spontaneously *anticipate* as occurring next as we continue our movements within them that matters to us. We thus have our existence within an unfolding

---

[18] In Shotter (1984) I wrote: 'Our accounts of ourselves must clearly be situated in the world to which we owe our being as we understand it, i.e. in the world of our everyday social life. But what is that world? It is, I shall maintain, a world consisting not only of socially "constructed" institutions, continually reproduced (and transformed) by the accountable activities occurring within them, but also of a larger social process out of which such institutions arise, a process which I have called our social ecology' (p. x).

process in time in which *differences* as such are continually happening to us, some of them as the incoming results of our own outgoing actions, and some of which just come to us 'unbidden'. Merleau-Ponty (1964) describes the importance of our spontaneous anticipation of the *relations* between such differences as they occur as follows:

> There is that which is to be said, and which is as yet no more than a precise uneasiness in the world of things said [i.e., the anticipations aroused by what is said]. Expression is a matter of acting in such a way that the two gather one another in or cross one another. I would never take a step if my faraway view of the goal did not find in my body a natural art of transforming it into an approaching view. My thought could not advance a step if the horizon of meaning it opens up did not become, through speech, what is called in the theatre a *real* décor [i.e., a stage set resembling the real setting for the actors' moves] (p. 19).

Living bodies, ecological relations, and time: three things that the western philosophical tradition has ignored (among many others). By assuming reality only to consist in separate entities in movement according to already pre-established laws, that tradition has generally assumed that there is only one way in which we make things intelligible to ourselves: as conscious *subjects* with minds, that we set out in a deliberate fashion to understand the things around us, cognitively and conceptually, as *objects*—with our life as subjects radically split off from the 'dead' world of objects. In understanding the others and othernesses in our surroundings in this way, we only understand them 'from the outside', so to speak, and thus relate ourselves to them in terms of certain a priori categorical schematisms.

This is because, James (1996) suggests:

> the ruling tradition in philosophy has always been the Platonic and Aristotelian belief that fixity is a nobler and worthier thing than change. Reality must be one and unalterable. Concepts, being themselves fixities, agree best with this fixed nature of truth, so that for any knowledge of ours to be quite true it must be knowledge by universal concepts rather than by particular experiences, for these notoriously are mutable and corruptible' (p. 237).

But if what I have suggested above is the case, and our reality is a living, flowing and growing reality, continually in movement, then there is also another, very different kind of knowing which becomes available to us 'from within' our ongoing, dynamically unfolding involvements and engagements with the others and othernesses around us—an embodied knowing which, so to speak, has us more than we have it, which is of an implicit or tacit kind which makes itself known to us only *in our spontaneously responsive movements*.

But further, and most importantly, whether James is correct in his surmise about the nobility of fixed concepts or not, what we have seen above is that a universal concept of a descriptive kind can give us a stable point of entry for our inquiries into the diffusely organized nature of those otherwise unique ways of knowing that we exhibit in our movement around in the world—a form of inquiry that opens us up to a realm of influence of a kind quite different from that of intervening in the behaviour of others. As we have seen, it is a form of inquiry that gives us access to the 'inner' workings of a living reality, a reality of an altogether different kind to that we think of as familiar. James (1996) describes its nature in the following terms, within it:

> no element *there* cuts itself off from any other element, as concepts cut themselves from concepts. No part *there* is so small as not to be a place of conflux. No part there is not really *next* its neighbours; which means that there is literally nothing between; which means again that no part goes exactly so far and no farther; that no part absolutely excludes another, but that they compenetrate and are cohesive; that if you tear out one, its roots bring out more with them; that whatever is real is telescoped and diffused into other reals; that, in short, every minutest thing is already its hegelian 'own other,' in the fullest sense of the term (pp. 271–2).

In other words, what Seikkula's client expressed in her two seemingly contradictory statements, drew on what was in fact available for expression within the flow of her experiences. So, while her *expressions* may have *sounded* contradictory, if James is correct, then I think we must say that the contradiction results from the demand in our everyday lives that the flow of our experiences *must* be given a logically proper form of conceptual or discursive expression. Yet in reality, prior to their expression, the immediate facts of her experience don't *sound* contradictory at all; they simply *are* aspects of a complex whole until conceptualized and named vocally.

The peculiar nature of the 'inside' of this kind of dynamic reality, to which there is no 'outside', no alternative 'other reality' to which it can be compared, which thus contains its 'own others', is what is so difficult for us to accept. For we cannot 'grasp' it conceptually. It is radically strange to us—there is no denying it.

Yet, it is *this* dynamically unfolding reality that shapes our everyday spontaneous responses to events occurring around us, including our continuous and compulsive attempts in Social Theory to reduce the unfolding dynamic nature of social activity to fixed and namable forms. And it is this reduction that both misleads us into looking into the past for the influences at work shaping our activities (instead of the future), and also into thinking that we can change our ways of behaving by changing our ways of talking—a mistake that Nelson Goodman (1972) described some time ago in the following terms:

> Philosophers sometimes mistake features of discourse for features of the subject of discourse. We seldom conclude that the world consists of words just because a true description of it does, but we sometimes suppose that the structure of the world is the same as the structure of the description. This tendency may even reach the point of linguomorphism when we conceive the world as comprised of atomic objects corresponding to certain proper names, and of atomic objects corresponding to atomic sentences (p. 24).

As a consequence, not only are our living, spontaneously expressive and responsive bodies ignored, but more importantly, also ignored is the continuous *background flow* of reciprocally responsive activity occurring between ourselves and all the others and othernesses (things, events, etc.) around us from within which all our activities arise and into which they all return. Yet, as Lock and Strong (2010) show, in the works of Vico, Mead, and Vygotsky, but especially in the works of Wittgenstein and Bakhtin, we begin to move away from the Cartesian mechanical world of dead forms and structures, and begin to find ourselves face-to-face with a wholly new horizon, a new world of life and of living events and processes in continual living *intra*-action with each other. This changes everything. Nothing in it retains its old character, especially language. Thought of in terms of representations and interpretations of 'picturable' states of affairs, we now realize that the stiff and frozen forms of language in which we have 'clothed' our circumstances in the past have hidden from us all the ways in which we, and other such beings, all live in unceasing, spontaneously responsive, *living relations with each other*, relations in which, in our activities, we become, inevitably, intertwined or intermingled in with each other.

A major consequence of the move from 'dead' Cartesian changes (in which new patterns are formed from the rearrangement of old ones) to a dynamic, living world of emergent forms, is an unexpected focus on the uniquely new, on first-time, unrepeatable events that can emerge—a focus on *singularities* rather than repetitions. Another major shift is from events in the present being determined by occurrences in the past, to their being determined much more by *anticipations*, by their possible 'consummation' in the future. A third shift is the switch from space to *time* as the crucial dimension in psychological or mental phenomena. There is also the unavoidable *creativity* of all our *joint* or *dialogical* activities, and thus a shift from a concern with change to the difficulty of achieving stability—plus the fact that all this goes on in the background to all our more deliberate activities, *spontaneously*, without any of our overall individual intentions being able easily to 'shape' it. Finally, we must add that, although we possess an 'acutely discriminative sense' (James 1890, p. 253) of the anticipatory '*feelings of tendency*, often so vague that we are unable to name them at all' (p. 254); 'if we try to hold fast the feeling of direction' in order to name them, the 'feeling of direction is lost' (p. 253); the indivisibility of its continuous movement is reduced to a sequence of separated shapes or forms.

Social constructionism is still (often) presented as a *theory* (or metatheory) of *knowledge*.[19] And social constructions are generally understood to be the by-products of (often unintended or unconscious) human *choices* (as distinct from the products of natural laws or principles). Thus a socially constructed reality is seen as a process produced by people acting both on their *interpretations* of the realities they inhabit, and on the basis of their *knowledge* of how things might be caused to change within it. As a result, social constructionism focuses on language and other of our discursive practices as internally *representing* or 'picturing' states of affairs out in the world at large. But in still focusing in its theories and metatheories on knowledge as such, it still ends, as I see it, by conducting its inquiries in an essentially Cartesian world of mental events still thought of in mechanical, i.e. 'dead', cause-and-effect terms. Yet, as we have seen above, what is crucial in 'living realities' is how our embodied and active ways of

---

[19] Social constructionists are no longer interested in knowledge tout court, nor can social constructionism remain 'ontologically mute' (Gergen 1994, p.72). As Gergen (2009) now notes: 'From a relational perspective, growing plants, the firmament, and the economy are not facts of nature; rather, they have become "objects of study" through one's relational participation... Our departments of knowledge are not demanded by the contours of the world, but result from social agreements at a particular time in history in a particular culture' (p. 207), in terms of our own relational ways of being in the world.

relating ourselves to our surroundings can give rise to anticipatory tensions as to what we might next encounter, as we bodily move around in them, and it is the fluctuations occurring in these tensions in relation to our movements that we can use to guide our own immediate actions—and which we can also use in 'calibrating' ourselves bodily to re-act 'automatically' in an optimum manner to certain kinds of crucial events.

In attending, then, both to the *social ecology* of our everyday activities, and to our own social *ontology*—to our ways of *being* a different kind of person with different sensitivities to different dimensions of difference in our surroundings—I have been concerned to bring into view—or better, into felt experience—the not-so-easily-noticed background to, or *provenance* for, our more self-consciously intentional social constructions; for it is only from within our bodily relations to that background that our real *needs* can become known to us, otherwise we are working merely with our intellectualized *desires* (Shotter 2009; Todes 2001).

I would like to end with some accounts by Tom Andersen (2007) of the radically strange, yet crucially important nature of events that can happen within such lived and felt inner realities, events that occurred around 1985, when the reflecting process was still being conducted by simply reversing the 'one-way' screen effect between the therapy room and the team room: 'There were many crossroads at that time—for example, the moment I stood in the door and said, "Would you like to listen to us?" Then the therapist got up in the usual way; he thought he should go along with us, just as we'd always done before. But I said, "You belong here". It was almost like having the feeling that we had abandoned him—he was left alone and abandoned. It was very unpleasant as well, but it had to be that way' (p. 162). Later, he realized that while the therapist belonged to one system—amongst those who talked in relation to the client's difficulties—those behind the screen who talked about *their* way of talking about difficulties, belonged to a different system. 'But when it happened, along came the words, "No, you belong here", completely by themselves. It was only long after that I understood it. But the spontaneous came from what is felt in the body' (p. 162). And later, in answer to Per Jensen's question: *Is there an ethical principle you refer to with this?,*" he replied: 'Yes, what I think is that what is unpleasant is to orient oneself away from participation in relationships the whole time. To feel the discomfort and of course think that this is an uncomfortable situation for others as well. So I believe I would say that it is to dare to take seriously that which one feels—what one feels with the body and in the body. [But then] we were nearing a new crossroads . . . we were very rational and sensible, with almost military interventions . . . But when one feels that this unpleasant, and can't manage to deal with it, then one has to adjust oneself to accommodate it—then one can deal with it [i.e. understand it] afterwards. Don't wait to deal with things rationally first' (p. 163). It is in our acting that we come to our first understandings, vague though they may be.

References

Andersen, T. (1992). Reflections on reflecting with families. In S. McNamee and K.J. Gergen (Eds.) *Social Constructionism as Therapy*, pp. 54–68. Sage, London.

Andersen, T. (2007). Crossroads: Tom Andersen in conversation with Per Jensen. In H. Anderson and P. Jensen (Eds.) *Innovations in the Reflecting Process*, pp. 158–74. Karnac Books, London.

Andersen, T. (2008). Reflecting talks: my version. In K. Jordan (Ed.) *The Quick Theory Reference Guide: A Resource for Expert and Novice Mental Health Professionals*, pp. 427–43. Nova Publishers, New York.

Anderson, H. and Jensen, P. (2007). *Innovations in the Reflecting Process*. Karnac Books, London.

Austin, J. (1962). *How to do Things with Words*. Clarendon Press, Oxford.

Bakhtin, M. M. (1981). *The Dialogical Imagination* (M. Holquist, Ed.; C. Emerson and M. Holquist, Trans.). University of Texas Press, Austin, TX.

Bakhtin, M. M. (1984). *Problems of Dostoevsky's Poetics* (C. Emerson, Ed., and Trans.). University of Minnesota Press, Minneapolis, MN.

Bakhtin, M. M. (1986). *Speech Genres and Other Late Essays* (V. W. McGee, Trans.). University of Texas Press, Austin, TX.

Bakhtin, M. M. (1993). *Toward a Philosophy of the Act* (V. Lianpov, Trans.; M. Holquist, Ed.). University of Texas Press, Austin, TX.

Bateson, G. (1973). *Steps to an Ecology of Mind*. Paladin, London.

Bergson, H. (1896/1911). *Matter and Memory*. Allen and Unwin, London.

Corcoran, T. (2009). Second nature. *British Journal of Social Psychology*, **48**, 375–88.

Garfinkel, H. (2002). *Ethnomethodology's Program: Working out Durkheim's Aphorism* (A. Warefield Rawls, Ed.). Rowman & Littlefield Publishers, New York & Oxford.

Gergen, K.J. (1994). *Realities and Relationships: Soundings in Social Construction*. Harvard University Press, Cambridge, MA.

Gergen, K.J. (2009). *Relational Being: Beyond Self and Community*. Oxford University Press, Oxford & New York.

Gibson, J.J. (1979). *The Ecological Approach to Visual Perception*. Houghton Mifflin, London.

Goodman, N. (1972). *Problems and projects*. Bobbs-Merrill, New York.

James, W. (1890). *Principles of Psychology*, vols. 1 & 2. Macmillan, London.

James, W. (1996). *A Pluralistic Universe: Hibbert Lectures at Manchester College on the Present Situation in Philsophy*. University of Nebraska Press, Lincoln and London. [First published 1909.]

Lock, A. and Strong, T. (2010). *Social Constructionism: Sources and Stirrings in Theory and Practice*. Cambridge University Press, Cambridge.

Merleau-Ponty, M. (1962). *Phenomenology of Perception* (C. Smith, Trans.). Routledge and Kegan Paul, London.

Merleau-Ponty, M. (1964). *Signs* (R. M. McCleary, Trans.). Northwestern University Press, Evanston, IL.

Nussbaum, M. (2001). *Upheavals of Thought: the Intelligence of Emotions*. Cambridge University Press, Cambridge.

Polanyi, M. (1958). *Personal Knowledge: Towards a Post-Critical Philosophy*. Routledge and Kegan Paul, London [Also Harper and Row Torchbook, New York, 1962.]

Polanyi, M. (1967). *The Tacit Dimension*. Routledge and Kegan Paul, London.

Ryle, G. (1949). *The Concept of Mind*. Methuen, London.

Seikkkula, J. (2009). Polyphonic dialogues–generating words for the not yet spoken, plenary at EBTA Conference, 'Imagine'. Helsinki, Finland, 4–6 Sept, 2009. http://www.ebta2009.com/attachments/044_EBTA2009-imagine%20Jaakko%20Seikkula%20Plenary.pdf [Accessed 16 July, 2010.]

Senge, P., Scharmer, O.C., Jaworski, J. and Flowers, B.S. (2006). *Presence: Exploring Profound Change in People, Organizations and Society*. Nicolas Brealey Publications, London.

Shotter, J. (1984). *Social Accountability and Selfhood*. Blackwell, Oxford.

Shotter, J. (1993). *Cultural Politics of Everyday Life: Social Constructionism, Rhetoric, and Knowing of the Third Kind*. Open University Press, Milton Keynes.

Shotter, J. (2005). Inside processes: transitory understandings, action guiding anticipations, and witness thinking. *International Journal of Action Research*, **11**, 157–89.

Shotter, J. (2008). *Conversational Realities Revisited: Life, Language, Body, and World*. Taos Publications, Inc., Chagrin Falls, OH.

Shotter, J. (2009). Moments of common reference in dialogic communication: a basis for unconfused collaboration in unique contexts. *International Journal of Collaborative Practices*, **11**, 1–23.

Shotter, J. (2010). Movements of feeling and moments of judgement: towards an ontological social constructionism. *International Journal of Action Research*, **61**, 1–27.

Todes, S. (2001). *Body and World* (H. L. Dreyfus and P. Hoffman, Introductions). MIT Press, Cambridge, MA.

Vygotsky, L.S. (1966). Development of the higher mental functions. In A.N. Leontyev, A.R. Luria, and A. Smirnov Eds., *Psychological Research in the USSR*. Progress Publishers, Moscow, pp.11–46.

Vygotsky, L.S. (1978). *Mind in Society: the Development of Higher Psychological Processes*. Edited by M. Cole, V. John-Steiner, S. Scribner, and E. Souberman (Eds.). Harvard University Press, Cambridge, MA.

Vygotsky, L.S. (1986). *Thought and Language* (Trans. newly revised by A. Kozulin). MIT Press, Cambridge, MA.

Vygotsky, L.S. (1987). *Thinking and Speech*. In *The Collected Works of L.S. Vygotsky: Vol.1* (R.W. Rieber and A.S. Carton, Eds.; N. Minick, Trans.). Plenum Press, New York.

Wittgenstein, L. (1953). *Philosophical Investigations* (G.E.M. Anscombe, Trans.). Blackwell, Oxford.

Wittgenstein, L. (1965). *The Blue and the Brown Books*. Harper Torch Books, New York.

Wittgenstein, L. (1969) *On Certainty* (G.E.M. Anscombe and G.H. von Wright, Eds.; D. Paul and G.E.M Anscombe, Trans.). Blackwell, Oxford.

Wittgenstein, L. (1980). *Culture and Value* (G. Von Wright, Introduction; P. Winch, Trans.). Blackwell, Oxford.

Chapter 6

Narrative therapy: challenges and communities of practice

Susanna Chamberlain

The person's not the problem. The problem is the problem

Erik Sween (1998).

Narrative therapy has been, from its inception, a practice-based therapy that is continually subject to a post hoc analysis of the practices and conceptualizations which are effective for the client and ethically sound for the therapist. From the early 1980s when both David Epston and Michael White were working in hospitals as clinical social workers, a critique of the effectiveness of accepted clinical practices was being developed. The focus of this critique was on what actually worked rather than upon what was ineffective.

In this chapter, I have chosen to examine the narrative therapy (Epston and White 1989, 1992; Epston 1989, 1998; Combs and Freedman 1998; Freedman and Combs 1996; Denborough 1996, 2008; Monks et al. 1997; Nicholson 1995; Tomm 1998; Weingarten 1998; C. White and Denborough 1998; M. White and Epston 1990, 1992; M. White 1980, 1984a,b, 1986a,b,c, 1988a,b, 1989, 1995, 1997, 2000a,b, 2001a, 2004, 2005, 2007) developed in Australia and New Zealand.

The following is a selection of stories or tales about narrative therapy, and some observations upon the development of particular ideas and practices. The first segment deals with the therapeutic context from which narrative therapy emerged. Following that is a brief review of the influences of postmodern theories upon the ideas in narrative therapy. After briefly touching upon the core collaborations which have created this approach, I then explore three aspects of narrative therapy: the challenges, the counselling models, and the community practices.

Narrative therapy in a therapeutic context

Narrative therapy emerged from the confluence of the anti-psychiatry movement, existentialist approaches to persons, and family therapy, and was very powerfully influenced by the ideas of postmodern philosophers, particularly Michel Foucault (1979, 1980, 1984). As early as 1946, challenges to the paradigm of the essentialist internalized Self began appearing in the field of psychology. This section briefly explores some of the ideas and theorists from within therapeutic fields who refuted the conceptualization of the self as an object and provided a context for the development of narrative ideas.

Viktor Frankl, a Jewish psychiatrist, emerged from a wartime concentration camp with the recognition that all of his psychiatric training had served little purpose in contributing to his or his fellow prisoners' survival. He realized that his survival had depended upon the development and sustaining, on a daily basis, of meaning in his life. Frankl's book *Man's Search For Meaning* (1959) issued a challenge to the understandings of the essentialist self which had developed in psychology in the early part of the 20th century. Frankl's work was to become highly influential over the latter decades of the century as alternative views to the dominant paradigm were increasingly sought, and among his early writings, Michael White indicates that Frankl was an influence on his thinking.

Frankl's work is often termed 'existential' and it certainly does share some resonances with the French post-war existentialism of Sartre, de Beauvoir, Camus, and Genet. The parallels are most apparent when we consider that 'logotherapy' and 'existentialism' take as the basis of their ontologies the being of the individual and the creation of a worldview from the perspective of that individual. Each is concerned with meaning or meaninglessness; each emphasizes the isolation of the individual and the consequent responsibility of all for individual political action.

In the late 1960s and early 1970s the impact of existentialism began to emerge in psychological circles in Britain (Laing and Esterson 1964/1970; Laing 1960/1972, 1967/1972, 1969; Boyers and Orrill 1972; Capra 1982; Szasz 1972). R.D. Laing, and later others, began to question the sanctity of the model of the essentialist self as it was employed within psychiatry. Laing's books influenced many practitioners, particularly psychologists and social workers, and the themes of challenge to the established order and the possibility of alternative interpretations of self were taken up to be explored in training courses and universities. Although White and Epston do not appear to derive their work from that of Laing, it was in the atmosphere of a questioning of the traditional models and the dominance of psychiatry that their stance of challenge emerged.

Among the people influenced by Laing's work was Gregory Bateson, anthropologist, research psychologist, and polymath. Bateson's early ethnographic explorations in New Guinea resulted in an ethnography (Bateson 1958) and papers that described interpersonal relationships in terms of relations of power (symmetry and complementarity). Bateson developed a significant interest in identifying the processes of human interactional systems, producing papers on double description, schizmogenesis, and 'ecology of mind'. He rejected the 'internalized self' in one particular paper (Bateson 1972, p. 318) where he talks about 'the dividing line between internal and external'—indicating that such a division is neither possible nor useful.

Bateson was to have a considerable influence, particularly in family therapy where his work was taken up by such diverse practitioners as Jay Haley and Michael White. Bateson implies a great deal about his conceptualizations in *Mind and Nature* (1979), and in *Steps to an Ecology of Mind* (1972, p. 319) clearly states his position on the concept of self: 'The system is not a transcendant entity as the "self" is commonly supposed to be.'

These ideas stand in clear opposition to the dominant stories of the self at the time Bateson was writing. Similarly, his models of presentation of serious material (for example the father–daughter conversations or the 'sketches') also offer clear alternatives to the usually prescribed methods of presenting weighty academic arguments in a dry manner within rigid constraints of particular disciplinary rhetorics. Bateson was practising what he espoused, the 'embodiment of the self', i.e. he wrote according to his own self-concept rather than being constrained by social or academic pressures.

The development of what has come to be called 'family therapy' is itself an interesting story. Until the late 1960s all therapy in Europe, North America, and a few periphery outposts was undertaken with individuals. As the psychoanalytic model developed into the dominant paradigm of psychiatry, it also became part of popular culture. Educated white Western people spoke confidently of the 'unconscious', Oedipus complexes, introversion or extraversion, neuroses and psychoses, the ego, and the 'death wish'. Even detective storywriters (like Dorothy L. Sayers or Dashiell Hammett) postulated complex psychological theories as 'motivation' for their characters' behaviours or actions.

It was common practice to see clients as isolated entities, devoid of context, and driven by unconscious motivations to which they were unknowing slaves. The stance of the practitioners was that of 'expert', he who has the template by which the world and the person may be judged, evaluated, and found wanting. This stance incorporated a negative worldview which privileged notions of the 'normal' (which was unattainable) while elucidating only that which was 'abnormal', pathologizing the person rather than the illness, issue or problem.

In the USA, Murray Bowen began to question the isolation of clients. His psychoanalytic work (Bowen 1978) had shown that parental and sibling relationships had an impact upon the psychic development of an individual, leaving the apparent adult either enmeshed or disengaged from his family of origin. For Bowen, the person was still driven by an ungovernable unconscious; the self was created within the family system, and played out the dramas of repeated patterns of relationships derived from several generations of the family of origin. The self was only truly independent once it became individuated and gave up being enmeshed with parents/grandparents/family system dynamics.

Bowen's family systems theory (1978), as it came to be called, was a significant challenge to the dominant story of the time because what Bowen had done was to contextualize the person within a system. The individual self was removed from its essentialist isolation and placed, in the eyes of the therapeutic field, within a framework of other persons. The self became interactive, at least during the developmental period (which could be the entire lifetime in Bowen's frame of analysis) and family therapy, sprung from originally Freudian notions of self, diversified dramatically over the next three decades (Bandler et al. 1976; Berne 1961, 1964; Boscolo et al. 1987; Boscolo and Bertrando 1993; de Shazer 1982, 1985; Guerin 1976; Haley 1973, 1976, 1980, 1971; Haley and Hoffman 1967; Handel 1968; Hoffman 1981; Horewitz 1977; L'Abate et al. 1986; Leupnitz 1988; McGoldrick et al. 1989; McGoldrick and Gerson 1985; Mandanes 1981; Minuchin 1974/1977, 1998; Minuchin and Fishman 1981; Napier and Whitaker 1978; Satir 1972/1978; Selvini Palazzoli et al. 1978; Walrond-Skinner 1976; Walters et al. 1988; Watzlawick et al. 1974; Weeks and L'Abate 1982; Whitaker and Bumberry 1988; Woollams and Brown 1978; Worden 1994).

The breakthrough was in the shift of emphasis from the individual focus to the systemic or structural. General systems theory was being developed in other contexts during this period. Anthropology and sociology had begun to view humans as contextualized social beings from the turn of the 20th century when Durkheim had written about social systems and the role of the individual (1915/1982, 1951), whether in the division of labour, the religious life, or in the incidence of suicide.

The social construction of the individual was being explored by Goffman as Bowen was developing his systemic approach.

> When we allow that the individual projects a definition of the situation when he appears before others, we must also see that the others, however passive their role may seem to be, will themselves project a definition of the situation by virtue of their responses to the individual and by virtue of any lines of action they initiate to him
>
> (Goffman 1959/1984, p. 20).

Here Goffman was arguing that persons are constituted in interaction with others. Much of his seminal analysis of the presentation of self was concerned with arguing for a socially constructed self, present in performance and ultimately not essentialist. Goffman's work was also an early influence on narrative therapy and the burgeoning narrative epistemology of the last decade of the 20th century, particularly when combined with Bakhtinian notions of performance, narrative, and heteroglossia and Foucault's postmodern challenges to power structures.

Collaboration

Narrative therapy has a long history of collaboration and is the result of the work of many people. These include Michael White and David Epston who provided the initial and later guiding ideas; Cheryl White whose publishing house (Dulwich Centre Publications) and conferences offered the opportunity for many practitioners to publish narrative inspired practices; and a range of therapists and teachers from around the world. These include: Steven Madigan, Jill Freedman and Gene Combs, Karl Tomm, Walter Behran, Lisa Berndt, Jenny Freeman, Kaethe Weingarten, Barb Wingard, Daf Hewson, Johnella Bird, John Winslade, Wendy Drewery, and the enormous number of practitioners who have contributed their work and ideas over the last two decades.

Initially, during the late 1970s and early 1980s, both Epston and White's work centred on the ideas that were being developed within family therapy. Michael White was a founding member of the Australia and New Zealand Family Therapy Association, and the first editor of its journal. Both White and Epston explored the systemic work that was being created by the Milan school, the structuralist model developed by Minuchin, and even touched on the strategic approach of Jay Haley and others. Until the mid 1980s these ways of working formed an important part of the practice of therapy, and some of the early papers published, particularly by White, show this to be the case. In 1984, when White resigned as editor of the *Australia and New Zealand Family Therapy Journal*, he also began to explore alternatives in practice. He was particularly interested in some of the political pressures that existed in everyday life and how these became enmeshed in the problems experienced by clients. He and his wife

Cheryl had long been engaged in trying to raise a consciousness of gender issues in the family therapy field, and this formed the basis of what was to become an ongoing practice of highlighting issues of power and dominance.

At the same time in New Zealand, David Epston was making a transition from his formative theoretical experiences with anthropology and exploring the practices available to social workers within the hospital system. This was something the Whites and David Epston had in common—the experience of the constraints and pathologizing approaches within the mental health field in the 1980s, and it was their independent but common striving to discover new ways of working that helped to forge narrative therapy.

For two and half decades, both David Epston and Michael White took their ideas around the world, teaching health and allied professionals in many countries, and developing a following for narrative approaches to therapy. In later years, Cheryl White and David Denborough would continue the work of teaching community practice, often in developing countries and remote settlements. Of the team, White was the most prolific writer, publishing many articles, and through Cheryl's publishing house, quite a few books. David Epston has been a prolific teacher and communicator, however, his publications have been rarer over the years.

Challenges

One of the core characteristics of narrative therapy has been the stance of challenge that is offered to dominant structures and discourse of power. In this section, I am interested in examining briefly how the taken-for-granted concepts of psychology and family therapy were challenged, and which challenges continue to be raised.

The practice of narrative therapy began as clinical work in which the driving force was the empowerment of the client and the privileging of the client's interpretation of his or her own life over the interpretations available from the 'expert' analysis offered by contemporary psychological theory. Originally located within the framework of systemic family therapy, White and Epston separately began to challenge the systems of power in which current models of family therapy were embedded. David Epston was developing the use of story and letter-writing as therapeutic practice, while Michael White was beginning to work on 'externalizing the problem' and exploring the significance of power in relationships. Their collaboration dates from the mid 1980s when they found that their ideas were parallel and cross-fertilizing of each other's work. It is important to note that their collaboration was a result of each reading and hearing the work of the other and joining forces in discussing issues and ideas on a continuous and sporadic fashion for over 20 years. The two men were not just supported, but also challenged at an intellectual level by their wives (Cheryl White and Anne Epston) who were strong feminist professionals in their own right.

Early interest in the work of Gregory Bateson (M. White 1986a, 1989, 2001b) led to an ongoing inclusion of ideas from social anthropology, including the concepts of 'rich' or 'thick' description from Clifford Geertz (M. White 1989, 1991, 2001b), principles of liminality and communitas drawn from Victor Turner's work (M. White 1989, 2001), and the self-reflexivity and collaboration with others from Marcus,

Fischer, Clifford, and the 'new ethnographers' (see Chamberlain 1990). In addition, narrative therapy has incorporated ideas from social constructionist psychology ([White and Epston 1989; M. White 2001a], Goffman [White and Epston 1989, 2001], E. Bruner [Epston and White 1989]; J. Bruner [White and Epston 1989]; Meyerhoff [M. White 1989; 1997, 2001a]). This is a thin description of what has become a rich and thick text of engagement with these theoreticians and thinkers over the past two decades.

In 1989 White and Epston drew upon the 'text analogy'—a concept which they utilized, drawing from the anthropological writings of Edward Bruner (1986), Clifford Geertz (1973, 1983, 1986, 1988), and the philosophical work of Michel Foucault. As White and Epston (1989, p. 21) wrote:

> In two senses, the text analogy introduces us to an intertextual world. In the first sense, it proposes that person's lives are situated in texts within texts. In the second sense, every telling or retelling of a story, through its performance, is a new telling that encapsulates, and expands upon, the previous telling.

From this time forward, the guiding principles of narrative therapy were located within postmodern theoretical understandings, particularly the work of Michel Foucault (see M. White 1989, 1991, 1992, 1995, 1997, 2000a, 2000b, 2001a), as well as Pierre Bourdieu (M. White 1992, 2001b), Derrida (M. White 1992), Bachelard (M. White 1989, 1997), Vygotsky, and at the last White was beginning to explore Deleuze. In reality, the ideas were developed in practice, and as post hoc analysis was applied, the theoretical conceptualizations drawn from postmodernism were applied to what was already working in the clinical setting. It was this constant seeking for a way to explain and develop the practice that led to narrative therapy exploring ideas from such a diverse range of thinkers.

In later writings (M. White 1989/1990, 1991) there is a drawing upon Derrida's (1981) conceptualization of all human experience, all transactions that are embedded in language, as being 'text' of one genre or another, and therefore open to deconstruction. There is a concern with authenticity:

> Thus, the idea that lives are situated in texts or stories implies a particular notion of authenticity – that a person arrives at a sense of authenticity in life through the performance of texts. This notion of authenticity may be affronting to many a cherished belief that carries propositions about the "truth" of personhood or of human nature; those beliefs that suggest that, under particular and ideal circumstances of life, persons will be 'released' and thus become truly who they are – authentic!
>
> (M. White 1989/1990, p. 31).

The key practices of narrative therapy in the late 1990s included some ideas which were developed in the late 1980s, such as the key notion of 'externalizing the problem'. As Sween (1998) points out, if narrative therapy were to have a slogan it would be: 'The person's not the problem. The problem is the problem.' This stance of separating issues from persons has led to practices such as invoking resistance to the power of problems, or to describing the problem being faced as though it were an entity. For example, David Epston created the Anti-Anorexia Leagues in New Zealand and North America which are associations of persons who are actively resisting the influence of Anorexia, or the anti-bullying practices in schools invoke participation of groups of school attendees in standing up to harassment. In each case the problem is seen as being external to the person who experiences the detrimental effects of the problem, and therefore the persons are capable of maintaining or developing a positive sense of themselves while attempting to deal with an issue, a problem, a story which is not useful. This practice inverts the dominant practice of pathologizing the individual, perceiving the person as the problem, or at least as the container of the problem, and actively engages persons in joint action against common problems.

In the early texts which began to explore what became known as narrative therapy, the term 'alternative stories' (Epston and White 1989) built upon the possibilities originally opened up by the use of Bateson's 'double description' (M. White 1986b). By 1988, the term used was 'redescription' (M. White 1988, in 1989, p. 39) or 'alternative descriptions':

> One category of such questions invites family members to participate in the construction of alternative self-definitions, self-definitions not determined by prevailing specifications for personhood
>
> (M. White 1989, p. 53).

At this same time, the focus of narrative practice was on exploring 'unique outcomes' (M. White 1989 p. 18) and on developing the 'narrative mode':

> The narrative mode locates a person as a protagonist or participant in a world that s/he is continually acting in and upon. This is a world of interpretive acts, a world in which every retelling of a story is a new telling, a world in which persons participate with others in the 're-authoring' and, thus, in the shaping of their lives and relationships
>
> (Epston and White 1989, p. 48)

The challenge here was to the simple acceptance of the received story or description of the problem. For the practitioner, the challenge is to find another way of describing, or of working with the client to co-create an alternative description of the set of circumstances. The core idea was to extricate the person from the problem, to identify the issue as being separate from the lived experience or subjective reality, so that the problem itself could be examined. The shift was from 'I'm stupid/mad/bad or stuck' to 'I have an issue to resolve'. This was a significant challenge to the psychiatric stance of the internalized condition. People with mental illness were seen as being separate from their illness, not overwhelmingly identified and somehow absorbed by their diagnosis. The challenge was to reject totalizing descriptions and incidentally, to reject the systems that demanded totalizing practices.

One of the more significant elements of the early work was the stand taken on the issue of power. White (M. White 1989) wanted to explore how to identify and challenge the dominant ideology, or the structures of power, in which the client was embedded. In part, this was a social and political challenge to the inequities of the culture or society in which people lived; as such the stance of challenge to the dominant discourse continues in the stream of community work which is the most significant element of the application of narrative principles today. As Denborough (2008) pointed out, issues of gender and equity had been highlighted by papers published by White as early as 1984 in the ANZJFT, and the Dulwich Centre Review (a forerunner to the current *Journal of Narrative Therapy and Community Work*) was publishing papers which raised challenges around gender and dominance from its inception in 1987.

The other core aspect of this challenging stance was to actually examine the inherent power relationship within the therapy context itself. The relationship between client and therapist was subject to a scrutiny from which arose ideas such as the client being the expert on their own life, while the therapist was there to facilitate rather than direct the process. Many of the later ideas, such as the use of 'consultants' (others who had similar experiences or family members who could be witnesses—insiders and outsiders) had their genesis in this stance of challenges to power.

Counselling models

The early years of narrative therapy saw the introduction of a number of innovative therapeutic practices. The practice of using written material as therapeutic intervention was developed by White and Epston in the 1980s and continues to be utilized today. Whether the written document is a letter, a certificate of achievement (e.g. the now famous 'Monster-taming Certificates' [M. White and Epston 1990]), a sophisticated document of identity (co-created with a person who is standing up to voices, mental illness, or disabling practices such as 'harassment' or 'malice'), the use of literary texts as therapeutic practice is still recognized and considered useful. This was an area which David Epston had pioneered, and continued to refine over the years. For quite some time, his practice not only centred on the subtleties of the therapeutic responses derived from the impact of receiving letters, but also explored the ways in which the creation of text was an action of redefinition of identity.

By 1992, when the idea of landscapes of action and consciousness were introduced, the key term appears to be 're-authoring' (M. White 1992a, p. 127), although we also find 'alternative preferences' in the same year (Epston and White 1992). It is also in the early 1990s that issues of 'agency' were raised:

> Those therapeutic practices that I refer to as 'deconstructive' assist in establishing, for persons, a sense of 'agency'. This sense is derived from the experience of escaping 'passengerhood' in life, and from the sense of being able to play an active role in the shaping of one's life – possessing the capacity to influence developments in one's life according to one's purposes and to the extent of bringing about preferred outcomes
>
> (M. White 1992, pp. 145–6 in Epston and White 1992).

In narrative terms, agency is the ability to direct one's own life and the outcomes of one's endeavours. The idea of preferences, or 'preferred outcomes', is already entrenched in the thinking.

One of the key practices was the use of sophisticated questioning techniques to draw out meaning or implications for persons of the stories of their lives. Particular significance was placed by the therapist on answers which produce 'news of difference' or 'unique outcomes', and the practice of questioning was regarded as 'opening space' for the person's own stories and interpretations. The primacy given to the therapist's interpretation in other therapeutic discourses was challenged with Narrative Therapy; here the emphasis is on the meaning for the client of the story she tells. As Freedman and Combs (1996, p. 44) summarized:

> In spite of all our education telling us that we do know, we try to listen for what we don't know.

The idea of 'news of difference' was an early practice in which any change in story or behaviour was noted and greeted with recognition that some aspect of the overwhelming problem had altered or was capable of being altered. Often this reflected to the client a possibility that had not been previously visible and signalled that some potential alternative may exist. The term 'opening space' was adopted precisely to create the framework into which new approaches could be invested. The term reflected an understanding that the constraints that bound the client or their situation were not permanent and invincible.

Embedded within the emerging narrative practices was an approach based on what was termed 'curiosity', and which involved the development of a range of questions. These were founded in an attitude that was at the same time exploratory and determinedly deconstructive. Each aspect of an established story would be examined to see how it fitted within the dominant discourse—what was socially acceptable in the particular context of the person's life—and subjected to scrutiny to uncover those unique outcomes or sparkling moments in which the client acted in a way that was different from, or stood up to, the usual practice. While narrative therapy was undoubtedly influenced by the questioning models developed by the Milan school, and formed versions of the circular questioning they favoured, it is also the case that they went on to create a repertoire of types of questions that have been adopted by narrative therapists as core practice. Some of the notable forms of questions included those used to 'externalize', to contextualize, to deconstruct, to explore for 'unique outcomes' or 'sparkling moments', to make visible new-old stories, or what White called the 'experience of experience' questions.

The practice of externalizing the problem is one in which the issue or problem facing the client is first identified as external to the person and then examined as if it were a separate entity. Externalizing questions are used to help externalize problems, restraints or processes which may not be useful. For example:

- What name would you give to this problem?
- So, what has X tried to talk you into about yourself?
- How has X tried to take over your life?
- When did X first enter your life?

The technique of externalizing the problem developed into a sophisticated and complex practice, where White initially, and later both therapeutic and community practitioners, interviewed the problem. The problem could be identified in the clients own terms (fear, anger, alcohol, misery or grief), or the practitioner may offer terms such as self-doubt, or self-loathing. A notable example of this has been in the anti-bullying work (Anti-Harassment Team of Selwyn College 1998) where Bullying was interviewed, along with his companions Fear and Anger. This interview in the round, the interrogation of the problem, allowed for the deconstruction of the complexity of the issue while enabling the client to create a sense of self-reliance and strength. This is encouraged in the practice of 'standing up to' or 'taking a stand against' in which the now externalized problem is seen as a visible enemy against which the client can mount a campaign of resistance. The language used often had a slightly military flavour, with people being asked how they can to be 'recruited' or how they would 'fight', but this was more to do with the political context of Foucault's own work.

Both the externalizing questions and those of contextualization reflect the strong influence of the postmodern concern with the structures of power; in particular the discourses of dominance of Foucault, which White found useful therapeutically. The range of contextualizing questions helped to locate the stories of persons' lives within multiple contexts: race, class, gender, culture, sexual preferences, language, workplace/profession, education, family, networks, religion, geographical location. The purpose of these questions was to determine how people arrived at the meaning they give to their stories. For example:

- What have you learnt which enables this story to be important in your life?
- Where did you learn that this was important?

There are two links to these questions within the narrative frame—the practice of deconstruction, and the idea of the intertwining landscapes of action and meaning. The practice of deconstruction required an approach which would rigorously expose beliefs and assumptions. Key questions could be:

- What are the assumptions which enable this story to make sense?
- What are the ideas that might explain how people are acting and speaking?
- What are some of the taken-for-granted ways of being that are connected with the problem?
- When did you first think that you might be heterosexual? (Hewson 1991)

It is important to note that in both White and Epston's practice the use of exploratory and probing questions was already deeply embedded before they began to use the postmodern discourse of deconstruction to explicate what their practice was achieving. When, in 1989, *Literate Means to Therapeutic Ends* was first published (later named *Narrative Means to Therapeutic Ends* by the publishers), the practice of asking those questions which could locate a person's problem within the practices of gender dominance or the then current inequities of the mental health system was flourishing. The ideas offered by Foucault, Lyotard, et al., enabled a more sophisticated understanding that the inequities of the social world could be themselves oppressive, and that some of the issues faced by persons may have more to do with their social and political location than be the result of any flaw within themselves. This was to become startlingly apparent as Dulwich Centre Publications (under the leadership of Cheryl White) began to discover and support community projects across the world in which the cultural, social and racial issues of dominance and oppression provided the key to understanding what needed to be done for whole communities to throw off significant problems. While Michael White was concentrating on deconstructing individual and family therapeutic practices, Cheryl and her team were taking the exploration into a broader context.

One of the notable counselling practices was the discovery of what were termed 'unique outcomes' or 'sparkling moments'. These are events or ideas which stand outside of the dominant story in the opinion of the client. They are not merely positives or simple exceptions, but incidences of an alternative way of being or thinking. For example:

- I was curious to hear that you did/thought X, does that indicate that there is already a part of your experience in which the dominant story (or X problem) has been challenged?
- Can you think of a time when you were able to do something different?

Experience of experience questions invite persons to express forgotten or neglected elements of their experience and invite them into imaginative exploration of alternative stories. Many of these were developed as a means of inviting the client to take a distant view of their own lives, or to find the point of view of others. While this form of the narrative question first appeared in the early 1990s, it was to become the source of inspiration for later conceptualizations, such as the insider/outsider witnesses of the early 2000s (White 2001b). The experience of experience questions could include, for example:

- If I had been watching you as a younger person, what do you think I might have witnessed that would allow me to understand your recent achievements?
- Who would be able to tell me about times when you have successfully challenged difficulties in your life?
- Who would be least surprised about your creation of a new story for yourself?

The idea that persons were multi-storied was an early challenge to the view that there was only one coherent interpretation available to the therapist. The inclusion in narrative practice of the ideas of the alternative or preferred stories allowed for the possibility of change and a resistance to the dominant story, the oppressive discourse or the overwhelming problem-saturated story. One issue which often arose in the therapy room was that of linkage—how could the therapist and client find a way to make the new story manifest? And what could be done to leave the old story behind. Daphne Hewson raised these issues in 1991 and provided some useful clues. Questions which help to link the old and the alternative stories are called New/Old Story Questions (Hewson 1991). For example:

- If you had already achieved the life you want and you were to look back to today, what steps would you be able to see that you had taken to get from here to there?
- When you knew that you were ready, what steps would you have taken to become ready?
- How will you know when you have done X for long enough?

Narrative therapy has at various times identified a whole range of other question types, such as:

- Orientation questions (If I was meeting with someone who had the problem you stood up to, what advice would you want to give them?).
- Circulation questions (Now that you have reached this point, who else should know about it? What difference will this news make to their attitude towards you?).
- Insider and outsider witness questions (Who has been inspired by your efforts? Who has inspired you to make these efforts?).

The lives of persons were seen to be multi-storied, i.e. have many possible narratives, and indeed, many coexisting narratives, some of which have been useful to the person, others of which have acted as constraints. For some time in the early 1990s, the notion of restraint (drawn originally from Bateson) provided a rich field for exploration in clinical practice. The questions that investigated: 'What prevented you?', 'What held you back from . . .?', addressed the idea that within each story there were factors that acted as restraints against action or ideation.

Another of the practices of narrative therapy which addresses this multi-storied existence is that of 'Re-membering', i.e. putting together in new ways expressions or stories, memories or dreams in relationships with others. Drawn originally from the work of Barbara Meyerhoff amongst elderly people, White defined the steps in re-membering as consisting of seeing life as a member of a community, exploring alternative stories of that membership, creating a sense of multiple perspectives and engaging in reflection upon the life from the range of possible viewpoints (M. White 2005).

Reflecting teams were initially developed by Tom Andersen who focused upon reflections on the language used within the therapy room. White incorporated into and extended the practice of using 'reflecting teams' (M. White 1995, 2000b) to situations other than the therapy room. One of the first instances of this usage was at Camp Coorong, where a group of therapists and team members from Dulwich centre provided reflections to the aboriginal community as they explored the grief of loss through aboriginal deaths in custody. Today, reflecting teams are used in training situations, in working with accountability groups, cross-cultural or anti-racism workshops, or in a variety of practice locales. Further development has been explored in the notion of insider/outsider witnesses, in which persons are asked to reflect upon the ideas or views of those who know them either very well or not well (M. White 1999).

The idea of creating maps and scaffolding (M. White 2007) developed from earlier ideas on landscapes. Drawing from Jerome Bruner's (1986) concept of landscapes, White developed a way of conceptually mapping the life experience of persons, and the meanings associated with those experiences. Narrative uses the term landscape to refer to ways of orienting the person to their actions, experiences and identity. Questions were developed to evoke the specific landscape.

Questions regarding landscapes of action refer to the past, the present or the future, and often focus on the alternative stories. For example:

- Where were you when this (the unique outcome) happened?
- What was the context (persons, place, situation, ideas)?
- What were the steps that led to you doing this?
- What are the steps you might have to take to get to a place where you would be living your alternative story?

The landscape of experience questions were concerned with finding the meanings a person may have for their actions. For example:

- What do you think this action means for your life?
- What did it take for you to do this? (Personal ability.)

- What were your intentions in doing this?
- What beliefs did you hold which enabled you to do or think this?

Although these maps were generally only concerned with the interplay of landscapes of action and experience, a number of other landscapes have been suggested as well. For example, in examining a landscape of identity, the questions focus upon the ways in which persons derive their identity from their relationships with others. For example:

- Who knows what it has taken for you to be here?
- What does it say about you as a person that you would do this?
- Who would be most/least surprised about your action/achievement?

The practice of building a map which traced the experiences of the person, examining the meaning ascribed to actions, and the possibilities of alternative stories was a post hoc analysis of what had happened during workshops and clinical experience. White (M. White 2005, 2007) reflected upon the questions posed to him and the answers that he had developed which showed how he navigated his way through clinical practice.

Community practice

From the very early years, when Michael and Cheryl White and David and Anne Epston were young social workers at the brink of their careers, they shared a passion for social justice and human rights. The story is that Michael and Cheryl actually met during a demonstration against the Vietnam War and formed then a partnership which lasted for over 37 years. In developing the work which became known as narrative therapy, these people were deeply determined to create a new way of working which would address inequity and injustice. The exploration of power and its effect on lives came after some years of trying to develop a gender-equitable therapy approach; and the willingness to become involved with marginalized communities in Australia showed that this determination did not flag.

In the early 1990s, the Dulwich Centre became involved in a landmark project (Camp Coorong) which attempted to address the toll on aboriginal people of the investigations into Aboriginal Deaths in Custody. This was just the beginning of an ongoing series of community workshops and collaborative community healing practices across Australia. At the same time as this stream was being developed, Cheryl White with her team at Dulwich Publications were travelling the world, seeing and hearing from community groups who were using narrative ideas or developing parallel practices in their own local environments. There had been for some years a strong association of mutual support with the Family Centre of New Zealand before Dulwich Publications published *Just Therapy* in the early 1990s.

Because of its strong social justice orientation, narrative therapy has been taken up by various ethnic groups such as Aboriginal people in Australia, Latino communities in California, people of colour in a number of countries, and by communities of common experience, such as young people who oppose bullying, pro-feminist men's organizations, people with disabilities, person who are lesbian, homosexual, or of bisexual orientation. Some organizations are now requiring narrative therapy training of recruits within Australia, and there is widespread support for the use of narrative community practices amongst indigenous peoples. Narrative therapy has been teaching and developing community practices in Israel, Rwanda, South Africa, Hong Kong, Colombia, Palestine, Mexico, Norway, Nigeria, Vietnam, Brazil, Denmark, Malawi, Singapore, Bosnia, Argentina, as well as Australia, New Zealand, Canada, USA, and the United Kingdom for two decades.

Today the practice of narrative therapy has spread beyond the narrow frame of clinical practice and is being incorporated into a diverse range of areas such as: social work, community work, schools, workplaces, community health and mental health programmes, training, and mediation. The range of clinical issues addressed extends from anorexia and bulimia, to grief and loss, sexual and other forms of child abuse, domestic violence, HIV/AIDS, addiction, schizophrenia and other mental health disorders, relationship difficulties, bedwetting and tantrums, as well as family problems.

Perhaps more significant is the spread of narrative therapy outside of the clinical realm into the area of social justice and activism (e.g. M. White 2003). From an early concern with gender, and the influence of feminist writers and clinicians, narrative therapy has provided an accessible analysis of structures of power and the constraints of political and social power that impinge on persons' lives. Within the literature of the field, and in the practices of narrative therapists, a wide range of social and political issues are being examined. These include: gender politics, heterosexual dominance, bisexuality, men's culture, women's culture, racism, racial and cultural political location, the needs of indigenous people, or people of colour, the rights of consumers of mental health provision, issues around ageing or disability, class, children and young people's issues, poverty and deprivation, therapeutic and other forms of abuse.

While narrative therapy has drawn heavily from postmodern thought for the explanation and analysis of practices, there has also been an element of the generative, the creative. This generative approach springs from finding the possibility of liberation that Foucault wrote of (in Rabinow, 1984), and which is the opening needed by people in order to make a difference in their lives.

The latest offerings from Dulwich Publications have tended to focus on the community approaches which are currently being developed by Cheryl White, David Denborough, and a team of teachers. Denborough's 2008 *Collective Narrative Practice: Responding to individuals, groups and communities who have experienced trauma* is described as introducing:

> . . . a range of hopeful methodologies to respond to individuals, groups, and communities who are experiencing hardship. These approaches are deliberately easy to engage with and can be used with children, young people, and adults. The methodologies described include: Collective narrative documents, Enabling contributions through exchanging messages and convening definitional ceremonies, The Tree of Life: responding to vulnerable children, The Team of Life: giving young people a sporting chance, Checklists of social and psychological resistance, Collective narrative timelines, Maps of history, and Songs of sustenance. To illustrate these approaches, stories are shared from Australia, Southern Africa, Israel, Ireland, USA, Palestine, Rwanda, and elsewhere.

One of the most interesting developments in narrative community practice is the 'Tree of Life', originally created in response to the therapeutic needs of children whose lives had been decimated by AIDS (Ncube 2006) in Africa. It has subsequently been adapted for use in aboriginal communities by local indigenous health workers (Stow and Johnson-Koomatrie 2009):

> This approach involves children drawing their roots (where they come from), their ground (where they live and what they do each day), their trunk (special skills and abilities), their branches (hopes and dreams), their leaves (special people), and their fruit (gifts). Groups of children then join their individual trees into a collective 'Forest of Life'.

In a similar vein, David Denborough (2008) noticed in a refugee camp that boys from differing tribes and potentially opposing factions would forego the expected stances in order to participate in a game of scratch football. From this observation he has developed a community collaboration method which uses games to develop alternative stories for young people.

Conclusion

What I have tried to show in this chapter is that narrative therapy emerged at a time when there was an undercurrent of dissatisfaction with the standard psychiatric approaches towards mental illness and personal problems. In the late 1970s, family therapy flourished as it attempted to incorporate the individual within a broader context, and as it dealt with problems as concerning the whole family, rather than focusing upon the individual as the entire limit of his own experience. The Whites and the Epstons engaged with the political ideas of the era, became engaged in the family therapy field, and began to correspond with their separate innovations, in the process influencing each other, and ultimately a whole field of endeavour.

The postmodern writings of theorists such as Foucault provided both a language with which to describe and analyse the practices that had proved effective in the therapy arena, and as support for the stance of challenge of the dominant orders, the hegemonies of everyday life, which became a significant part of both the therapy and the community work. Whether the oppressive regime was one of gender, race, heterosexual dominance, or ableism, each was to be challenged and deconstructed. More than this, alternatives were to be discovered and co-created in a practice Epston referred to as co-research, where client and therapist entered into a collaboration in developing alternatives stories and preferred lives.

The counselling practices included a wide range of innovative and useful techniques, ranging from a repertoire of incisive and interrogative questions to the encouragement of creative expressions. The central concept that the 'person's not the problem, the problem's the problem' enabled the 'externalizing of the problem', to the extent that the problem itself could be interviewed, its motives and gains discovered, and the person could choose whether to remain recruited by the externalized problem or not.

Drawing from a range of anthropologists, White and Epston developed a number of concepts: Bateson provided the inspiration for double descriptions, Geertz offered the ideas of thick and thin descriptions, Myerhoff indicated the possibilities of re-membering persons within communities (1982, 1986), Vygotsky showed that learning theory could be incorporated into therapy (1986), and Bruner provided the language of landscapes which became developed into ways of mapping aspects of life and meaning.

What is particularly interesting in the community approaches is that every one of the innovations that narrative therapy developed over the years is utilized in ways that lead to practices which form the basis for the community to address problems and find alternative ways of being. The documents of identity, the letters and certificates once confined to the family, individual, or therapy room, now find a place within a community arena. The reflecting team which enables a group of caseworkers to come together, sharing their differing perspective on and with the client in therapy, becomes an opportunity for some parts of a community to listen and respond to a particular group. The maps which serve the purpose of locating an individual within their own landscapes of action and experience here help to develop a clear picture for the community to come together with a new picture of itself.

Narrative therapy is the result of a number of collaborations over the last three decades—collaborations between Epston and White to provide the early and continuing development of key ideas, between Michael and Cheryl White in disseminating and facilitating the work being done in the field, between a huge range of teachers and therapists with each other, and more importantly with their clients and communities.

References

Aboriginal Health Council (1995). *Reclaiming our stories, reclaiming our minds.* Dulwich Centre Publications, Adelaide.

Anti-Harassment Team of Selwyn College, Lewis, D., and Cheshire, A. (1998). The team in action. *Dulwich Centre Journal*, **2**(3), 4–18.

Bandler, R., Grinder, J. and Satir V. (1976). *Changing with families.* Science and Behavior Books, Palo Alto, CA.

Bateson, G. (1958) *Naven: A survey of the problems suggested by a composite picture of the culture of a New Guinea tribe drawn from three points of view.* Stanford University Press, Stanford, CA.

Bateson, G. (1972). *Steps to an ecology of mind.* Ballantine, New York.

Bateson, G. (1979). *Mind and nature: A necessary unity.* Dutton, New York.

Berne, E. (1961). *Transactional Analysis in Psychotherapy.* Grove Press, New York

Berne, E. (1964). *Games People Play.* Castle Books, New York.

Boscolo, L., Cecchin, G., Hoffman, L., and Penn, P. (1987). *Milan systemic family therapy.* Basic Books, New York.

Boscolo, L. and Bertrando, P. (1993). *The Times of time: A new perspective in systemic therapy and consultation.* W. W. Norton, New York.

Bowen, M. (1978). *Family therapy in clinical practice.* Aronson, New York.

Boyers, R. and Orrill R. (1972). *Laing and anti-psychiatry.* Penguin Books, Middlesex.

Capra, F. (1982). *The turning point.* Flamingo/Fontana, London.

Bruner, J. (1986). *Actual minds, possible worlds.* Harvard University Press, Cambridge, MA.

Chamberlain, S. (1986). The "I" is silent as in ideology: an exploration of some shared cultural assumptions. *Dulwich Centre Review*, pp. 66–76. Dulwich Centre Publications, Adelaide.

Chamberlain, S. (1990). The new ethnography: windmills and giants. *Dulwich Centre Newsletter: Research and Family Therapy*, **2**, 39–46.

Combs, G. and Freedman, J. (1998). Tellings and retellings. *Journal of Marital and Family Therapy*, **24**(4), 405–8.

Denborough, D. (Ed.) (1996). *Beyond the prison: Gathering dreams of freedom*. Dulwich Centre Publications, Adelaide.

Denborough, D. (Ed.) (2001). *Family therapy: Exploring the field's past, present and possible futures*. Dulwich Centre Publications, Adelaide.

Denborough, D. (2008). *Collective narrative practice: Responding to individuals, groups and communities who have experienced trauma*. Dulwich Centre Publications, Adelaide.

Denborough, D., Freedman, J., and White, C. (2008). *Strengthening resistance: Narrative practices in responding to genocide survivors*. Dulwich Centre Foundation, Adelaide.

Derrida, J. (1981). *Positions*. University of Chicago Press, Chicago, IL.

de Shazer, S. (1982). *Patterns of brief family therapy: an ecosystemic approach*, New York, Guilford Press.

de Shazer, S. (1985). *Keys to solution in brief therapy*, New York, W. W. Norton.

Durkheim, E. (1915/1982). *The Elementary Forms of the Religious Life*. George Allen & Unwin, London

Durkheim, E. (1951). *Suicide: a Study in Sociology*. The Free Press, Glencoe, IL

Epston, D. (1989). *Collected papers*. Dulwich Centre Publications, Adelaide.

Epston, D. (1998). *Catching up with David Epston: A collection of narrative practice-based papers published between 1991 & 1996*. Dulwich Centre Publications, Adelaide.

Epston, D. and White, M. (1990). Consulting your consultants: The documentation of alternative knowledges. *Dulwich Centre Newsletter*, **4**, 25–35.

Epston, D. and White, M. (1992). *Experience, contradiction, narrative and imagination: Selected papers of David Epston and Michael White, 1989–1991*. Dulwich Centre Publications, Adelaide.

Foucault, M. (1979). *Discipline and punish: The birth of the prison*. Peregrine Books, Middlesex.

Foucault, M. (1980). *Power/knowledge: Selected interviews and other writings*. Pantheon Books, New York.

Foucault, M. (1984). *The history of sexuality*. Peregrine Books, London.

Frankl, V. E. (1959). *Man's search for meaning: an introduction to logotherapy*. Hodder & Stoughton, London.

Frankl, V. E. (1967). *Psychotherapy and existentialism*. Touchstone, New York.

Freedman, J. and Combs, G. (1996). *Narrative therapy: The social construction of preferred realities*. W. W. Norton, New York.

Geertz, C. (1973). *The interpretation of cultures*. Basic Books, New York.

Geertz, C. (1983). *Local knowledge: Further essays in interpretive anthropology*. Basic Books, New York.

Geertz, C. (1986). Making experiences, authoring selves. In V. Turner and E. Bruner (Eds.) *The anthropology of experience*, pp. 373–80. Chicago University Press, Chicago, IL.

Geertz, C. (1988). *Works and Lives: The anthropologist as Author*. Stanford University Press, Stanford, CA.

Goffman, E. (1959/1984). *The Presentation of Self in Everyday Life*. Penguin, Middlesex.

Guerin, P. J. (Ed.) (1976). *Family Therapy: Theory and Practice*. Gardner Press, New York.

Haley, J. (1973). *Uncommon therapy: The psychiatric techniques of Milton H. Erickson*. W. W. Norton, New York.

Haley, J. (1976) *Problem-solving therapy*. Jossey-Bass Publishers, San Francisco, CA.

Haley J. (1980). *Leaving home.* McGraw-Hill Book Co, New York.
Haley, J. (Ed.) (1971). *Changing families: A family therapy reader.* Grune & Stratton, Orlando, FL.
Haley, J. and Hoffman, L. (1967). *Techniques of family therapy.* Basic Books, New York.
Handel, G. (1968). *The Psychosocial Interior of the Family.* George Allen & Unwin, London
Hewson, D. (1991). From laboratory to therapy room: Prediction questions for Reconstructing the "New-old" story. *Dulwich Centre Newsletter,* **3**, 5–12.
Hoffman, L. (1981). *Foundations of family therapy: A conceptual framework for systems change.* Basic Books, New York.
Horewitz, J. S. (1977). *Family Therapy and Transactional Analysis.* Jason Aronson, New York
L'Abate, L., Ganahl, G., and Hansen, J. C. (1986). *Methods of family therapy.* Prentice-Hall, Englewood Cliffs, NJ
Laing, R. D. (1969) *Self and others.* Penguin, Harmondsworth.
Laing, R. D. (1960/1972). *The divided self: An existential study in sanity and madness.* Penguin, Middlesex.
Laing, R. D. (1967/1972). *The politics of experience and the bird of paradise.* Penguin, Middlesex.
Laing, R. D. and Esterson, A. (1964/1970) *Sanity, madness and the family.* Penguin Books, Middlesex.
Leupnitz, D. A. (1988). *The Family Interpreted: Feminist Theory in Clinical Practice.* Basic Books, New York.
Mandanes, C. (1981). *Strategic Family Therapy.* Jossey-Bass, San Francisco, CA.
McGoldrick, M. and Gerson, R. (1985). *Genograms in family assessment.* W. W. Norton, New York.
McGoldrick M., Anderson, C. M., and Walsh F. (Eds.) (1989). *Women in families: A framework for family therapy.* W. W. Norton, New York.
Minuchin, S. (1974/1977). *Families and family therapy.* Tavistock Publications, London.
Minuchin, S.(1998). Where is the family in narrative family therapy? *Journal of Marital and Family Therapy,* **24**(4), 397–403.
Minuchin, S. and Fishman, H. C. (1981). *Family therapy techniques.* Harvard University Press, Cambridge, MA.
Monk, G., Winslade, J., Crocket, K., and Epston, D. (Eds.) (1997). *Narrative therapy in practice: The archaeology of hope.* Jossey-Bass Publishers, San Francisco, CA.
Myerhoff, B. (1982). Life history among the elderly: Performance, visibility and remembering. In J. Ruby (Ed), *A crack in the mirror: Reflexive perspectives in anthropology,* pp. 99–117. University of Pennsylvania Press, Philadelphia, PA.
Myerhoff, B. (1986). Life not death in Venice: Its second life. In V. Turner and E. Bruner (Eds) *The anthropology of experience,* pp. 261–86. University of Illinois Press, Chicago, IL.
Napier, A. Y. and Whitaker, Carl, (1978). *The family crucible.* Bantam Books, Toronto.
Ncube, N, (2006). The tree of life project: Using narrative ideas in work with vulnerable children in South Africa. *International Journal of Narrative Therapy and Community Work,* **1**, 3–16.
Nicholson, S, (1995). The narrative dance: A practice map for White's therapy' *Australia and New Zealand Journal of Family Therapy,* **16**(1), 23–28.
Rabinow, P. (Ed.) (1984). *The Foucault reader.* Pantheon, New York.
Satir, V., (1972/1978). *Peoplemaking.* Condor, Suffolk.
Selvini Palazzoli, M. S., Cecchin, G., Boscolo, L. and Prata, G. (1978). *Paradox and counterparadox.* Aronson, New York.

Stow, C. and Johnson-Koomatrie, C. (2009). *Finding hidden stories of strengths and skills: using the tree of life with Aboriginal and Torres Strait Islander children.* Dulwich Centre Publications, PAL DVD, Adelaide.

Sween, E. (1998). The one-minute question: What is narrative therapy? *Gecko*, **2**(3), 55–67.

Szasz, T. (1972). *The myth of mental illness.* Paladin, Suffolk.

Tomm, K. (1998). A question of perspective. *Journal of Marital and Family Therapy*, **24**(4), 409–13.

Vygotsky, L. (1986) *Thought and language.* MIT Press, Cambridge, MA.

Walrond-Skinner, S. (1976). *Family Therapy: The treatment of natural systems.* Routledge & Kegan Paul, London.

Walters, M., Carter, R., Papp, P., and Silverstein, O. (1988). *The Invisible Web: Gender patterns in family relationships.* Guilford Press, New York.

Watzlawick, P., Weakland, J. and Fisch, R. (1974). *Change: Principles of problem formation and problem resolution.* W. W. Norton, Adelaide.

Weeks, G. R. and L'Abate, L. (1982). *Paradoxical Psychotherapy: Theory and Practice with Individuals, Couples, and Families.* Brunner/Mazel Publishers, New York.

Weingarten, K. (1998). The small and the ordinary: The daily practice of a postmodern family therapy. *Family Process*, **37**, 3–15.

Whitaker, C. A. and Bumberry, W. M. (1988). *Dancing with the Family: A symbolic-experiential approach.* Brunner/Mazel, New York.

White, C. (Ed.) (1995). Speaking out and being heard. *Dulwich Centre Newsletter*, **4**, 7–9.

White, C. and Denborough, D. (Eds.) (1998). *Introducing narrative therapy: A collection of practice-based writings.* Adelaide: Dulwich Centre Publications.

White, M. (1980). Systemic task setting in family therapy. *Australian Journal of Family Therapy*, **1**(4), 172–82.

White, M. (1984a). Marital therapy-practical approaches to longstanding problems. *Australian Journal of Family Therapy*, **6**, 1.

White, M. (1984b). Pseudo-encopresis: From avalanche to victory, from vicious to virtuous cycles. *Family Systems Medicine*, **2**, 2.

White, M. (1985). Fear busting and monster taming. *Dulwich Centre Review*, Adelaide, Dulwich Centre Publications.

White, M. (1986a). Anorexia nervosa: A cybernetic perspective. *Dulwich Centre Review*, Adelaide: Dulwich Centre Publications.

White, M. (1986b). Negative explanation, restraint & double description: a template for family therapy. *Family Process*, **25**, 2.

White, M. (1986c). Ritual of inclusion: An approach to extreme uncontrolled behaviour in children and young adolescents. *Dulwich Centre Review*, Dulwich Centre Publications, Adelaide.

White, M. (1988). The process of questioning: a therapy of literary merit? *Dulwich Centre Newsletter*, **Winter**, 8–15.

White, M. (1988). Saying hullo again: The incorporation of the lost relationship in the resolution of grief. *Dulwich Centre Newsletter*, **Spring**.

White, M. (1988/9). The externalizing of the problem and the re-authoring of lives and relationships. *Dulwich Centre Newsletter*, **Summer**.

White, M. (1989). *Selected Papers.* Dulwich Centre Publications, Adelaide.

White, M. (1989/90). Family therapy training and supervision in a world of experience and narrative. Dulwich Centre Newsletter, **Summer**, 27–38.

White, M. (1991). Deconstruction and therapy. *Dulwich Centre Newsletter*, **3**, 21–40.

White, M. (1992). Men's culture, the men's movement and the constitution of men's lives. *Dulwich Centre Newsletter*, **3&4**.

White, M. (1994). A conversation about accountability. *Dulwich Centre Newsletter*, **2**, 3.

White, M. (1995). *Re-authoring Lives: Interviews & Essay*. Dulwich Centre Publications, Adelaide.

White, M. (1997) *Narratives of Therapists' Lives*. Dulwich Centre Publications, Adelaide.

White, M. (1998). Notes on narrative metaphor and narrative therapy. In C. White and D. Denborough (Eds.) *Introducing narrative therapy: A collection of practice-based writings*. Dulwich Centre Publications, Adelaide.

White, M. (1999). Reflecting-team work as definitional ceremony revisited. *Gecko*, **2**, 55–82.

White, M. (2000a). *Reflections on narrative practice: Essays & interviews*. Dulwich Centre Publications, Adelaide.

White, M. (2000b) Direction and discovery: A conversation about power and politics in narrative therapy. An interview by Michael Hoyt and Jeff Zimmerman. In M. White (Ed.) *Reflections on narrative practice*, pp. 97–116. Dulwich Centre Publications, Adelaide.

White, M. (2001). Folk psychology and narrative practice. *Dulwich Centre Journal*, **2**, 3–36.

White, M. (2001a). Narrative practice and the unpacking of identity conclusions. *Gecko*, **1**, 28–55.

White, M. (2003). Narrative practice and community assignments. *The International Journal of Narrative Therapy & Community Work*, **2**, 17–55.

White, M. (2004). Working with people who are suffering the consequences of multiple trauma: A narrative perspective. *The International Journal of Narrative Therapy and Community Work*, **1**, 45–76.

White, M. (2005). Children, trauma and subordinate storyline development. *The International Journal of Narrative Therapy & Community Work*, **3**, 4.

White, M. (2007). *Maps of narrative practice*. W. W. Norton, New York.

White, M. and Epston, D. (1989). *Literate means to therapeutic ends*. Dulwich Centre Publications, Adelaide.

White, M. and Epston, D. (1990). *Narrative means to therapeutic ends*. W. W. Norton, New York.

White, M. and Epston, D. (1992). *A conversation about AIDS and dying in Experience, contradiction, narrative and imagination*, pp. 27–36. Dulwich Centre Publications, Adelaide.

White, M. and Morgan, A. (2006). *Narrative therapy with children and their families*. Dulwich Centre Publications, Adelaide.

Woollams, S. Brown, M. (1978). *Transactional Analysis*. Huron Valley Institute Press, Dexter, MI.

Worden, M. (1994). *Family Therapy Basics*. Brooks/Cole, Pacific Grove, CA.

Chapter 7

Collaborative therapy: performing reflective and dialogical relationships

Sue Levin and Saliha Bava

Introduction

Collaborative therapy, a social constructionist approach, is a dialogical, reflective, relational approach to social, communal, and mental health, which can be applied in varied settings such as academic, community, business, and research (Anderson and Goolishian 1986; Anderson and Levin 1998; Bava and Levin 2007; Gehart et al. 2007; London and Rodriguez-Jazcilevich 2007; Wagner 2007). In constructing this chapter our ideas may be read as if they are static and finished, rather than that the process of collaborative therapy, and the definition of such, is fluid and evolving. We construct this approach within a theoretical and clinical context, focusing on conversations about suicide as primary case dialogues since these are considered the most challenging of clinical conversations. In this chapter we write our ideas in two sections. In the first section we describe the context that is historically and philosophically located at the Houston Galveston Institute, and reflections on current practices of collaboration. In the second section we elaborate on how we practice the philosophy of collaborative therapy and give case examples.

Locating our context

History and discourse

Originating with multiple impact therapy (McGregor et al. 1964), the founders were part of the child psychiatry department, at the University of Texas Medical Branch (UTMB), in Galveston. One such example of the many ways in which they contributed to current practices is illustrated in a story the late Harry Goolishian tells in a video (http://www.balmbra.no/Videos.htm) about how his curiosity led to him to violate the current practice standards maintaining the transference between therapist and client.[1] Harry experimented with meeting the spouse of his client and found that

---

[1] The terms 'therapist' and 'client' are used throughout the paper to refer to the discourse in the mental health field, however we attempt to interact as human beings and stay reflexive about the limitations of this language.

the client's reports of his wife's behaviour were completely different than how he experienced her. This early experiment is one of the steps in the creation of family therapy practice.

Harry Goolishian, Harlene Anderson, George Pulliam, and Paul Dell separated from UTMB and started the Galveston Family Institute in 1979. GFI, as it was known, became the Houston Galveston Institute (HGI) in 1990. This organization was founded to further the development of family therapy ideas emerging from systemic thinking and cybernetics. A seminal work, Anderson and Goolishian's classic 1988 paper, 'Human systems as linguistic systems', set HGI's practices apart from other family therapy ideas as rooted in problem-determined language systems rather than family systems. Therapy needed to address the system of people who coalesced around particular [sets of] problems; who were working and talking to each other for this purpose.

HGI began using the term collaboration in the late 1990s to emphasize the difference between joining as a strategy versus a value. Strategic/brief therapy models promoted 'using the client's language' to gain his/her confidence enough to be able to get him/her to change. This was seen as manipulative and unethical, particularly by the feminist family therapy movement (Hare-Mustin 1987; Rampage 1988). As we explored the critiques and implications of this approach to joining—which we might now call engaging or connecting with the client—we began to use the word collaborate to describe our view of our work *with* clients as a partnership, a shared journey in which the client–therapist team works together to re-solve the issues which the client defines as the focus of therapy.

The lessons that HGI carries forward to current practice are: 1) that any standard practices should be critiqued to ask 'should we be continuing to do what we currently are doing as therapists?' and 2) the stories that we hear from clients are based in their realities and perspectives and not 'the Truth', but rather 'their truth'. A wide range of influences contributed to a shift to language and conversational systems, the current focus of therapy. Some of those involved in making this shift include: Tom Andersen (1991) and his colleagues in Norway who developed the reflecting team idea, Ken Gergen, Sheila McNamee, and other founders of the Taos Institute who contributed to social constructionist theory (Gergen 1997; McNamee and Gergen 1992, 1998); Sally Ann Roth and her colleagues at the Cambridge Family Institute who began the Public Conversations Project (Roth et al. 1992); Steve de Shazer (1985), Insoo Kim Berg (1994, 2000), Eve Lipschik (2002), and others who created solution-focused therapy; and Michael White, David Epston, and their colleagues at the Dulwich Centre who developed narrative therapy (White 2007; White and Epston 1990). Many others with whom we have been in conversation should be acknowledged, but space does not allow; we hope they know that they are part of our story about our history.

Today, we refer to these innovative ideas of practice as collaborative therapy (Anderson and Gehart 2007) which has its roots in systems theory, constructivism, hermeneutics, and constructionism. Elements of these influential theories are seen in the emphasis on conversation, attention to the client's language and narrative/story, a shared search for meaning, and an orientation towards expansion of possibilities and meaning (Anderson 1993, 2007; Anderson and Goolishian 1992; Anderson and Levin 1997; Goolishian and Anderson 1990).

Reflections on performing collaboration

One way in which we have explored expanding possibilities in practice is through studying performance (Bava 2005; Carlson 1996; Denzin 2003; Horsfall 2008; Pelias 1999; Schechner 2002). Goffman (1959) refers to our everyday life as a performance. What we do and the ways we are being and becoming are all performances. We use the language of performance, rather than behaviour, to emphasize collaborative ways of being that are flexible, relational and improvisational (Bava and Levin 2007).

The process of being or becoming someone (Anderson 1990) is situated within sociocultural, political, historical, and contextual discourses. We perform and are shaped by these discourses and in turn shape them. Performance, though often associated with critical cultural or social and dramaturgical theory (Carlson 1996; Schechner 2002), is transdisciplinary like collaboration. Our view is that it is not nested within any one discipline rather it is a way of constructing our experiences.

Doing therapy and becoming a therapist is a professional performance. As therapists and supervisors we act and improvise upon scripts that are shaped through our training and theory. Collaborative, dialogical, reflective, and relational practices are generative and performative and there are multiple ways in which these constructs are enacted. We present this script to illustrate one of our performances as collaborative therapists.

Currently, the use of the word collaboration has become very common and the multiple uses and demonstrations of collaboration that we have encountered, do not match our interpretation and meaning. Often the term, collaboration is applied to any kind of partnership. Organizations say they are collaborating (Frydman et al. 2000). Therapists say they are collaborating. Co-authors and co-presenters say they are collaborating. Wile (1999, 2002), who has written about collaborative couples therapy (or CCT), seems to use collaboration as a technique in which one is able to step into the clients shoes and world-views. A description of the collaborative treatment method calls it 'a unique model for psychiatric, psychological, neuropsychological, and neurological evaluation and treatment'.[2] Narrative therapy has recently been labelled a collaborative therapy.[3] These multiple meanings and actions indicate the inevitable need for new language, some of which you may begin to see in this chapter. We perform our specific expression and practice of collaboration in multiple contexts, such as therapy, training, organizational, and community, as well as others. It is situated in the postmodern and social constructionist stream of thinking.

We are constructing our meaning of collaboration, which we are also performing with each other and with the reader, as we write this chapter. Each of us, including our clients, is positioned within the intersections of multiple social locations (Brown 2009) which shape our understandings of language and making meaning. This is a process of unfolding and creating ideas and understandings. Since people have varying meanings for collaboration, it is important to explore the meanings and expectations of the participants, thus creating the space for the process to be collaborative. Rather than use collaboration as a noun, we emphasize the action and active construction of

---

[2] http://www.collaborativepsychology.com/services.html.
[3] http://www.thewindsofchange.ca/index.php.

the collaborative process that keeps it as an active verb; a way of being and doing. Further, the emphasis then is not on the name or the label for the process, rather it is on the act of co-creating, what we collectively can call collaboration.

Collaborative approach: practising a philosophical stance

Collaborative therapy is not a formulaic or mechanistic model or set of techniques (Anderson 2007). Rather it is a way of being, a philosophical stance we take in conversations and relationships, with intentions that are specific to the context and purpose that brings people together as dialogical partners for change or action. The central focus is on the use of dialogue to facilitate the desired change as per the client's expectations. What distinguishes such a conversation from any other conversation is that it is a reflexive process; it is the continued building and exploring of and how to talk about the purpose of this therapeutic interaction. The focus is on the relational process where the person(s) within the relationships and context are central (Gergen 2009a, 2009b). The therapist and client work together to create a relational space in which the client has a sense of belonging and shared responsibility.

We will illustrate this philosophical stance by interweaving clinical examples with theoretical guideposts. We will discuss two clients[4] we have worked with, Tim who worked with Saliha[5] and Linda who worked with Sue. We will use additional examples of working with other people who are suicidal, as we both have had intense experiences with this issue. We hope it will demonstrate that having a collaborative conversation which some label 'just talking' is transformative. Often, it seems, professionals think that talk therapy is okay for some issues but not for others; that 'serious' problems require medical intervention, such as psychopharmacology and/or hospitalization. Since suicide talk is considered one of the most challenging of clinical conversations, we will use that as our contextual base to discuss collaborative therapy, with the assumption that the practices that we describe here are applicable to other clinical issues as well. Collaborative therapy when we are talking about suicide, and all other issues that we work with, is based on a relational partnership between the therapist and client, one in which both participate to define the problem and co-evolve solutions.

Opening conversations: introductions and expectations

Setting the stage for therapy is the building of the relationship. We believe that this occurs when the client calls to make an appointment, not when they come in. Clients who call HGI speak to a therapist to set the appointment, not an intake person or a scheduler. This offers the therapist and client the earliest options for marking their

---

[4] The clients' identities, as well as that of Tim's referring therapist, have been protected by changing their names and other significant identifying information.
[5] Rabia was a regular co-therapist with Saliha after the first year of work with Tim. We acknowledge that much of the writing about this work reflects the many conversations that Saliha and Rabia had together.

conversations and relationship as important. The therapist is able to ascertain such important information as: whose idea therapy is (someone else or the person calling)?; how and when the idea of starting therapy began?; who else is involved (or might want to be) in discussion?; etc. This conversation and initial understanding can create invitations to the therapy (and to defining the therapy) that the caller (and potential client) had not entertained. The relationship is in the process of being defined by both the client and the therapist. We believe we are each more than a client and therapist, we are also two *people* who are entering a relationship in which we are performing certain roles. How do we both want to be in this relationship?

An illustration of how we enter and perform beginning relationships follows. In my (Saliha's) initial phone conversation with Tim to set up our appointment, he chose how he wanted to introduce himself to me. He requested that I ask his previous therapist to give me a summary of his presenting issues. Most clients do not make such a request; rather such information is usually shared by the referral source. I respected Tim's wish that I learn about him this way and I also wished to honour my way of meeting people, that is, to hear their stories directly from them. So when he asked if Julie, his previous therapist, had told me about him, I suggested that I recap what I heard and that he fill me in more about what else is important for me to know. I also inquired why it was important that Julie tell me his story before I met him. I learned that he felt more comfortable knowing that I had his background information before we met. This was the beginning of a 4-year relationship with Tim. Today as we write about this journey, he says this about our first meeting: 'On the day of my first appointment I was nervous of course, but when my name was called and I turned my head to see a beautiful welcoming smile, I immediately felt relieved and at ease'. In the next section we continue to explore how we perform meaning-making and others aspects of the therapeutic relationship.

Ways of generating meaning: language, listening, hearing, and reflecting

Our language becomes generative within a relational process of meaning making, which Shotter (1984) refers to as 'joint action' and Gergen (2009a) refers to as 'co-action'. Words have meaning within a sociocultural-temporal context. Their usage within specific communities of practice creates certain realities. Thus, we experience ourselves performing different meanings of collaboration due to our sociocultural-temporal spaces, which might overlap but are not identical. In joint action with each other we create and improvise new conversations within this way of being (Anderson 2007), being-in-collaboration; a new form of life (Wittgenstein 1973). This relationally-responsive or 'spontaneously responsive' (Shotter 2003, 2007) activity shapes the performance of our relationships to be generative and us as meaning-generating beings.

We find listening, hearing, and reflecting as meaning-making practices that keep us in a collaborative stance, in a collaborative relationship. Typically, therapists are trained to listen objectively for the purpose of diagnosing and intervening, using theoretical frameworks rather than creating understandings with the client. One of the goals of collaboration is to hear (Levin 1991); to understand our clients the way they want us to, including how they design, organize and live their lives.

We would like to illustrate the meaning-making process with clients who think about and attempt suicide. As therapists we have the opportunity to hear and understand the subtle messages and meanings that include 'wanting to kill oneself', 'wanting to die', and 'not wanting to live'. Each of these is a different way of enacting a life. Though each of the statements refers to an ending, not all are about death. It is at this crucial choice point, where the 'conversational partners' (Anderson 2007, p. 45) explore how to act into the unfolding of the story. According to Shotter (2007) this is the process of joint action, where in dialogue we create together the next action.

For instance, Sue's client recently announced that she would consider 'ending it all in 2 weeks'. Her message is about how tired she is of the intestinal pain she has suffered for the last three months, and is still undiagnosed and untreated. We ask ourselves, and our clients, the question, 'What is this conversation about?'. Is it about ending one's life or about ending one's pain and seeking relief? Through the joint action of creating understanding new forms of life emerge (Wittgenstein 1973).

In addition to our joint actions with clients, we also attend to our own ideas and stories about what we are hearing and what we are not hearing. This cultivates the practice of reflexivity. It is a process for reflecting not only *what* we are hearing when the client speaks, but also draws attention to *how* we are hearing it. We listen for both content and process; it is a way of holding dual attention. We reflexively hear our client's ways of making sense and our own ways of making sense of the client's sense-making as we attend to what is being created between us.

Our intention as collaborative therapists is to listen to what the client *wants us* to hear while also attending to our professional discourse(s), which is likely to slow down the conversational process. We want to make conversational space for the client and their story to be present. The therapist offers reflections and multiple perspectives in the conversation. We engage with the idea of assessment for suicide as one of the possibilities for conversation but not the most important idea.

For example, a client who has had suicide as an option for many years, brings various stories to therapy based on what is happening from session to session and within each session. If the therapist focuses on assessing and managing suicide, the possibilities for conversational space are limited and directed by the therapist. However a therapist who appreciates that the client's life includes more than the 'single story' (TED 2009), can create space for multiple perspectives and actions to unfold.

Managing suicide is usually approached using biomedical discourses, which we listen to and reflect upon as sociocultural practices. We do not define mental health as mental illness; rather we locate it as construction consisting of multiple discourses that may be grouped within the larger discourses of human wellness. Human wellness is another construction which we can locate within the discourses of social meaning-making.

Performing client–therapist relationships

A person tells a story about a problem, e.g. depression, and we are curious why he/she chose to tell us only that story. Is there anything else in addition that we should learn about them? We attempt to open the space and the possibility that there are other stories that could, would and/or might be told. This type of respectful inquiry is a way of performing curiosity and possibility, which are hallmarks of collaborative therapy. Tim said he had to perform like a depressed person so I (SB) would take him seriously, to which I inquired about whether it was possible for both his performance of depression and of humour to be present, so I could learn more about him as a person.

We continue to be reflexive, as we build the relationship by thinking about the following questions: How do we enter into a relationship with clients? What are our preconceived ideas of how to be a therapist? How to 'treat' a client? What are the 'appropriate ways' to be in relationship with clients? These questions may or may not be explicit in our internal and external dialogue, but they are part of our discourses of what it means to act as a 'therapist.'

The therapist is more than a role. The therapist is a person who is situated in social, cultural, political, and historical contexts. These social locations intersect with each other (Brown 2009) making unique performances. Similarly the client brings into play his or her unique performance. The intersection of these two performances is where the client–therapist relationship plays out. This relationship gets improvised within each conversational space and turn. Thus, we are enacting situated practices.

In the introduction of Tim, we described how he chose how to perform as a client—a depressed client and how I invited him to expand the performance. Though Tim states that he does not remember this conversation, it was a turning point for me, in negotiating how we would work together in therapy. Tim remembers how I greeted him and my approaching him with a warm smile. These moments, though each of us remembered different moments, are relational and performative moments which opened up possibilities for partnership as therapist and client.

Conversational partners creating hope and possibility

We think it is possible to have collaborative relationships and conversations with clients—even ones who are thinking about suicide. Even in the worst of times, it is possible that people can construct themselves in ways that they are capable of, and might even be able to enjoy things. This can open possibilities that would otherwise be ignored. These can be intensely *hopeful* rather than only intensely *difficult* conversations.

So, the questions become, how is it possible to invite people who are very depressed and suicidal to be[come] conversational partners with their therapist? How can we share responsibility with our clients for 'treatment' and 'progress'? Many people, would be likely to say that someone who is thinking about suicide is clearly 'out of his/her mind' and needs someone to take control and keep him/her safe.

Some think that talking about suicide with a person who is at risk could 'push them over the edge'. During the two times that Linda has been severely suicidal since I (Sue) have worked with her, we have had many challenging, difficult, and hopeful conversations. Often, I would talk with Linda and ask, 'Is it okay for me to say something that you might not like?' Or, 'I know that you are going to disagree with this because you are so against going to a hospital, but is it okay if I explain why I think it is an option you should consider?'. I define these conversations as challenging because they ask her to think about some things that she does not want to think about. They are also difficult as I consider them a potential threat to the relationship that I had formed with

Linda. She fears and distrusts most people (for good reasons) and it was critical at these times that she recognize that I wanted her *permission* to explore things that she typically would not consider. Additionally, I believe that performing as a therapist that sees Linda as responsible for her own safety and future provides a context for hopefulness.

At the time of this writing, Linda reported the possibility of shifting her performance into this hopeful and resourceful way of being. This was a shift in which she appeared curious and open to accept the existence of an identity that she does not always see. Further, she said, 'What I'd like to learn is how I can see in myself the things you see'.

In our experience, the ability to work with clients to create openings for hopefulness and possibilities includes a network of conversational partners. Anderson talks about exploring the clients' conversational partners in terms of who, when, where and how (2007). Just as it is important to recognize that clients have many conversations with people in their ordinary lives about these issues, so do we, as therapists. A network of supportive, conversational partners creates possibilities and hopefulness for the therapist as well. One of the reasons that we want to write about these experiences with Tim and Linda is that we have had many conversations with each other and with our colleagues at HGI, both formal and informal, about how to keep creating possibilities and hopefulness. Tim and Linda have also been invited into these conversations, including in some training seminars and consultations.

The process of creating conversational partnership is an ongoing part of therapy that involves how we position ourselves from the beginning and then throughout the therapeutic relationship, as well as within our network of relationships. It involves how we think about ourselves, about our clients and their performance of problems, the way we think about our roles and our ideas of change and healing. The process involves how we perform and play these ideas, and how we talk about our work with and without the client present. Simply put it is about intentionality and reflective practices.

Belongingness: a shift away from power and fear

It is challenging but critical, when working with people who are suicidal to construct conversations in which they feel they belong. The therapist's expertise lies in not rushing to view the client as being helpless but drawing on the client's history and resources that he/she may not be accessing for competency. During a crisis, the client's view may be limited by his or her perception of the issue. Likewise, the therapist may be limited by his or her fear. Sometimes, responding/reacting to fear leads therapists to construct a position of power in the relationship (Figure 7.1).

Power is dynamic and created, not just applied. We believe that when suicide becomes an issue in therapy the performance of power imbalances can become extreme. In response to their own fears, sometimes therapists inadvertently perform 'knowledge' in a way that exacerbates the client's feelings of powerlessness and reduces his/her options. Joiner and colleagues (2009) report that one of the most important factors in good therapy when a client is suicidal is the therapist–client relationship and that relatedness is critical to client success. In collaborative therapy, which also promotes the importance of the relational partnership, therapists must focus on the

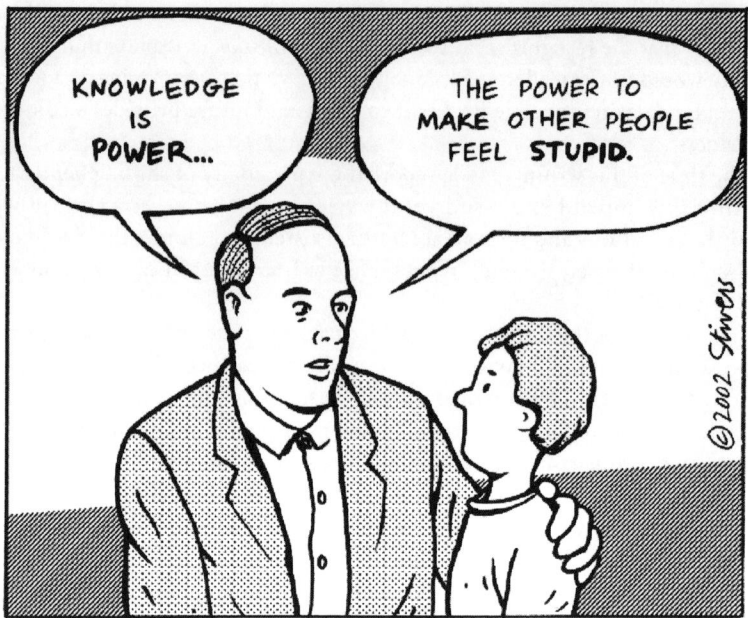

Figure 7.1 Remembering that 'The Client is the Expert' helps avoid this talk. Reproduced with permission of Mark Stivers © 2002.

relationship between their own fears and client engagement. This fosters a creative conversational process, which maintains connection and shared power between the therapist and client.

Collaborative therapy values curiosity, exploring options, shared responsibility and decision-making which are important when someone is considering suicide. Though each situation is different and unique, people often feel that they are out of options when they consider suicide. Taking over, as a therapist, and making decisions and giving recommendations, cements the idea that the client is incompetent to think about his/her life and death. The therapist becomes the one who 'knows best'. The client no longer belongs as a partner in the decision-making.

Van Orden, et al. (2008) make this point as they report on research that indicates that clients who feel a low 'sense of belonging' along with a high 'sense of burdensomeness' are at high risk of suicide. They promote, as we do, the practice of creating caring and connected therapeutic relationships. We expand, below, on the challenges and opportunities in our performance of connection with our clients.

Staying in connection

When we find ourselves in challenging situations and relationships, there may be a tendency to pullback, to care for one's self. The challenge is how to stay in connection *and* take care of self? How do we stay in dialogue, i.e. be open to the plurality of ideas and possibilities rather than a singularity of focus?

We believe that staying engaged and talking to clients about suicide impacts the risk of suicide completions. Figure 7.2 visually illustrates this hypothesis. In our experience, the more and 'better' that one is talking about suicide, the less risk of actually committing this, there is. By 'better' we refer to the creation of 'thick' descriptions (Geertz 1973) through conversations (Anderson 1997) that construct new meanings and understandings. It is important to recognize that being in conversation with a therapist does not totally eliminate risk. When someone is determined to commit suicide they will (Szasz 1999), and they may be willing to discuss their determination if the therapist is open to that conversation. If a therapist is able to engage someone in this conversation, about how determined they are to die, the discussion itself creates the possibility to be able to explore other potential outcomes. Also in this process, meanings are explored and created, thus offering the possibility that new directions might emerge. Being in conversation with someone about suicide means that there is a connection, and we assume that the person considering suicide is interested in having a discussion about it, for some reason.

Having these conversations, hearing others' stories of pain and hoping to die can be difficult (Levin 1991). As therapists we sometimes are not prepared for these intense conversations (Levin 2009). This can lead us to disconnect from people by changing the topic, trying to intervene (by listening to our professional discourses) or 'just' not listening to the client. As the flowchart shows, finding ways to stay engaged and connected with clients through this challenging and uncertain process can play an important part in reducing the risk of suicide.

Some clients are uncertain whether it is 'safe' to discuss suicide with their therapist for fear of there being consequences. 'Will it get reported (to my parents, or to my psychiatrist)?' 'Will it be in my record?' 'Will I be sent to the hospital?' 'Will the therapist judge me?' Many clients are afraid that these thoughts indicate that they are 'crazy' and they don't want to be diagnosed, hospitalized, and/or stigmatized.

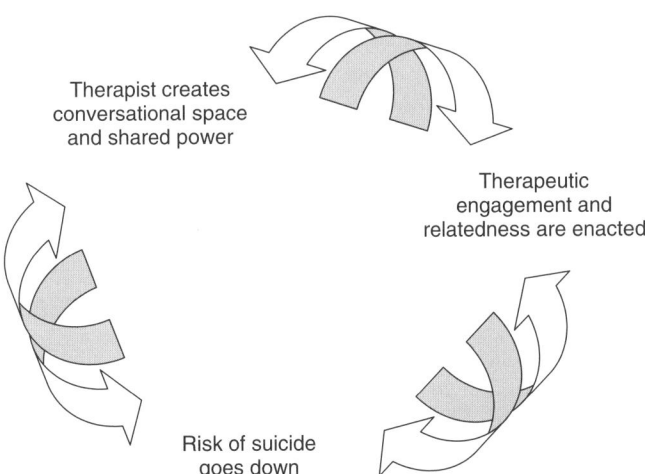

Figure 7.2 The flow of conversation and risk of suicide.

One client, named Michael, came to me (Sue) to find out if he was crazy for thinking about suicide. He arrived in an electric wheelchair, barely mobile. He was a victim of ALS (amyotrophic lateral sclerosis), a progressive muscular dystrophy that would eventually kill him after paralysing more and more of his musculature. Was he crazy to consider suicide in this condition? Being able to discuss this and how he would make decisions to continue his life as long as possible, versus choosing to end it, was incredibly comforting to him. The relational partnership that I had with this man was important. He was able to know that he was not crazy and that I understood his decision to consider suicide as an option. He told me that he was not able to have these conversations in other relationships in his life.

People in pain need connection. We can be bridges for people who are suicidal to move from one 'space' to another; to move from spaces of pain, anger, and isolation to spaces of hope, connection, and confidence. Though Michael did not give up his ideas about suicide, space was created for him in which he felt supported and more in control when facing his disease and the rest of his life. This anecdote is one of many that have informed the creation of the ideas that are illustrated in Figure 7.2.

To have these conversations, a therapist has to be willing to entertain that the idea of dying is not a crazy idea—or should only be available to people with terminal medical illnesses. Though some of us have not personally had these thoughts and feelings (at least not seriously), our clients have. We should be willing to accept their stories and experience and wishes as serious. In Western culture, from a legal and medical standpoint, suicide is indicative of psychological pathology. The legalization and medicalization of suicide can keep us from staying connected with our clients.

Connecting with uncertainty: a not-knowing stance

Curiosity, a key stance in collaborative therapy, keeps us on the way to mutual understanding in therapy. A curious or not-knowing stance (Anderson 2007) positions the therapist as a learner, with the goal of understanding the meanings and context in which the client's story and situation have emerged. London (2009) states, '[Not-knowing] does not mean that you do not know anything. On the contrary, it invites you to offer your ideas, as many as possible, carefully and tentatively allowing the other person to think with, or without you, about the relevance each utterance has in his or her own life'.

Ideas are offered to facilitate conversation, and as Norwegian psychiatrist Tom Andersen has said, to help people talk with themselves and with each other in a way that they have not been able to do before. In other words, the focus is on the process of the conversation more so than its content. Not-knowing requires us to offer our utterances in a tentative manner, not expecting that the other will accept or agree with them, and to be open to being challenged (see Anderson 2009).

'Uncertainty, curiosity, humbleness and creativity naturally flow from the not-knowing position' (London 2009). This position also keeps the therapist in a non-expert stance and focused on the client rather than on the therapist's internal and professional discourses. The not-knowing stance generates space in the dialogue for both the therapist and the client to co-create possibilities and connections where none seem to exist.

Conversations that create connections in the face of isolation and pain carry the possibility of hope. One of the most challenging conversations, which is also a way of connecting, is about uncertainty. Therapists may grasp for direction and something to do when faced with immediate threat and risk. The challenge is for the therapist to stay present in the face of threat, risk, fear, and uncertainty. We practise 'going slow', not rushing in to find a solution, or a fix, or to do something. We must sit with both our client's desire to die and our fear and uncertainty about what will happen next. Shifting our attention to risk-reduction while not connecting with the client can lead to missing possibilities within the conversation.

So what do we mean by connecting through uncertainty? Connecting through uncertainty means being open to new ways of having this conversation; being okay that you may not know what is coming next; being open about the possibilities of where this conversation could go next; of checking in with the client about the next steps, rather than assuming that he or she cannot make choices for him/herself. In the final analysis, it is being okay with the possibility that the client will choose to die, and not judging oneself as lacking in compassion or not being empathic for holding this position. We see this as a moral stance that is not limited to discussions of empathy and compassion.

Reflecting on the therapist's uncertainty

Tim says his suicidal thoughts return when he is unable to 'juggle the balls' and they are crashing down around him. When he comes to see me (Saliha), he may present with 'suicidal ideation'. This is when I have learned to sit with uncertainty and connect with him and his story. Through his story I can learn in what context the current story of suicide is emerging. I also remind myself that suicide is a part of his larger narrative and not the only narrative.

One of the larger narratives that I've learned from my past work with Tim, is that when he is overwhelmed he 'feels like the rope around his neck is tightening'. He interprets that feeling as meaning that he is suicidal and this expands to other thoughts of suicide. One thing that has emerged in our work together that has been helpful when he feels overwhelmed is for us to make a to-do list and write it out on a flip chart. Tim has always used lists to organize himself. I take this approach with him, when I am convinced he is unable to self-organize.

Even if Tim presents with the idea that he is feeling suicidal, I do not begin with the assumption that he is overwhelmed or cannot think for himself. I calibrate my performance to his performance of helplessness and distress. He may present as unable to think and as a helpless child, saying 'You fix this, you are the professional'. Even in a situation in which he presents this way, I choose to stay in connection and create a conversational space where we both can continue working in spite of the feeling that he has given up and I am alone.

I work hard at: 1) seeking his permission to be of help, 2) seeking his agreement to work together (to lessen his feeling that the 'balls are all going to crash around me') and, 3) seeking his agreement to explore other ways of creating a sense of relief (as an alternative to suicide). I get up to write, uncertain what I am going to write, except for the idea it might need to be a list that will give him some focus. Sometimes, the lists have had to do with current work projects, while at other times the list has been focused on what he had to do to get his papers in order, so that he could die. Having the conversation of putting his papers in order feels like a risky conversation to have, yet what I do not know is the power of that conversation. And, not to have that conversation is not to connect with him.

Being public creates shared responsibility

It is helpful to have conversations that are usually unspoken, about our concerns, fears, and hopes for clients. Being public about these concerns, fears and hopes can offer opportunity to connect with clients in new ways. In our experience, offering our inner dialogues (Anderson 2007) is a way of inviting shared responsibility and creating space for creative conversations.

In addition to being public with our clients about inner struggles and unease with their suicide talk, we can explore ideas and be supported through supervision and peer consultation. We, as therapists, work to create relationships in which we can have these conversations, and to have colleagues who can support us being in connection and partnership with our clients. These conversations make the unspoken and the yet-to-be-spoken public and create another layer of shared responsibility with our every-day working colleagues. This process parallels what we do with our clients, as the following example illustrates:

After Linda's suicide attempt a year before this writing, I (Sue) told her that even though I understood her desire to end her suffering, I wasn't sure that I could handle going through the process with her again. During the time up to that attempt, I was very available and present with her, talking often on the phone after work, while she was also having 2–3 sessions per week. My ability and my decision to be available and present to Linda was because my intention was to listen to her and not to professional discourses related to diagnosis and pathology. On the night when she took pills, I spoke to her about her making the final decision to die. Once I decided that there was no more that I could say, I said goodbye, telling her, 'I hope you get through this, but this is your choice and only you can decide what to do'.[6]

Linda survived and continued to work with me. She says that one reason she survived is that she couldn't swallow as many pills as she needed and wanted to. Her throat 'closed up'. She believes that her body wouldn't let her die. She called me when she woke up and decided to go to the emergency room. I met Linda at the emergency room and helped her decide to go to a psychiatric hospital for several weeks. We stayed connected through this ordeal, including several more hospital visits [sessions].

I do not believe that Linda would have continued working with me if I had called her [estranged] family or the authorities and had her hospitalized against her will. These were considerations that I discussed with her in much detail in the months prior

---

[6] In Texas, where HGI is located, the law states that therapists may violate confidentiality to call authorities when someone endangers themselves or others (Texas Health & Safety Code 611.004). Just as there are many factors that influence how therapists choose to manage themselves and their clients when dealing with suicide, the law is one factor which must be considered.

to her attempt. She stated appreciation that I respected her wishes and her ability to have control over her life.

Following her discharge from the psychiatric hospital, Linda agreed to try medication. She decided to try to live. Despite the new direction in therapy, she has periodically wanted to stop taking her medication for 'bi-polar' disorder. She discusses this in our sessions. One of her current and important goals is not to go back to the [psychiatric] hospital, especially not involuntarily. When she talks about stopping her medication, I share my concern that her history has shown that stopping her medication increases the chances that she'll attempt suicide and end up back in the hospital. At the same time I acknowledge that I can't forecast anything for sure and this time maybe different.

At the time of this writing, after a brief period where she stopped taking medication, Linda has approached this issue very differently. As part of our evolving conversations about the pros and cons and side effects, which have led to weight-gain and pre-diabetic and other medical issues for Linda, she has decided that it is time to go back on the medications. Linda has, for the first time in the 3 years that I have worked with her, made this decision without having to go through a hospitalization first.

Though the example of Sue's work with Linda, above, can be considered unconventional, it is in keeping with our beliefs that actions and meanings emerge from within relationships and conversations. Such actions and meanings create possibilities rather than following current conventions of practice. Though there is risk in sharing these alternative ways of working, we hope that they invite reflection and create new possibilities for the field.

Conclusion

In this chapter we have talked about collaborative therapy as a social-constructionist, relational approach to mental health practice. Taking a reflective position we have looked at our history and the field of mental health and the notion of collaboration. One of the ways in which we have expanded our practice is to understand it as a performance. From this perspective we view clients and therapists as human beings performing in conversations and relationships around issues of concern. These performances are on a continuum of ordinary, everyday conversations about hopes and concerns to extraordinary and unspoken conversations about issues such as suicide.

We use the stories of clients who are (or have been) suicidal to illustrate the ways in which collaboration offers powerful possibilities that keep clients and therapists connected towards the design of new lives. The collaborative process gives the client and therapist permission to talk in ways that are not familiar (Andersen 1991). The not-knowing stance keeps the therapist from grabbing onto the right protocol, a medication solution, or a stop-suicide intervention. Though not-knowing is risky, as there may end up being a death when someone decides they want to die, honouring that possibility and exploring it also offers genuine respect, concern, and interest in the client's reality and current experience. Such a conversation is difficult to have because as therapists we are also human; we care about our clients, have values and are challenged by uncertainties.

Being human allows us to feel the depth of the concern and respect and not stay distant in our 'professionalism.' As active participants in collaboration we bring our fears, concerns, and values into the interplay of our relationship. This bi-directional connection, human being to human being and therapist to client, in conversation offers hope and possibilities.

Acknowledgement

We deeply appreciate our clients with whom we learn and feel honoured to accompany them on their life journey. Special thanks to Tim and Linda for giving us permission to share their stories. We thank our colleagues, learners and family who support and grow the work that we do, and Carolyn Callahan, PhD for her ongoing support and proofing of the chapter. And Saliha appreciates Rabia's partnership on their co-therapy journeys.

References

Andersen, T. (1991). *The reflecting team: Dialogues and dialogues about the dialogues.* W.W. Norton & Co., New York.

Anderson, A. (1990). *Reality isn't what it used to be.* Harper & Row Publishers, San Francisco.

Anderson, H. (1993). On a roller coaster: A collaborative language systems approach to therapy. In S. Friedman (Ed.) *The new language of change: Constructive collaboration in psychotherapy,* pp. 323–44. Guilford, New York.

Anderson, H. (2007). The heart and spirit of collaborative therapy: The philosophical stance— "A way of being" in relationship and conversation. In H. Anderson and D. Gehart (Eds.) *Collaborative therapy: Conversations and relationships that make a difference,* pp. 43–59. Brunner-Routledge, New York.

Anderson, H. (2009). FAQ. *International Journal of Collaborative Practices* 1. [online]. http://collaborative-practices.com/faq/#3. [Accessed 30 November 2009.]

Anderson, H. and Gehart, D. (Eds.) (2007). *Collaborative therapy: Conversations and relationships that make a difference.* Brunner-Routledge, New York.

Anderson, H. and Goolishian, H. (1986). Systems consultation to agencies dealing with domestic violence. In L. Wynne, S. McDaniel, and T. Weber (Eds.) *The family therapist as systems consultant,* pp. 284–99. Guilford Press, New York.

Anderson, H. and Goolishian, H. A. (1988). Human systems as linguistic systems: Preliminary and evolving ideas about the implications for clinical theory. *Family Process,* **27**(4), 317–93.

Anderson, H., and Goolishian, H. (1992). The client is the expert: A not-knowing approach to therapy. In S. McNamee and K. Gergen (Eds.) *Therapy as social construction,* pp.25–39. Sage, Newbury Park, CA.

Anderson, H. and Levin, S.B. (1998). Generative conversations: A postmodern approach to conceptualizing and working with human systems. In M. Hoyt (Ed.) *The handbook of constructive therapies: Innovative approaches from leading practitioners,* pp. 46–67. Jossey-Bass, San Francisco, CA.

Anderson, H., and Levin, S. B. (1997). Collaborative conversations with children: Country clothes and city clothes. In C. Smith and D. Nylund (Eds.) *Narrative therapies with children,* pp. 255–81. Guilford Press, New York.

Bava, S. (2005). Performance Methodology: Constructing Discourses and Discursive Practices in Family Therapy Research. In D. Sprenkle and F. Piercy (Eds.) *Research methods in family therapy* (2nd Ed.), pp. 170–90. Guilford Press, New York.

Bava, S. and Levin, S. (2007). Collaborative disaster response: Setting-up mental health services in a Mega-shelter. In *AFTA Monograph Series: Systemic Responses to Disaster: Stories of the Aftermath of Hurricane Katrina*, pp. 7–15. American Family Therapy Academy, Washington, DC.

Berg, I. K. (1994). *Family based services: A solution-based approach.* W.W. Norton & Co., New York.

Berg, I. K. (2000). *Building solutions in child protective services.* W.W. Norton & Co., New York.

Brown, L. (2009). Cultural competence: A new way of thinking about integration in therapy', *Journal of Psychotherapy Integration,* **19**(4), 340–53.

Carlson, M. (1996). *Performance: A critical introduction.* Routledge, New York.

Denzin, N. K. (2003). *Performance ethnography: Critical pedagogy and the politics of culture.* Sage Publications, Thousand Oaks, CA.

de Shazer, S. (1985). *Keys to solution in brief therapy.* W.W. Norton & Co., New York.

Frydman, B., Wilson, I. M., Wyer, J. (2000). *The power of collaborative leadership: Lessons for the learning organization.* Butterworth-Heinemann, Oxford.

Geertz, C. (1973). *The interpretation of cultures.* Basic Books, New York.

Gehart, D., Tarragona, M., and Bava, S. (2007). A collaborative approach to research and inquiry. In Anderson, H. and Gehart, D. (Eds.) *Collaborative therapy: Conversations and relationships that make a difference*, pp. 367–87. Brunner-Routledge, New York.

Gergen, K. (1997). *Realities and relationships: Soundings in social construction*, Harvard University Press, Cambridge, MA.

Gergen, K. (2009a). *An invitation to social construction.* Sage, Newbury Park, CA.

Gergen, K. (2009b). *Relational being: Beyond self and community.* Oxford University Press, Oxford.

Goffman E, (1959). *The presentation of self in everyday life.* Anchor Books, New York.

Goolishian, H., and Anderson, H. (1990). Understanding the therapeutic process: From individuals and families to systems in language. In F. Kaslow (Ed.) *Voices in family psychology,* pp. 91–113. Sage Publications, Newbury Park, CA

Hare-Mustin. R. T. (1987). The problem of gender in family therapy theory. *Family Process,* **26**, 15–27.

Horsfall, D. (2008). Performing communit(y)ies [51 paragraphs]. *Forum Qualitative Sozialforschung/Forum: Qualitative Social Research,* **9**(2), 57.

Joiner, T. E., Van Orden, K.A., Witte, T. K., and Rudd, M. D. (2009). *The interpersonal theory of suicide: Guidance for working with suicidal clients.* The American Psychological Association, Washington, D.C.

Levin, S. (1991). Hearing the unheard: Women's stories about being battered. PhD dissertation, Union Institute, Cincinnati, OH.

Levin, S. (2009). Intense Conversations: Hearing about Trauma, Violence & Suicide [Course notes], Contemporary Therapeutic Perspectives, Massey University, New Zealand.

Lipchik, E. (2002). *Beyond technique in solution-focused therapy: Working with emotions and the therapeutic relationship.* Guilford Press, New York.

London, S. (2009). FAQ. *International Journal of Collaborative Practices* [online]. http://collaborative-practices.com/faq/#2. [Accessed 30 November 2009.]

London, S. and Rodriguez-Jazcilevich, I. (2007). The development of a collaborative learning and therapy community in an educational setting: From alienation to invitation.

In H. Anderson and D. Gehart (Eds.) *Collaborative therapy: Conversations and relationships that make a difference*, pp. 235–49. Brunner-Routledge, New York.

McGregor, R., Ritchie, A., Serrano, A., Schuster, F., and Goolishian, H. (1964). *Multiple impact therapy with families*. McGraw-Hill, New York.

McNamee, S. and Gergen, K. (1992). *Therapy as social construction*. Sage, Newbury Park, CA.

McNamee, S. and Gergen, K. (Eds.) (1998). *Relational responsibility: Resources for sustainable dialogue*. Sage, Newbury Park, CA.

Pelias, R. J. (1999). *Writing performance: Poeticizing the researcher's body*. Carbondale, Southern Illinois University Press, IL.

Rampage, C., Goodrich, T. J., Halstead, K., and Ellman, B. (1988). *Feminist family therapy: A casebook*. W.W. Norton, New York.

Roth, S., Becker, C., Herzig, M., Chasin, L., and Chasin, R. (1992). Creating conditions for dialogue on the abortion issue: A report from the public conversations project. *Ki Notes*, **4**, 3–4.

Schechner, R. (2002). *Performance studies: An introduction*. Routledge, New York.

Shotter, J. (1984). *Social accountability and selfhood*, Blackwell, Oxford.

Shotter, J. (2003). Cartesian change, chiasmic change: The power of living expression. *Janus Head*, **6**(1), 6–29.

Shotter, J. (2007). Getting it: Withness thinking and the dialogical . . . in practice, K.C.C. Consultants, London. [See also http://pubpages.unh.edu/~jds/Kentmgt2005.htm.]

Szasz, T. S. (1999). *Fatal freedom: The ethics and politics of suicide*. Praeger, Westport, CT.

TED, (2009). *Chimamanda Adichie: The danger of a single story*. http://www.ted.com/talks/chimamanda_adichie_the_danger_of_a_single_story.html. [Accessed January 2010.]

Texas Health & Safety Code 611.004, Texas Health & Safety Code—Chapter 611. Available at http://www.statutes.legis.state.tx.us/Docs/HS/htm/HS.611.htm

Van Orden, K.A., Witte, T.K., Gordon, K.H., Bender, T.W., and Joiner, T.E. (2008). Suicidal desire and the capability for suicide: Tests of the interpersonal-psychological theory of suicidal behavior among adults. *Journal of Consulting and Clinical Psychology*, **76**, 72–83.

Wagner, J. (2007). Trialogues: A means to answerability and dialogue in a prison setting. In H. Anderson and D. Gehart (Eds.) *Collaborative therapy: Conversations and relationships that make a difference*, pp. 203–20. Brunner-Routledge, New York.

White, M. (2007). *Maps of narrative practice*. W.W. Norton & Co, New York.

White, M. and Epston, D. (1990). *Narrative means to therapeutic ends*. W.W. Norton & Co., New York.

Wile, D. B. (1999). Collaborative couple therapy. In J. Donovan (Ed.) *Short-term couple therapy*, pp. 201–25. Guilford, New York.

Wile, D. B. (2002). Collaborative couple therapy. In A. S. Gurman and N. S. Jacobson (Eds.) *Clinical handbook of couple therapy* (3rd ed.). Guilford, New York.

Wittgenstein, L. (1973). *Philosophical investigations*, Prentice Hall, Englewood Cliffs, NJ.

Chapter 8

Solution-focused brief therapy: listening in the present with an ear toward the future

Maureen Duffy

The beginnings of SFBT

Solution-focused brief therapy (SFBT) was developed from the work of Steve de Shazer (1982, 1985, 1988, 1991, 1994) and Insoo Kim Berg (Berg 1994; Berg and Cauffman 2003; Berg and Dolan 2001; Berg and Miller 1992; Berg and Steiner 2003) and their colleagues at the non-profit Brief Family Therapy Center in Milwaukee, Wisconsin during the 1980s. The centre later became known as the Milwaukee Brief Family Therapy Center (BFTC). Other early and influential members of the BFTC who worked together on the development of the original ideas and guiding principles of what was to become known as SFBT were Eve Lipchik, Elam Nunnally, Alex Molnar, and Michelle Weiner Davis. They collaborated with de Shazer and Berg on the first journal article (de Shazer et al.1986) to set forth the SFBT ideas that continue to evolve. The influence and popularity of SFBT has spread throughout the world and today is practised worldwide (Kim 2008; Miller et al. 1996; Trepper et al. 2006).

The developers of brief therapy were clearly more interested in finding out what worked for their clients than in spending time exploring what wasn't working. De Shazer talked about the early days in the development of SFBT (Hoyt 1994) and commented on how surprised he was about some of the things that he and his team were observing in therapy that were working for their clients. It was during these early days that they began to put together their SFBT model that didn't centre on presenting problems, aetiologies, and symptoms in the way that over a hundred years of psychotherapy had done since the time of Freud. To emphasize how different the SFBT model was, de Shazer reported in 1992 (Hoyt 1994) how he began every training workshop with the following statement: 'If somebody had told me about this model 15 years ago, I would have called the men in the white coats. This can't work. And everyday I'm surprised, but it does work. And I still am. It's not logical in some way' (p. 24). In this same conversation, de Shazer mentioned something that I believe is still important to remember; namely, that most of us get married to our theories to some degree but that it's important to keep looking at what's working for our clients because it might not fit our theories and, if we pay attention to our clients, we might be surprised.

Applications of the SFBT model

SFBT has been used to address a wide array of clinical problems and has also been used as a consulting and educational model in a variety of larger systems contexts and in business. Among the range of clinical issues to which SFBT has been applied are problem drinking and substance abuse (Berg and Miller 1992; McCollum and Trepper 2001; Pichot 2001), grieving (Peller and Walter 1992/93), depression (Johnson and Miller 1994), suicide (Sharry et al. 2002), sexual abuse (Dolan 1991), post-traumatic stress disorders (Dolan 1991), chronic severe mental illness (Eakes et al. 1997), and bullying (Young and Holdore 2003), to name just a sample. In addition, some master practitioners of SFBT are making efforts to apply findings from neuroscience that emphasize the importance of emotion in their clinical work (Lipchik 2002).

SFBT has been used in a variety of larger system contexts, such as school settings (Franklin et al. 2008; Kral 1995; Metcalf 2002), prison settings (Lindforss and Magnusson 1997), human service agencies (Berg 1994; Pichot and Dolan 2003) and in adult psychiatric settings (Macdonald 1994, 1997). The influence of solution-focused approaches has also extended into the business world in the areas of management and coaching (Berg and Cauffman 2003; Cauffman 2003) and mediation (Bannink 2006). Solution-focused brief therapists work with individuals (Lipchik 2002), couples (Murray and Murray 2004; Zimmerman et al. 1997), families (McCollum and Trepper 2001), groups (Newsome 2004; Sharry 2001), and with people of all ages (Berg and Steiner 2003; Macdonald 1994, 1997; Newsome 2004; Selekman 1993, 1997).

An overview of the SFBT model

SFBT places high value on the experiential world of the client and engages the services of a therapist in the co-inquiring of what works in the client's experiential world and how it works when it does. SFBT has become attractive to the managed care mental health model because of its relative brevity and cost-effectiveness. As a result, SFBT is practised widely and, often, without an understanding of the radical shift that its philosophical and discursive positioning represents. In this section of the chapter, I will review the key ideas and practices associated with SFBT and, later, in the chapter, discuss more fully how those ideas and practices are reflective of the discursive traditions with which they are associated. Kim (2008) in a recent meta-analysis examining the effectiveness of SFBT described the model as 'a strengths-based intervention that is founded in the belief that clients have the knowledge and solutions to solve their problems. Collaboration and co-construction of answers are important components of the change process used by the practitioner' (p. 107). The following are ten key ideas and techniques central to the philosophical standpoint and practice of SFBT:

- Solution-focused brief therapists draw an important distinction in their work between problems and solutions, where problems reflect deficit positions and solutions reflect preferred futures. Problems and solutions are regarded as complementarities with one always invoking the other.
- Solution-focused brief therapists assume an intentional non-pathologizing stance with respect to their clients and their clients' lives and problems.

- Knowing details about the client(s)' presenting problem is not necessary nor is the taking of psychosocial histories or exploration of the past.
- SFBT engages clients in a collaborative exploration of what is already working in their lives and of what their ideas for their preferred futures are.
- Solution-focused brief therapists orient themselves to helping clients identify and realize their visions of a preferred future.
- Clients possess strengths, resiliencies, and resources that are identified and utilized in therapy.
- Solution-focused brief therapists assume an influential but not expert role in the conduct of therapy and operate well from positions of uncertainty and curiosity.
- Small changes can make a big difference and are acknowledged and valued in SFBT.
- SFBT is a questioning model that utilizes a series of specific questions, in particular, exception questions, coping questions, scaling questions, and the miracle question. Pre-session change questions, competence and resource questions, and future-oriented questions are also frequently used.
- Solution-focused brief therapists give clients compliments and 'pats on the back'.

For those unfamiliar with the SFBT model, Simon (1996) provides the following examples of the basic questions used by SFBT therapists that she learned in her training and work with Steve de Shazer, Insoo Kim Berg, and Eve Lipchik:

> Exception questions
> 'What's different when the problem is not occurring?'
> Coping questions
> 'With all the terrible things you've been through, what has kept you from becoming a stark raving lunatic?'
> Scaling questions
> 'On a scale from one to ten, with one being the way you felt when you called to make the appointment and ten being feeling great, how are you doing right now?'
> The miracle question
> 'Suppose tonight while you are sleeping a miracle occurs, and the problem you came here to deal with is no longer a problem. But because the miracle happened while you were sleeping, you didn't know it happened. What would be the first thing you would notice after you woke up that would tell you the miracle happened?'
> Future-oriented questions
> 'What will you do with all the time you save when you no longer have the problem?'
> Competence and/or resource questions
> 'How did you do that?'
> 'How did you figure that out?' (p. 54).

The above ten key ideas and Simon's examples of the common questions asked in SFBT provide a brief but descriptive overview of the model, its operating assumptions, and its set of therapeutic practices. How these operating assumptions and therapeutic practices in SFBT differ from those of traditional therapies is summarized in Table 8.1.

Table 8.1 Therapeutic discourse

Traditional	Solution-focused
Static (Newtonian)	Dynamic (quantum)
Normative	Non-normative
Therapist as expert knower	Therapist as co-constructor and co-researcher
Problem saturated	Solution and exception saturated
Pathology oriented	Strengths oriented
Importance of the past	Pull of the future
Ecologically disruptive interventions	Ecologically mindful interventions
Large-scale change	Small scaled or minimal change
Goal setting and problem solving	Equifinality (Many paths to desired goal/solution)
Conscious purpose	Emergence (Novel forms of self-organization)

Problem-solving versus solution-focused: a very short story

Bannink (2007) in contrasting solution-focused approaches with traditional problem-solving approaches proposes that:

> Psychotherapy should no longer be considered as a group of methods that makes use of psychologically validated knowledge *to reduce emotional problems.* The time is ripe for a positive objective. Instead of reducing problems it is possible to ask the solution-focused question: 'What would you rather have instead?' The positively formulated answer of most clients will be: happiness in a satisfying and productive life (p. 93).

This focus on how clients would want their lives to be different as opposed to how they might go about reducing problems or symptoms is the heart of the solution-focused approach in therapy. One of the stand-out moments for me in my own training that helped me understand the difference between problem-solving or symptom reduction and focusing on solutions occurred as I was watching a videotape of an interview with Insoo Kim Berg. In the video, Insoo was responding to concerns that the solution-focused approach would not be appropriate for clients in life-threatening situations. Insoo described consulting on a case in London of a man who was dying of AIDS. Insoo's question to him was simply 'What would a good death be for you?'. The question wasn't about delving into his fears or into the issue of relationship repairs that he may have wanted to address before his death. It was about what his best imagined future might look like, however brief that future was going to be. Hearing the question was like being transported to Oz where Dorothy, the Tin Man, the Scarecrow, and the Lion learned that they already had the power they were looking for, that the power didn't reside with the Wizard (Baum and Denslow 1900/2000). The dying man was invited to consider what, uniquely for him, would constitute a good death—what that might look and feel like for him. The solution was having a good death and doing the things that having a good death required.

The SFBT model of therapy: underlying assumptions

While SFBT includes a set of questioning techniques that have come to be very much associated with the model, SFBT can never be reduced to set of techniques without violating the underlying philosophical assumptions of the model. Those assumptions have to do with a particular view of the nature of reality and the epistemological standpoint of the therapist. SFBT is a non-normative clinical model, meaning that there is no particular view of what is normal, healthy, or good for a person that is built in to the structure of the model. Clients, in linguistic partnership with their therapists, develop their own understandings of what might be good or appropriate for them at a particular point in time, even if those understandings are at odds with prevailing cultural perspectives and norms.

The following is an example of a verbal exchange during therapy between a couple experiencing marital problems who had consulted a solution-focused brief therapist. The exchange could understandably raise ire and eyebrows in a number of different quarters. But the meanings that came out of the exchange, even though some of the words were far from respectful or even civil, worked well for the particular couple involved. A couple sought therapy because they said that their marriage was falling apart. She wanted out of the marriage. He wanted peace and quiet and his wife back the way she was before she became unhappy with things. Both were terrified of getting a divorce and both were angry. She didn't feel appreciated and he felt overwhelmed. In the therapy session, they were arguing. Very uncharacteristically, the husband yelled at his wife and said 'you're a fucking bitch'. Calmly, the wife looked at him and said, 'that's the sexiest thing you've ever said to me'. Inexplicably, he started laughing, she started laughing, and the therapist started laughing. The desired future that both wanted was a way to express and manage anger without becoming overwhelmed and a way to express affection and be sexy with each other.

There is no question that the phrase 'you're a fucking bitch', uttered by a male towards a female goes against most of our understandings of what constitutes respect, gender equity, and common decency. Out of respect for women, many therapists would be quick to challenge the use of such a phrase in therapy and in life. In this particular case, the husband said that hearing himself use such an objectionable phrase helped him realize that he needed to find different ways of expressing anger and to develop a wider repertoire for inviting his wife to be affectionate with him. His wife said she wanted more affection from him and what he wanted was his marriage to continue. In the moments surrounding that exchange, the job of the solution-focused therapist was to recognize what was working and stay out of the way and that's exactly what the therapist did. To paraphrase de Shazer, it is in many ways illogical to think that the husband calling his wife a 'fucking bitch' would lead him almost instantaneously to recognize that continuing to be angry in the way that he had was not going to get him what he wanted and that he needed to start doing things differently. But that is exactly what happened and the therapist was wise enough to see it.

The therapist utilized the opening in the conversation and immediately followed-up with a competence-based question and asked the husband 'How did you come to the recognition that you needed to develop more ways of being affectionate with your wife when you heard yourself saying those derogatory words to her?'. And then, 'What is your wife going to notice first as you begin to explore new ways of showing affection to her?'. The therapist then followed with the reciprocal question to the wife 'What small signs will you notice that will let you know that your husband is on the right track with you and that things are improving in your relationship?'. To the wife, the therapist also asked, 'How were you able to take those words of your husband and see something else in them besides anger?'. All of these questions were predicated on the therapist noticing and acknowledging that the couple was dealing quite well with an angry exchange and then building on that demonstrated competence. In terms of the SFBT model, the questions can be classified as competence questions and questions that broke down the miracle question into small parts focusing on what small indicators each partner would notice as things began to move in their preferred directions.

In addition to being a non-normative model, SFBT rests on an ontological view of the world as being socially constructed (Bannink 2007). Social constructionism suggests that what we decide, individually and collectively, to agree on as 'real' is a result of the co-creation of shared meanings in and through language. The problems and solutions we develop and name are likewise the result of this same activity of bringing forth meanings that together we share and agree upon. A number of years ago in a psychopathology course I was teaching, an English professor from another university took the class. One of the assignments was a very straightforward one; namely, to develop a clinical case presentation of a client with a symptom set and an associated diagnosis. The English professor presented his case of a young pallid woman swooning against an elaborately carved and brocaded upright couch in her parlour. A male physician was attending to her with smelling salts. The wealthy young woman had a history of defying rules and regulations and had become involved with a group of suffragettes. The English professor's diagnosis: the vapours. The treatment regimen recommended for the vapours was rest, smelling salts as needed, water massage, and isolation from the suffragettes since one of the symptoms of the vapours was a tendency to cause trouble (Maines 1999). The young woman lived, of course, at the end of the 1800s during the height of the Victorian era. The other students in the class were mesmerized listening to the English professor present his case complete with diagnosis and treatment recommendations. Their attention was caught between the sexual undertones of the treatment protocols of Victorian England and its view of women as weak and hysterical and the absurdity, viewed from their time and place, of a diagnosis like 'the vapors'. One thing, however, was quite clear—that the vapours was a medical construction that incorporated a view of women as weak, whose place was in the home, and who, under no circumstances, should challenge authority. Being assigned a diagnosis like 'the vapours' also organized a set of potential actions including enforced rest, dosing with smelling salts, close surveillance to prevent associating with 'troublemakers,' and various forms of pelvic massage by male physicians who were assured steady work since 'the vapours' was a chronic condition requiring regular medical intervention (Maines 1999). The English professor in my course, whose professional interest was Victorian literature, demonstrated through his presentation of the case of 'the vapours' the socially constructed nature of diagnoses, mental illness, problem descriptions, treatments, remedies, and solutions in such a vivid way that most of the students became quite sceptical about all of the psychopathological diagnoses they encountered throughout the remainder of the course. What became clear was that a name is not just a name—that a world view and set of actions become associated with the name. What also became clear was the social and participatory nature of the act of naming itself—and the attendant ethical responsibilities involved in the act of naming.

In thinking about their own thinking about the relationship between language, meaning, and action, Walter and Peller (1996), highly skilled solution-focused therapists, traced their changes in understanding about the significance of language. They said:

> When we were using a brief strategic therapy model, we commonly thought of words and distinctions as *frames*. We spoke of behaviors being defined by the meaning or frame we placed around them. We considered words like 'good' or 'bad' to be the meaning surrounding the behaviors. The implication of separating behavior and meaning is that the behavior is somehow real and the meaning is subjective. Language as creational includes more than interpretation and framing. Language *creates* the experience of bad behavior. The behavior is not separated from the interpretation of 'badness' (pp. 12–13).

Walter and Peller had embraced the critical constructionist idea that has become part of modern quantum physics, namely, that observation is creation (Wolf 1989). The quantum physics world suggests that we bring forth into reality that which we observe and to which we pay attention. In therapy, if we pay attention to problem descriptions we will bring them forth in increasing detail with their associated collectively agreed upon range of attendant meanings and actions. We think and act quite differently about 'a marriage that is falling apart in which the wife wants out', than we do about a marriage in which the husband has decided that he 'needs to develop a wider repertoire for inviting his wife to be affectionate with him because that is what she wants'. It's the same marriage but radically different descriptions that bring forth radically different understandings and that organize radically different action potentials. The solution-focused brief therapist wisely co-participates in bringing forth the description that contains the image of the client's preferred future.

When lessons about social constructionism start showing up in newspapers, magazines, and airports we can safely assume that social constructionism has left the academy and gone mainstream. The idea of reality as socially constructed and as reflective of personal and social values and norms has been powerfully illuminated by the 'Your Pont of View' ad campaign initiated in October, 2008 by HSBC Bank (HSBC Bank 2008). In the ads, the same image appears in succession with an entirely different 'point of view' descriptor written across the image. One image, for example, identically reproduced three times in a row, is of the back of a shaved head and is aptly entitled 'Shaved Head.' The observer can decide if the head is male or female or even if the distinction is important. What is so powerful are the different descriptive words written across each of three identical shaved heads. The first descriptor is 'style', the second is 'soldier', and the third is 'survivor'. As an observer, I react to the shaved head with the word 'style' on it in a particular way. My reaction is light and I consider whether I think shaved heads are attractive or not. When I move to the same image with the word 'survivor' written on it, my reaction is entirely different. I feel my skin prickling and the concept of 'torture' overwhelms me momentarily. Then I shift again and think that the survivor might be a cancer survivor who had undergone chemotherapy or radiation treatment. When I move to the image that says 'soldier' on it I think of the dozens of young people in uniform I have just seen walking around the airport and wonder what their futures hold for them. It is hard to come up with a more vivid example of the social constructionist perspective that meanings are culturally created in language and dependent upon perspective and point of view. The same image can have multiple and dramatically different meanings. The HSBC Bank ad campaign 'Your Point of View' has made walking down an aircraft jet way where the images are frequently displayed an exciting and thought-filled activity.

For therapists, the implications of assuming a social constructionist standpoint involve both their own thinking and ways of looking at the world and their actual practices in therapy. Thinking and acting are not dichotomous activities but rather are mutually influential. However, for heuristic purposes only and to illustrate the implications for thinking and acting of embracing a social constructionist perspective in SFBT, I will consider separately the implications of social constructionism for thinking and for acting in the next sections of this chapter.

The solution-focused brief therapist's standpoint: influences from social constructionism

In this section, I will present what seem to me to be some basic and important implications of holding a social constructionist ontology for thinking about therapy that are relevant for the SFBT therapist. The social constructionist perspectives identified here as important for the SFBT therapist can be developed and practised over time.

1. It makes sense for the SFBT therapist to practice looking at a set of data or information from many different perspectives—not in the interest of finding the 'right' or 'correct' perspective but in the interests of learning how to pick up ideas, leave them aside, and then pick up other ideas. Really getting the idea that the world consists of multiple views of it that are linguistically, situationally, culturally, time, and place influenced is a basic aptitude in developing a finely honed social constructionist standpoint.

2. Becoming comfortable with ambiguity, uncertainty, and even confusion is also another therapist standpoint skill that will hold an SFBT therapist in good stead. Appreciating the possibilities inherent in ambiguity and uncertainty will help the SFBT therapist develop a sense of curiosity that is necessary if one is to engage with clients authentically and in detail about preferred futures, exceptions, and actions that are making a positive difference in their lives now.

3. Seeing clients as resourceful and as making every effort to do the best they can at any moment in time helps the SFBT therapist to bypass blaming and pathologizing and to stay focused on the abilities that clients are demonstrating in their lives, even if those abilities are denied by most observers. In my own training, I remember either reading about or seeing Insoo Kim Berg, while training and working with children and family services personnel in Milwaukee, respond in the middle of the

night with a family services worker to a call about a mother who was reportedly abusing her child. As I recall the story, a mother was screaming at her young adolescent son and slapping him for being out too late or for some other rule violation. Insoo went up to the mother and gently said. 'You must love your son very much'. The story blew me away and Insoo's comment made perfect sense to me even though, from one perspective, the mother could have been and maybe was charged with child abuse. That mother could not have been so engaged with that boy and expending all that energy on him if she didn't have some hopes for a positive future for him that in her mind her son was at risk of throwing down the drain. With those six words 'You must love your son very much', Insoo demonstrated the magic of seeing things differently.

4. For me, the most important derivative of social constructionism in terms of one's therapeutic thinking and standpoint is the ethical obligations it imposes to be mindful of the implications of bringing forth any particular description of a person, situation, event, or other aspect of the nature of things in the world. There's no neutral ground to stand on, so every description brings forth certain realities attendant with truckloads of real world implications as does intentional avoidance of bringing forth particular descriptions. Mindfulness of our own participation in the bringing forth of particular descriptions and attentiveness to the effects of descriptions on our clients seems to me to be the basic ethical obligation for a social constructionist-oriented therapist.

Therapists who adopt a constructionist standpoint are themselves challenged to continuously look at their own looking at in order to identify the values and beliefs that permeate their choices of perspective. In the following section, I will shift to looking at praxis—the interweaving of theory and practice and the influence of social constructionism on how solution-focused brief therapists do what they actually do and say in the therapy room. Their doing is connected to their philosophical standpoint, so there will be some folding back on the above section about therapists' standpoints in order to illustrate practices.

The practice of SFBT: influences from social constructionism

This section will focus on some important implications of holding a social constructionist perspective for clinical practice for SFBT practitioners.

1. Marking distinctions between problems and solutions is a central therapeutic activity in SFBT. It is a way of playing with complementarities. In 1992, in a conversation with Michael Hoyt and John Weakland, de Shazer responded to Hoyt's question 'What do you think is the essence of being a brief therapist?'. De Shazer replied, 'My first immediate thought is that "essence" is a muddling word. Because when you talk "essence" that means you also talk something about "nonessence."'(Hoyt 1994, p. 12). For the quantum physicist, Niels Bohr, reality was composed of complementarities—invoking one side of a distinction simultaneously invokes the other. Invoking 'absence' suggests 'presence', invoking 'problem'

suggests 'solution', and, of course, vice versa. For Bohr, reality was always both under and over determined (Bohr 1937; Brody and Oppenheim 1969; Folse 1985). For the SFBT therapist, this playing with complementarities is focused on the side of the distinction that emphasizes 'solution' or 'preferred future' and the ethics of SFBT require the amplifying of what the clients want for themselves and what their visions of their preferred futures are as opposed to amplifying their problem-saturated stories of their lives.

2. SFBT therapists engage collaboratively with their clients and honour their clients' perspectives by asking a lot of questions. The kinds of questions asked by SFBT therapists are described in the earlier section entitled 'An overview of the SFBT model'. While questions, like declaratory statements, are never neutral, they serve the purpose of eliciting the client's perspective so that it becomes central to the therapeutic dialogue. How a client responds to an SFBT question often reveals strengths and resourceful ways of looking at or handling situations that may never have surfaced had the question not been asked. Such resourceful responses can then be further used by the SFBT therapist to advance the client's movement in the direction of their (not the therapist's) desired goals and solutions.

3. In SFBT, therapists do occasionally make declarative statements. These statements often take the form of brief exclamatory compliments (Simon 1996) like 'Wow that was amazing that you were able to do that under those circumstances' or 'You're hanging in like that with your job and your academic work is impressive'. Such compliments serve as validation and encouragement of the changes and movement that the client is making toward desired goals. The compliments are part of the larger set of actions by the solution-focused brief therapist to amplify the resourceful, solution side of any problem/solution complementarity.

4. Actions are also manifest in restraint and in actions in which one intentionally chooses not to participate. The actions that solution-focused brief therapists commonly refrain from doing are asking about the history of the problem, exploring a client's past, and pathologizing or otherwise negatively labelling a client or another in the client's life. To do so would be to participate in the bringing forth or social construction of a story of the client and/or others as troubled, as troublemakers, or as part of a thinly described heroes and villains story. From my perspective, participating in the pathologizing of clients, their family members, and others in their social network represents an ethical violation for a solution-focused brief therapist. Therapists, even those who practice from a decentred position, as do solution-focused brief therapists are still influential and clinical ethics requires accounting for how that influence is used.

Solution-focused brief therapists whose actions are guided to greater or lesser degrees by theory, like other practitioners, do not always think and act congruently. Espoused theories and theories in use are frequently inconsistent (Argyris 1991). The following example is illustrative and I include it to raise the ethical questions of whether the theoretical standpoint of a solution-focused brief therapist is limited to the therapy room or whether it should extend to more general positioning in life. Ponder the case of a professional woman who was having both marital and family difficulties.

She sought therapy from a discursively-oriented therapist who, based on a discursive theoretical standpoint, eschewed both pathologizing and advising people about what decisions they should make with regard to particular questions and issues in their lives. In the therapy room, the therapist performed fairly congruently within the context of the relevant espoused theory. Outside of the therapy room, the therapist discussed the case with other professionals in what was framed as consultation but in ways that could also be described as gossipy. Additionally, outside of the therapy room, the therapist took a vocal position that the woman's husband was irredeemably insensitive and that she and her children would be better off were she to divorce him. The therapist's behaviour outside of the therapy room was theoretically incongruent with the therapist's espoused discursive position and was therefore quite surprising. The example is included here to raise the following ethical question for consideration. Should assumption of a SFBT or other discursive standpoint reflect professional behaviour only or extend more generally into a therapist's life as a theoretical standpoint and as a basis for broader action? There is scant therapeutic literature of which I am aware that addresses this intriguing question.

Reflections on SFBT and the discursive traditions

In this section I will reflect on features of the SFBT model, described above, in order to summarize some of its signature characteristics within the brief and discursive traditions of psychotherapy. Important aspects of the SFBT model are (a) taking what the client says seriously, (b) marking a distinction between problems and solutions, and (c) not conflating descriptions with prescriptions. De Shazer (Hoyt 1994) explains these ideas well:

> I know what I don't want, and that's for anybody to develop some sort of rigid orthodoxies. I'm afraid of that. I'm always afraid of that. For me, it's a big point of concern. That there's a right way to do this and this. And to see my descriptions—and they've done this to me; I've probably done this to myself—to see my descriptions as prescriptions. So what I'd like, I suppose, is what I said earlier about listen and take them seriously. The 'take them seriously' part. That's what I want people to take out of it is to take it seriously. And I suppose that the break between 'problems' and 'solutions,' certainly that part (p. 39).

In addition to the three characteristics of a solution-focused therapeutic stance described above, Trepper et al. (2006) note that 'SFBT focuses on client strengths and resiliencies examining previous solutions and exceptions to the problem, and then, through a series of interventions, encouraging clients to do more of those behaviors' (p. 134). We might, therefore, summarize the orienting posture of the solution-focused brief therapist as one in which the therapist is: (a) taking what the client says seriously, (b) marking a distinction between problems and solutions, (c) not conflating descriptions with prescriptions, and (d) focusing on clients' strengths and resiliencies. Taking what the client says seriously and not conflating descriptions with prescriptions are particularly congruent therapist orientations within the world of discursive psychotherapy. Marking a distinction between problems and solutions is equally a discursive activity in that the differences are identified in language between conversational partners, in this case, between therapist and client(s), as they together generate the meanings of problems versus solutions. Such meanings are not given or pre-ordained. They are created in dialogue within a particular context, in this case, within the context of therapy. The particular therapeutic context, of course, is influenced by larger contexts of culture, knowledge, and power. Focusing on clients' strengths and resiliencies renders the therapist important and influential but at the same time relieves the therapist of the role of expert conductor of the therapeutic session. Sutherland (2007) explains the preferences and standpoints of discursive therapists in this way:

> Discursive therapists share the preference for the metaphors of text, narrative, or discourse; skepticism with respect to discovering singular objective truths; an emphasis on the prominent role of language in the everyday constitution of meaning and action; the view of problems and solutions as evolving socio-cultural practices; and therapy as a process of mutual influence and transformation. These therapists advocate for a pragmatic and non-pathological approach to working with families. They respect clients' idiosyncrasies, preferences, and priorities and focus on clients' expertise and capacity to implement desired changes. Most importantly, discursive practitioners view their own use of language in therapy as constructive of the "reality" of clients' lives, identities, and relationships, rather than viewing it as objectively reflective of that reality (p. 195).

SFBT, in common with other discursive therapeutic approaches, when conducted with skill and elegance, opens up possibilities for ways of being that signify movement, positive change, and life for client and therapist alike. Appleby (2008) suggests that the closing off of possibilities is akin to death and that static understandings, descriptions, and definitions freeze and truncate possibilities for difference and newness; whereas, examining how meanings, descriptions, and definitions have come to be understood in the ways that they have gives rise to people, relationships, and words that 'are in a constant state of becoming' (p. 108). Given the choice, it is reasonable to assume that most therapists and clients alike would choose possibility, hope, and becoming over being boxed in and stuck.

It requires vigilance to avoid freezing words into static descriptions, or worse, into prescriptions and dogma. When words are fashioned into certain forms like problem statements, diagnoses, or even poetry they tend to develop a weightiness that is more difficult to ignore than if they were left as airy thoughts or ideas. When meanings are static, words become weighty and can be used to bludgeon. When meanings are open to interpretation, words are breezy and invite exploration and play. The short poem that follows by Billy Collins (1988), former Poet Laureate of the United States, and reprinted with permission of the University of Arkansas Press, presents a choice about how to approach words—a very similar choice that is also presented to therapists who must decide what they are to do with their tools of words and language.

> Introduction To Poetry
>   (Billy Collins, New York, USA)*
> I ask them to take a poem
> and hold it up to the light
> like a color slide

---

* **Credit:** Billy Collins, 'Introduction to Poetry' from *The Apple that Astonished Paris*. Copyright © 1988, 1996 by Billy Collins. Used by permission of the University of Arkansas Press, http://www.uapress.com.

or press an ear against its hive.
I say drop a mouse into a poem
and watch him probe his way out,
or walk inside the poem's room
and feel the walls for a light switch.
I want them to waterski
across the surface of a poem
waving at the author's name on the shore.
But all they want to do
is tie the poem to a chair with rope
and torture a confession out of it.
They begin beating it with a hose
to find out what it really means.

SFBT and bipolar disorder

I remember hearing Steve de Shazer say, when asked about whether SFBT could be used with people who had psychotic experiences, that he couldn't make hallucinations go away but that he could make them less bothersome to people. A part of my work involves working with people who have been diagnosed with bipolar disorder—many of whom have experience with hallucinations and/or delusions that are sometimes quite troubling to them. As part of this work I also consult with family members who have developed their own concerns around their loved one's bipolar condition. In this section of the chapter, I will provide a series of examples from my work with people diagnosed with bipolar disorder and their family members. I will also provide an example of how I used an SFBT perspective, focusing on exceptions, in a blog on PsychCentral that reaches a wide audience of people diagnosed with bipolar and their family members.

Vignette 1: a young man with auditory hallucinations

I had been consulted by a young man who had been diagnosed with bipolar disorder and who complained of intrusive auditory hallucinations. He had been prescribed lithium and an atypical antipsychotic medication to control his bipolar. He felt that he was 'going in circles' and that he wasn't achieving any of his goals for the future which included being able to concentrate better, finding a job, and, having a girlfriend. Although our work together also included focusing on concentration, getting a job, and finding a girlfriend, the following vignette deals only with the hallucinations.

What I didn't do

I didn't challenge the notion of mental illness or the construction of bipolar disorder. I also didn't question his medications.

What I did do

T: What is different between the times when your hallucinations are bothering you a lot and when they stay more in the background?
C: (Without hesitation) They bother me more when I haven't had enough sleep, when my medication isn't right, and when I'm not doing anything interesting.
T: How are the hallucinations different when they are not bothering you so much?

C: When they don't bother me so much, they're just like a low rumble or low buzz in the background that I can ignore. When they bother me a lot, I get confused about what to listen to—them or the person I'm talking to or what's on television. When they're bad, they distract me and get in my way. When they're not so bad, I can ignore them.

T: So it seems like you have a pretty good idea of what's going on in general when the hallucinations stay in the background. I'm wondering if it would be helpful to think about what small steps you can start to take every day to help the hallucinations stay there in the background.

C: Yeah, that would help. I need them to be in the background because they get in my way.

Vignette 2: a worried mother of a college-aged daughter with bipolar

A 65-year-old mother of a college aged daughter with bipolar consulted me about her fears and concerns for her daughter's welfare and future. Her daughter returned home from college 2 years previously after a serious suicide attempt in which she had suffered multiple injuries. The daughter was living in the house with her mother and father and the mother said she knew her daughter needed to be more independent but was terrified that she would try to kill herself again. The excerpt below focuses on what it might take for the mother to increase her own confidence in her daughter's ability to live independently.

What I didn't do

I didn't focus our therapeutic conversations on how well or how poorly the mother thought her daughter was doing. Nor did I engage the mother in conversation about the details of her daughter's past suicide attempt.

What I did do

T: What is it that you've noticed that leads you to believe your daughter needs more independence from you and her father?

C: She's cranky with me about how I do things around the house and she's bored with us and the things we talk about. I think she should be living on her own and she's said that she wants to, but I'm so afraid of what might happen to her. She's made a lot of progress but I don't know if it's the right time for her to move out or not.

T: What sorts of things might you start to notice that would give you more confidence about your daughter's ability to live on her own or with a friend?

C: That she would talk to me about it and that we would start to make plans and arrangements we could all live with.

T: When you think about it, in terms of your own confidence in your daughter's ability to live on her own, where would you rate yourself now on a scale from 1 to 10, with one being no confidence and ten being full confidence?

C: I guess I'd have to say a '6'. That's actually a surprise. I'm over the half-way mark.

T: If you wanted to move your confidence level up a half or full point what small steps might you take that would help move you in the direction you want?

C: Well I guess I could stop waiting for her to raise the issue of moving out and make it easier for her to talk with us about it. If I knew how she felt about it and more details about what she wanted to do it would make me feel better. I've just been so afraid. That would maybe get me half a point. If I wanted the full point, I'd have to take a deep breath and talk to her about how I needed to feel safe that she would reach out if she started to feel bad again.

Vignette 3: blogging for bipolar and asking about exceptions

What follows is my blog on PsychCentral entitled 'Coping with and Treating Bipolar: What Works for You?' (12 March 2010). This blog entry is part of 'The Bipolar Advantage' blog hosted by PsychCentral. John Grohol's PsychCentral is an award winning psychology and mental health website celebrating its 15th anniversary and has been named as an innovator organization of the Society for Participatory Medicine. PsychCentral and the Bipolar Advantage support the mission of the Society for Participatory Medicine which is to foster deep engagement of clients/patients with health care providers in all areas affecting their health. 'The Bipolar Advantage' blog is hosted by PsychCentral and was developed by Tom Wootton, a leading mental health consumer advocate and author (Wootton 2005, 2007, 2010). Wootton invites readers to consider alternative constructions of mental illness and of what it can mean in a life-enhancing way to live with such a diagnosis. The 'Bipolar Advantage' blog is read by people from around the world so the ideas and questions posed on it have quite a long reach. Most of the blog readers are either people diagnosed with a mental illness, family and friends, or mental health professionals. In the blog, which is reprinted here in its entirety, I focused on the complementarity that exists between 'problem' and 'solution' or 'exception' when dealing with the construction of 'bipolar disorder'. The central question that I posed in the blog is a solution-focused exception question. Hopefully, the participatory nature and tone of the blog is also evident.

Coping with and treating bipolar: what works for you?

I'm going to start this blog by making my operating assumption transparent. My assumption is that those who visit this site and read 'The Bipolar Advantage' blog entries are looking to improve the quality of their lives, whether they have bipolar or another condition or whether they love someone who does. There is much wisdom in what has been written on this blog by a team of talented and caring individuals. There is also much wisdom expressed by those who have commented. The result is the development of collective wisdom about what it means to live with bipolar or another condition that comes from the reflections of the writers and readers together—and all who participate here are both readers and writers.

Whether you are a person with bipolar or another condition or a loved one, it might be easier to recount the pain and struggles of daily life and finding help than it is to recount what has worked for you. The pain and struggles may indeed be part of the journey to finding help and more tranquility. In the 28 February, 2010 *New York Times Magazine*, Jonah Lehrer wrote a fascinating article entitled 'Depression's Upside'. (Sounds to me very like Tom Wotton's *The Depression Advantage*). In his article, Lehrer said that 'if depression didn't exist—if we didn't react to stress and trauma with endless ruminations—then we would be less likely to solve our predicaments. Wisdom isn't cheap and we pay for it with pain' (p. 41).

Finding solutions and what works taps one's creative resources and also requires investigating one's own trial and error efforts to create a personally satisfying life in order to separate what works from what doesn't work. Finding solutions and what works in one's own life is a form of artistry that can result in highly individual and unique solutions and outcomes. We would like to tap into the collective wisdom of those who come to this blog looking for a better quality of life by gathering together descriptions of what has been helpful for you as a person with bipolar or another condition or for you as a loved one or family member. To help us gather together the collective wisdom of those living every day with bipolar or another condition we are asking that you respond to the following question. You can be a person with bipolar or another condition or a loved one or family member. Here's the question to which we are inviting you to respond:

> What experiences and/or treatments have you as a person with a bipolar condition or other condition or you as a family member of a person with a bipolar condition found helpful in managing, coping with, and/or treating bipolar in you or a family member?

Remember the focus is on what has worked and what you have found to be helpful not on the opposite. There's a lot written already about the pain—this is about the pleasure of crafting solutions and building a life worth living, however challenging that may have been or be. You can respond to the question in the comments section. Remember your comments are available to all readers so only include information you are comfortable sharing with others. Also, please don't refer to a family member or treatment provider by name in your comments. By responding you can help us build the collective wisdom of what has worked and what has been helpful for people with bipolar or another condition and their loved ones. Send stories, vignettes, ways of thinking, ways of shifting your thinking, practices, treatments—anything and everything that has made a positive difference in your life. We'll put it all together and share it back with you.

Readers' responses

Since the blog was only published in mid-March, 2010, I have not had the opportunity yet to summarize and thematize the responses to it. Most of the responses came from individuals who had been diagnosed with bipolar disorder while a few came from family members. As we might expect from the solution-focused manner in which the question was posed, the readers responded to the question of 'What works for you?' in a wide variety of ways but almost universally focused on ways of thinking and acting that had helped them to manage or cope with bipolar more effectively than they had at some point in their pasts. There was clearly no 'one size fits all' way of managing or coping with bipolar, but, interestingly, a number of readers commented that reading material like 'The Bipolar Advantage' blog was reassuring and helped them to assess their own ways of thinking better. Staying connected to hopeful and more positive constructions of bipolar disorder was meaningful to a number of readers. Practices like gratitude, acceptance, and self-patience were also mentioned as very helpful.

Other practices, like developing a framework for looking at, questioning, and appraising one's own thoughts and reactions, was also mentioned. Some readers found medications helpful to essential; other readers found medications unhelpful and had given them up, at least at the time of their writing in to the blog.

Closing reflections

When talking in any way about the immense cultural construction of mental illness, it is more common to find discussions of how impossible and agonizing life is with a mental illness than it is to find discussions about what might be helpful or even advantageous. Such a skew in favour of negative and deficit perspectives has real implications for people diagnosed with a mental illness and for their family members. It's not hard to see how both those with a diagnosis of mental illness and their family members can be understood for feeling frightened and largely hopeless given the volume of gloomy information that exists about causes, aetiology, and prognoses. While no doubt well-intended, the information about how to deal with bipolar and other mental illnesses tends to reduces options and resources for thinking and acting creatively because it is so prescriptive, and so narrowly prescriptive at that. For a scared parent, an adult child who deviates from the narrowly prescriptive formula for living with bipolar or another mental illness can thrust a whole family into chaos and shift an attitude of mutual support and helpfulness to an unhelpful one of constant surveillance of one party over the other.

Hence the critical importance when dealing with mental illness of introducing variety and pushing out the boundaries of what works for people. The rationale for the blog 'What Works for You?' was to invite people to think about and share what they had done that had worked for them in terms of effectively living with and managing bipolar. The blog specifically asked people to share only their stories of what worked—not their broader life stories about what happened in their lives and how they came to be diagnosed. The goal was to provide a forum where people could share their own unique approaches and experiences in being at least comfortably and possibly satisfyingly bipolar. The principles of SFBT that emphasize the 'solution' side of the problem/solution complementarity can be put to good use in the area of what is called 'serious mental illness' because it is an area in which the constraints for thinking about and managing the set of disorders involved are typically quite narrow and rigid.

The techniques and practices of SFBT may seem deceptively simple. Their constructionist assumptions lead therapists who elect to practise from an SFBT perspective to listen in the present with an ear to the future and to co-create conversations that help people move into their preferred versions of their futures. Along with the excitement and creativity that is still a part of the SFBT community, there is now a sizable body of research that supports the effectiveness of SFBT for a wide variety of problems and in a wide range of populations.

References

Appleby, B. S. (2008). Trace and transference: Therapy in a post-structuralist era. *American Journal of Psychotherapy,* **62**(2), 103–115.

Argyris, C. (1991). Teaching smart people how to learn. *Harvard Business Review,* **69**, 99–109.
Bannink, F. P. (2006). Solution-focused mediation. *Journal of Conflict Management,* **7**, 143–45.
Bannink, F. P. (2007). Solution-focused brief therapy. *Journal of Contemporary Psychotherapy,* **37**, 87–94.
Baum, F. L. and Denslow, W. W. (1900, 2000). *The wonderful Wizard of Oz* (100th anniversary ed.). HarperCollins, New York.
Berg, I. K. (1994). *Family-based services: A solution-focused approach.* Norton, New York.
Berg, I. K. and Dolan, Y. (2001). *Tales of solution: A collection of hope inspiring stories.* Norton, New York.
Berg, I. K. and Cauffman, L. (2003). *Solution focused corporate coaching.* Lernende Organisation, Jänner, February, 1–5.
Berg, I. K. and Miller, S. D. (1992). *Working with the problem drinker: A solution-focused approach.* Norton, New York.
Berg, I. K. and Steiner, T. (2003). *Children's solution work.* Norton, New York.
Bohr, N. (1937). Causality and complementarity. *Philosophy of Science,* **4**(3), 289–98.
Brody, N. and Oppenheim, P. (1969). Application of Bohr's principle of complementarity to the mind-body problem. *The Journal of Philosophy,* **66**, 4, 97–113.
Cauffman, L. (2003). *Solution-focused management and coaching.* Lemma, Utrecht.
Collins, B. (1988). *The apple that astonished Paris.* The University of Arkansas Press, Fayetteville, AR.
de Shazer, S. (1982). *Patterns of brief family therapy: An ecosystemic approach.* New York: Guilford Press
de Shazer, S. (1985). *Keys to solution in brief therapy.* Norton, New York.
de Shazer, S. (1988). *Clues: investigating solutions in brief therapy.* Norton, New York.
de Shazer, S. (1991). *Putting difference to work.* Norton, New York.
de Shazer, S. (1994). *Words were originally magic.* Norton, New York.
de Shazer, S., Berg, I. K., Lipchik, E., Nunnally, E., Molnar, A., and Gingerich, W. (1986). Brief therapy: Focused solution development. *Family Process,* **25**(2), 207–21.
Dolan, Y. (1991). *Resolving sexual abuse: Solution-focused therapy and Ericksonian hypnosis for survivors.* Norton, New York.
Duffy, M. (2010). *Coping with and Treating Bipolar: What Works for You?* 12 March. http://blogs.psychcentral.com/bipolar-advantage/2010/03/what-works-for-you/ [Accessed 29 March 2010.]
Eakes, G., Walsh, S., Markowski, M., Cain, H., and Swanson, M. (1997). Family centered brief solution-focused therapy with chronic schizophrenia: A pilot study. *Journal of Family Therapy,* **19**, 145–58.
Folse, H. (1985). *The philosophy of Niels Bohr: The framework of complementarity.* North Holland, New York.
Franklin, C., Moore, K., and Hopson, L. (2008). Effectiveness of solution-focused brief therapy in a school setting. *Children and Schools,* **30**(1), 15–26.
Hoyt, M. F. (1994). On the importance of keeping it simple and taking the patient seriously: A conversation with Steve de Shazer and John Weakland. In M. F. Hoyt (Ed.) *Constructive therapies,* pp. 11–40. Guilford, New York.
HSBC Bank (2008). The evolution of 'Your Point of View' campaign, 20 October. http://www.hsbcusa.com/ourcompany/pressroom/2008/news_10292008_hsbc_campaign.html [Accessed 29 March 2010.]

Johnson, L. D. and Miller, S. D. (1994). Modification of depression risk factors: a solution-focused approach. *Psychotherapy: Theory, Research, Practice, Training*, **31**, 244–53.

Kim, J. S. (2008). Examining the effectiveness of solution-focused brief therapy: A meta-analysis. *Research on Social Work Practice*, **18**(2), 107–16.

Kral, R. (1995). *Solutions for schools*. Brief Family Therapy Center, Milwaukee, WI.

Lehrer, J. (2010). Depression's upside. *The New York Times Magazine*, 28 February, 38–44.

Lindforss, L. and Magnusson, D. (1997). Solution-focused therapy in prison. *Contemporary Family Therapy*, **19**, 89–104.

Lipchik, E. (2002). *Beyond technique in solution-focused therapy: Working with emotions and the therapeutic relationship*. New York: Guilford.

McCollum, E. E. and Trepper, T.S. (2001). *Creating family solutions for substance abuse*. Haworth Press, New York.

Macdonald, A. J. (1994) Brief therapy in adult psychiatry. *Journal of Family Therapy*, **16**, 415–26.

Macdonald, A. J. (1997). Brief therapy in adult psychiatry: further outcomes. *Journal of Family Therapy*, **19**, 13–22.

Maines, R. P. (1999). *The technology of orgasm:"Hysteria," the vibrator, and women's sexual satisfaction*. The Johns Hopkins University Press, Baltimore, MA.

Metcalf, L. (2002). *Counseling toward solutions: A practical solution-focused program for working with students, teachers, and parents*. Jossey-Bass, San Francisco, CA.

Miller, S. D., Hubble, M. A. and Duncan, B. L. (eds.). (1996). *Handbook of solution-focused brief therapy*. Jossey-Bass, San Francisco, CA.

Murray, C. E. and Murray, T. L. (2004). Solution-focused premarital counseling: Helping couples build a vision for their marriage. *Journal of Marital and Family Therapy*, **30**, 349–58.

Newsome, W. S. (2004). Solution-focused brief therapy (SFBT) groupwork with at-risk junior high school students: Enhancing the bottom-line. *Research on Social Work Practice*, **14**, 336–43.

Peller, J. and Walter, J. (1992/93). Celebrating the living: A solution-focused approach to the normal grieving process. *Family Therapy Case Studies*, **7**(2), 3–7

Pichot, T. (2001). Cocreating solutions for substance abuse. *Journal of Systemic Therapies*, **20**, 2, 1–23.

Pichot, T. and Dolan, Y. (2003). *Solution-focused brief therapy: Its effective use in agency settings*. Haworth Press, New York.

Selekman, M. D. (1993). *Pathways to change*. Guilford, New York.

Selekman, M. D. (1997). *Solution-focused therapy with children*. Guilford, New York.

Sharry, J. (2001). *Solution focused groupwork*. Sage, London.

Sharry, J., Darmody, M., and Madden, B. (2002). A solution-focused approach to working with clients who are suicidal. *British Journal of Guidance & Counselling*, **20**, 383–99.

Simon, D. (1996). Crafting consciousness through form: Solution-focused therapy as a spiritual path. In S. D. Miller, M. A. Hubble, & B. L. Duncan, (eds.). *Handbook of solution-focused brief therapy*, pp. 44–62, Jossey-Bass, San Francisco, CA.

Sutherland, O. (2007). Therapist positioning and power in discursive therapies: A comparative analysis. *Contemporary family therapy*, **29**, 193–209.

Trepper, T. S., Dolan, Y., McCollum, E. E., and Nelson, T. (2006). Steve de Shazer and the future of solution-focused therapy. *Journal of Marital and Family Therapy*, **32**(2), 133–9.

Young, S. and Holdore, G. (2003). Using solution-focused brief therapy in individual referrals for bullying. *Educational Psychology in Practice,* **19**, 271–82.

Walter, J. L. and Peller, J. E. (1996). Rethinking our assumptions: Assuming anew in a postmodern world. In S. D. Miller, M. A. Hubble, and B. L. Duncan, (eds.). *Handbook of solution-focused brief therapy,* pp. 9–26. Jossey-Bass, San Francisco, CA.

Wolf, F. A. (1989). *Taking the quantum leap: The new physics for nonscientists* (Rev. Ed.). Harper Perennial, New York.

Wootton, T. (2005). *The bipolar advantage.* Bipolar Advantage, San Francisco, CA.

Wootton, T. (2007). *The depression advantage.* Bipolar Advantage, San Francisco, CA.

Wootton, T. (2010). *Bipolar in order: Looking at depression, mania, hallucination, and delusion from the other side.* Bipolar Advantage, San Francisco, CA.

Zimmerman, T. S., Prest, L. A. and Wetzel, B. E. (1997). Solution-focused couples therapy groups: An empirical study. *Journal of Family Therapy,* **19**, 125–44.

Chapter 9

From Wittgenstein, complexity, and narrative emergence: discourse and solution-focused brief therapy

Gale Miller and Mark McKergow

> A living language is in a state far from equilibrium. It changes, it is in contact with other languages, it is abused and transformed. This does not mean that meaning is a random or arbitrary process. It means that **meaning** is a local phenomenon, valid in a certain frame of time and space . . . Above all, language is a system in which individual words do not have significance on their own. Meaning is only generated when individual words are caught in the play of the system
>
> *Complexity and postmodernism: Understanding complex systems,*
>
> Paul Cilliers (1998, p. 124).

Solution-focused brief therapy (SFBT) interactions are designed to facilitate change by assisting clients in clarifying how they would like their lives to be different, inviting new descriptions of what is possible in clients' lives, and by identifying resources that clients might use in changing their lives. There is a sense, then, in which change is 'talked into being' (Heritage 1984a) in SFBT interactions. This is not to say that change is an illusion or fiction that is unrelated to the practical events and relationships of clients' lives. It is, rather, to say that SFBT interactions provide clients with resources for seeing and acting on possibilities for change that are already, to some degree, present in their lives. Change in SFBT is a co-construction involving clients, therapists and others' in clients' lives. Put differently, change happens in social interactions occurring within therapy sessions and in clients' non-therapy lives. It is a social construction because change involves formulating and applying new orientations to self, others, and the future.

SFBT was initially developed by a group of therapists and academics associated with the Brief Family Therapy Center (Milwaukee, WI, USA) in the 1980s and 1990s. It emerged within a practical clinical context concerned with fostering effective and efficient change in the lives of a socially diverse population of clients (Miller 1997). The precursor to the approach was a variant of strategic therapy (de Shazer 1982) and, later, it evolved into contemporary SFBT (de Shazer 1988, 1991). The history of SFBT is a process of moving from a systemic perspective to a discursive orientation emphasizing how problems and solutions are organized within clients' use of language.

These changes were accompanied by evolving descriptions of observable interactional processes in therapy (Miller 1997, 2001).

The discursive emphases of SFBT became clear with the ascension of a Wittgensteinian (1958) perspective as the dominant descriptive language of the early solution-focused brief therapists (de Shazer 1988, 1991). They drew upon Wittgenstein in developing an interpretive framework for giving language to practice (Mattingly and Fleming 1994), that is, for seeing and talking about the otherwise unnoticed aspects of their interactions with clients. The therapists' interest in discourse went beyond the questions and other 'techniques' that are often associated with SFBT. They also included the 'philosophy' of SFBT, which consists of the assumptions and concerns that organize SFBT interactions.

We explore the philosophy and practice of SFBT in this essay. First, we discuss discursive themes at the centre of solution-focused brief therapists' conversations about their practices and relationships with clients. These conversations have implications for how SFBT is conceptualized in empirical studies. Our second purpose involves extending the conceptual reach of commentaries on SFBT and empirical studies of it by developing connections to complexity theory.

Complexity theory is concerned with the organization and operations of complex systems, which are defined by their ability to transform unstructured beginnings into new and more complex patterns of relationship (Cilliers 1998; Merry 1995; Stacey 2000; Waldrop 1992). Complex systems are said to be self-organizing because they have the capacity to adapt to unanticipated events and uncertain environments by transforming themselves (Griffin 2002; Shaw 2002). Thus, complex systems are sites of synergistic change that emerges as aspects of systems react to one another to produce new system relationships and possibilities. One such site consists of persons' uses of language within social interaction to produce new and unpredicted meanings and orientations to social reality. This is, of course, the focus of discursive therapies and of discursively-oriented studies of therapy.

> For discursive therapists, the therapeutic conversation is where and how change happens... When clients' presenting problems and solutions can be seen as discursively related to how they are regarded and talked about, therapy can be helpful insofar as it helps us put words to the inarticulable. However, it also can be helpful should it: dis-solve a concern...; generatively challenge our assumptions and introduce new perspectives, prompt aha's where we find our own solutions; or inspire us to look beyond our normal cognitive horizons. Thus, discursive therapy sees change occurring in the back and forth of communicative interaction (Strong and Lock 2005, p. 589).

We see complexity theory as a useful framework for describing SFBT practices and their implications for clients' lives. It is a standpoint for exploring the assumptions and practices of SFBT practitioners, and for refocusing conversations about SFBT in the future. Complexity theory also has implications for the kinds of questions that discursively-oriented researchers ask about SFBT, and what they treat as relevant data for their discursive analyses of it.

A major emphasis running through this essay is 'narrative emergence'. We use this term to call attention to several interrelated aspects of SFBT as a distinctive form of discursive therapy and complex system. The concerns include recognition that while the future is unknowable, it is an ever present possibility in the present. We continuously create and discover the future by engaging in self-organizing activities (particularly social interactions) that are, at least partly, improvised, and potentially transformative. Thus, the narratives emergent in our everyday lives are always under construction. They exist in our ongoing 'work' to make sense of and manage the exigencies of life. We take up these issues later in the essay. But, first, we turn to a Wittgensteinian understanding of SFBT.

A Wittgensteinian understanding

Aspects of the discursive approach to therapy abound in the evolution of SFBT. For example, the therapy practices developed by early solution-focused brief therapists emphasized how talk and social interaction are practical activities having consequences for persons' lives. The therapists treated solution-building in therapy as an interactional accomplishment that involved both clients and therapists. The therapists asked questions that were designed to help clients describe their past and present lives in new ways, and to articulate clear images of what their future lives will look like. Further, clients were cast as the ultimate authorities in determining the focus and goals of their therapy interactions. Therapists and clients initiated change by constructing circumstances that justified clients' saying that they knew how to go on with changing their lives (Wittgenstein 1958, nos. 154–55).

Problems and solutions as language games

A major move in solution-focused brief therapists' discursive turn was their use of Wittgenstein's concept of language game to differentiate between problems and solutions as forms of talk and orientations to life (de Shazer 1988, 1991). Language games are socially shared uses of verbal and nonverbal language that organize social settings, relationships and interactions as kinds of events (Wittgenstein 1958). Wittgenstein uses this metaphor to call attention to the game-like organization of such mundane human activities as telling jokes, expressing and accepting sympathy and reporting on events (Gill 1996). But he also uses it in discussing the social contexts in which people tell jokes, express and accept sympathy, report on events and otherwise use language to achieve their practical ends.

These aspects of language games are inextricably interconnected for Wittgenstein and solution-focused brief therapists. For example, what counts as a funny joke, credible expression of sympathy, or adequate report varies from one social context to another. But, at the same time, we distinguish between different kinds of social contexts by observing and interpreting people's activities within social interaction. We 'see' social contexts by noticing what kinds of jokes people laugh and don't laugh at, how they express and accept sympathy, and how they describe their experiences in the world. It is in the interplay between persons' concrete uses of language and the contexts that frame their interactions that meanings emerge, including people's senses of themselves as competent members of society, and of how their lives generally fit with the worlds in which they live. Hence, language games are homes for words and meanings (Pitkin 1972).

Solution-focused brief therapists treat problems and solutions as different ways of talking about how the events of clients' lives fit or do not fit with clients' preferred ways of life. The problems language game emphasizes what is out of sync in clients' lives, the ongoing negative consequences of their problems (including clients' fears, anxieties, and frustrations with their circumstances), and often on what might have caused clients' lives to go awry. Social interactions focused on such issues are contexts for selectively describing life as beyond clients' control. It is a language game of restricted personal agency and continuing disappointment, failure or worry. Therapy extends such talk by classifying clients' problems, and using problem categories to define clients' selves and life trajectories.

The solutions language game emphasizes clients' competencies, agency, and past successes in managing their lives. Solution-focused interactions orient to the future by treating clients' strengths and abilities as springboards for constructing new and better lives. Concern for identifying the causes of persons' problems and classifying the problems within diagnostic categories are replaced by questions about how clients are able to get by despite their problems, the times when clients' problems are less severe, and how clients will know that their lives have gotten a little bit better. Such topics are central to selective description in SFBT. These therapists draw upon the client depictions of themselves and their lives in developing parting messages that many solution-focused brief therapists give to clients at the end of therapy sessions. The messages consist of compliments and perhaps suggestions that clients might think about or do between therapy sessions. The messages are designed to link therapy with clients' non-therapy lives, thereby facilitating between session changes.

The idea that problems and solutions are language games has profound implications for therapists' orientations to therapy. It shifts attention away from such questions as, 'Does this client really suffer from a significant problem?', 'What kind of problem are we dealing with?', and 'What can I do to solve the client's problem?' Rather, the issues of concern centre on clients' use of language, particularly how therapists might help clients to leave problem talk and enter the discourse of solutions. This shift involves more than getting clients to use different words, because the logics of the problems and solutions language games are fundamentally different. Language games are homes for meaning because they are contexts of inference (Pitkin 1972; Sacks 1992; Wittgenstein 1958). As Levinson (1983) explains,

> understanding an utterance involves a great deal more than knowing the meanings of words uttered and the grammatical relations between them. Above all, understanding an utterance involves the making of *inferences* that will connect what is said to what is mutually assumed or what has been said before
>
> (Levinson 1983, p. 21).

In participating in problem- and solution-focused language games, then, we learn to make connections between issues and events that are spoken about and those that are left unsaid. The simultaneous processes of talk and interpretation that organize therapy form conditions of possibility for constructing accounts that assign coherence and direction to clients' lives.

SFBT as an interactional event

The idea that problems and solutions are language games lends itself to a variety of discursive strategies of observation, description, and analysis. Three popular and related strategies are conversation, rhetorical and narrative analyses. Each of them highlights aspects of SFBT sessions as interactional events. We use the term *interactional event* to stress how solution-focused brief and other therapy interactions are discrete, bounded, and socially recognized interactions that take place in identifiable times and places. While the interactions may orient to the past and project future lives for clients, they are organized around beginnings and endings with a limited array of activities occurring in between.

Conversational, rhetorical, and narrative approaches to SFBT emphasize how the problems and solutions language games are interactionally organized, the 'moves' available to 'players' (clients, therapists and other participants) within the language games and the storylines that the 'players' interactionally construct. Conversation analysis is designed to expose the machinery of social interactions (Sacks 1992), particularly the sequential or turn-taking organization of interactions, the interpretive methods used by participants in the interactions, and the inferences that they express in interaction. The machinery of social interaction forms a platform for the construction of therapy and other social realities.

For example, conversation analysts discuss how solution-focused brief therapists ask optimistic questions that call for answers describing clients' strengths, abilities, and successes (MacMartin 2008), express formulations that summarize and reframe selected aspects of clients' remarks (Bavelas et al 2000; Gale and Newfield 1992), and offer candidate answers to these questions (Gale 1991). We have observed a variety of other interactional moves by solution-focused therapists, including change-of-state tokens (Heritage 1984b) that mark clients' statements as significant and impressive (such as responding to clients' reports with 'Wow!'), and perspective display sequences (Maynard 1991) that begin with the therapists asking for clients' perspectives on an issue and then either asking for further elaboration or offering their own interpretations of the issue. Solution-focused brief therapists also use extreme case formulations (Pomerantz 1986) to highlight the extraordinary nature of clients' reports (e.g. 'So, this is a really big change for you?'), and in asking scaling and related questions (e.g. 'Think about a scale from 1–10. One is the worst that your life could possibly be and 10 is the day after your miracle happens, where are you on that scale right now?').

Solution-focused brief therapists' uses of language are also rhetorical moves. They are devices of persuasion that justify therapists' preference for interpreting clients' lives in solution-focused ways. So viewed, therapy interactions are micro-political processes in which therapists and clients negotiate the practical meaning of their relationship, the focus of each therapy session, and what needs to happen in order for the clients to say that therapy was helpful (Roy-Chowdbury 2006; Miller 1986). The conversational moves discussed above are, then, resources that solution-focused brief therapists selectively use to convince clients that their problems are not intractable, and that change is possible. Change-of-state tokens—such as 'wow'—are particularly interesting since they suggest that clients have reported something that has significantly impressed or otherwise altered their therapists' understanding of the issues at hand (Heritage 1984b). Of course, researchers might also consider how clients' answers are persuasive moves within this language game.

Another useful rhetorical approach involves analysing the structure of problems as forms of argumentation, and how solution-focused interactions undercut them. A useful starting point is Emerson's (1981) analysis of last resorts as arguments that cast problems as intractable and justifying extreme responses to them as well as feelings of despair and hopelessness (Järvinen and Miller 2010). Solution-focused interactions undercut last resort arguments by inviting clients to reflect on and describe the times when their problems have not been so overwhelming, the larger implications of making small changes in their lives, and how clients keep going despite their problems. Therapists' parting messages further amplify these themes.

The rhetorical processes embedded in SFBT interactions are also sources for constructing new narratives of self and life for clients (Miller 1997). While they are seldom fully developed as new life stories, these interactions unfold as storylines about clients as strong, intelligent, loving and resourceful people who live in social environments that offer some level of resources that clients might use in changing their lives. SFBT storylines also include depictions of the times when clients have used their personal agency to address problems, when clients' problems were not so severe, and what clients' lives will look like after a miracle happens. Narrative themes in SFBT might be analysed as alternatives to the chaotic, tragic, and disempowering storylines of the problems language game (Frank 1995; Miller and de Shazer 1991). Solution-focused brief therapists treat clients' depictions of their lives as 'evidence' justifying solution-focused storylines.

There are a variety of narrative perspectives available to researchers in explicating how solution-building is a form of story-telling. For example, interesting analyses might focus on the tropes used by therapists and clients to construct dramatic plots (White 1978), the embodied performance aspects of therapy interactions (Langellier and Peterson 2004), and how therapists and clients negotiate narrative paradigms for clients' lives (Roth 1989). We believe that a particularly useful approach is Burke's (1969) dramatistic perspective, which blends concern for narratives with attention to the importance of inference in telling convincing stories. Of special note is his claim that speakers and listeners orient to events, issues, and feelings as dramas involving characters, scenes, agents, forms of agency, and purposes. Burke's perspective suggests that effective narratives do not need to be expressed as full-fledged stories, a partially developed storyline is a sufficient invitation to listeners to elaborate it on their own.

Taken together, conversation, rhetorical and narrative analyses describe how solution-focused brief therapists and clients co-construct emergent narratives. The narratives emerge in their persuasive talk and stories about clients' strengths and abilities, past successes in problem solving, why it is reasonable to assume that clients' lives will change in the future. Narrative emergence is also facilitated by clients' depictions of how change might place in their lives and what the change will look like. We next turn to how this understanding of SFBT might be extended and even transformed within complexity theory.

A complexity perspective

Complexity, by that name and as an explicit topic of interest, has been a part of the intellectual landscape since the 1980s (Cilliers 1998, Merry 1995), particularly with the publication of Waldrop's *Complexity: The Emerging Science at the Edge of Order and Chaos* (1992). Interest spread rapidly into diverse fields, including biochemistry and physics, economics, computational science, sociology, political science, ecology, and management studies (Cilliers 2005; Gell-Mann 1994; Jantsch 1980; Lewin 1992; McKergow 1996; Ormerod 1998; Stacey 2007; Stein 1989). To define a complex system is not easy because these systems do not behave in the familiar manner of conventional thinking and analysis. This is why we begin by defining what complex systems are not, and then turn to how complexity theory is useful in understanding diverse conversations, including solution-focused interactions.

Complex systems need not be complicated. Complicated systems often appear to be complex because they consist of many specialized parts that are connected in linear relationships. The parts are, to varying degrees, dependent on each other for their proper functioning and designed to operate in recurring ways (Cilliers 1998). Thus, they lack the ability to learn or innovate. An example is the automobile, which is designed to accomplish a limited number of predictable actions. Indeed, unpredictability in complicated systems is a sign of trouble because system parts are linked together linearly. This makes it possible for us to describe them in the language of causality. If a car does not start and makes a particular kind of noise when we turn the ignition key, then we can say that the problem is probably caused by X, Y, or Z. Further, complicated-linear systems may be analytically parsed and represented as texts, pictures, formulas, or stories. For example, the circuit diagram of the car's electrical system will show all that is needed in order to use, build, and change it.

Aspects of complex systems

Complex systems usually include many interacting elements. The relationships among the elements often appear to be simple, but the multiple, self-referential, and rich nature of the interactions leads to behaviour that is both sensitive to small disturbances and yet robust to large infractions (Cilliers 1998). This robustness means it is very hard to 'break' or destroy a complex system, in contrast to a complicated one. It is ironic that many of us are reluctant to diagnose or repair problems with our cars, but we have no such hesitation about engaging in wide ranging conversations involving quite different speaker and listener positions, emergent rules about our own and others' behaviour, and unpredictable topics. Our typical orientation to conversation points to most people's competence at these complex, spontaneous, self-organizing interactional events. Thus, a complexity perspective on therapy calls attention to clients'—often unnoticed—conversational skills and knowledge.

A focus on complexity also points to the potential unpredictability of social interactions and of the ever present possibilities for change within them. Complex systems adapt, evolve, and may transform themselves in seemingly spontaneous ways as their elements interact with one another and with their environments. The interactions are 'rich' in the sense that they may convey multiple forms of information and meanings through various interactional means, all of which have potentially far-reaching implications for system operations and for the relationships among system elements and their environments. Consider, for example, the range and amount of information that is constructed and conveyed through verbal and nonverbal means in a dinner party interactions among friends, a metaphor introduced by Stacey (2007).

The information and meanings produced in complex system interactions are amplified, damped, and otherwise adjusted as the system elements process received information and meanings, and respond to one another. Put differently, the processes that organize particular complex systems feedback onto themselves, thereby creating conditions of possibility for the transformation of the systems. The future in complex systems emerges in ways that are neither pre-determined nor random. In the case of conversation, these feedback processes involve conversationalists' ongoing interpretations of their own and others' verbal and nonverbal actions, and adjustment of their subsequent actions in light of the interpretations. Thus, complexity and learning are built into the very act of social interaction. Stacey (2007) refers to this as 'complex responsive processes', stressing that all acts of conversation are taken in response to what has gone before and that the emergence of whatever order appears is a result of local conversational interaction between people.

Complex systems are open systems. They are so intermeshed with their environments that it is difficult—often impossible—to draw clear boundaries between the systems and their environments. Complex systems do not simply interact with their environments; they actively construct relevant environments and system-environment relations as they respond to diverse situations. Following Goodman (1978), we treat this aspect of social interaction as a world-making activity, meaning that people interactionally construct the environments to which their conversations orient. But, as Derrida (2004) points out, conversations are not built in isolation from events occurring 'outside' of the conversations. The meanings constructed in ongoing interactions include traces of other interactions that are reconstituted in the ongoing interactions. Derrida (2004, p. 23) explains:

> Whether in written or in spoken discourse, no element can function as a sign without relating to another element which itself is not simply present. This linkage means that each 'element'... is constituted with reference to the trace in it of the other elements of the sequence or system. This linkage, this weaving, is the text, which is produced only through the transformation of another text.

One implication that might be developed from Derrida's analysis is that narratives emergent in social interaction may simultaneously transform the past and orient to possible futures that are otherwise unknowable. Further, the outcomes of the self-organizing processes of complex systems are not analysable using currently available or indeed conceivable analytic methods (Richardson et al. 2001). While particular models and explanations of complex systems may be useful in representing some aspects of complex systems, they end up oversimplifying the interactional processes that make complex systems complex. Abstract models and explanations cannot anticipate how complex systems might innovate and may transform themselves—complex systems are said to be 'incompressible', and any summary or description will be incomplete, and will differ from the original in further unanalysable ways.

This is not to say that attempts at representation are without merit. As Cilliers (1998) recommends, the complexity that defines complex systems is most usefully addressed by developing diverse descriptions of complex systems operating at particular times and in particular places. He states that such descriptions can be compared, contrasted, and combined to develop multiple understandings of complex processes that are otherwise highly resistant to representation. This descriptive approach to complexity systems is a way of recognizing that all ways of knowing are partial and incomplete. They obscure even as they reveal.

Finally, aspects of complexity theory resonate with postmodernist activism. For example, both orientations to social life reject the pursuit of foundational, essentialist, and universal truths about people, social conditions, and knowledge. Rather, they focus on the diverse and shifting local contexts in which relative truths emerge and are applied. They also recognize that the application of socially constructed truths fosters potentially far-reaching changes by creating new and unpredictable contexts of action and meaning. Creating such conditions for change is a major focus of the 'intervention' strategies of affirmative activist postmodernists (Rosenau 1992). Affirmative activist postmodernism consists of a cluster of diverse optimistic, participative, and grass-roots orientations to social change. Affirmative activists use multiple discourses to generate diverse perspectives on seemingly settled realities, including narratives that might appear to belie their ideological interests (see, for example, Throgmorton 1996).

This is how affirmative postmodern activists embrace the ongoing 'politics of life,' which they treat as preferable to searching for emancipating solutions and cures to social problems (Rosenau 1992). The latter orientation is a defining feature of modernist approaches to change (Rosenau 1992). Cilliers (1998) depicts this orientation as accepting and cooperating with the complex, self-organizing processes that organize life in contemporary societies. The same language might be applied to the philosophy and practices of SFBT. Thus, the nexus of complexity theory and affirmative postmodernism forms a useful standpoint for reconsidering how SFBT is a discursive therapy.

Complexity in SFBT

Complexity theory and affirmative postmodernism are interpretive frameworks for understanding SFBT as a distinctive orientation to change. We have noted that solution-focused brief therapists reject diagnostic approaches to problems and the related assumption that problems classified in the same categories call for the same remedies. They state that diagnostic approaches over look the uniqueness of each client's life circumstances and marginalize clients' differing desires for the future. Looked at from the standpoints of complexity theory and affirmative postmodernism, solution-focused brief therapists' disinterest in diagnosis is an acknowledgement of the impossibility of reducing complex processes to therapy categories and a way of embracing the shifting politics of life.

We also see an affinity between complexity theory and SFBT in their shared emphasis on description as a world-making activity (Goodman 1978). Specifically solution-focused brief therapists treat their clients' solution-oriented descriptions as sources of change because they are alternative standpoints for engaging the shifting, non-linear complexities of life. It is significant that this approach to change does not involve developing systematic plans for transforming clients into new kinds of people. Rather, it consists of developing ideas about how clients might participate in their lives in new ways. The idea of participation, rather than intervention, is key. It recasts watching for times when one's problems are less severe, or absent and for signs that one's miracle might be happening as ways of engaging in life. Indeed, therapists participate along with clients in co-creating new significance and vitality to clients' life experiences. The focus on therapy as participation also displaces claims that therapists possess some kind of better or superior view on clients' lives.

This is how world-making is done in SFBT. It is an interactional process. The solution-focused approach to change stands in contrast to more mentalistic and biologically-oriented strategies, which emphasize how therapy interactions are occasions for assessing the underlying thoughts, emotions, beliefs, or urges that direct clients' perceptions and actions (Miller, de Shazer and De Jong 2001). Consistent with Lyotard's (1989) analysis of *The Postmodern Condition*, solution-focused brief therapists treat clients' talk as orientations to self, others, and the possibilities of their lives. Thus, change is an interactional process of refocusing clients' participation in the social relationships, communication networks, and language games of their everyday lives. It is organized within the emergent narratives constructed by therapists and clients inside and outside of therapy sessions.

Stacey (2007) discusses the difference between conversations which remain trapped in reproducing the same patterns of talk, and those which may foster the emergence of new knowledge. Following Shotter (1993) and Shaw (2002), Stacey (2007) states that:

> the thematic patterning of conversation is iterated over time as both repetition and potential transformation at the same time. However, this potential need not always be realized. . . . Change can only emerge in fluid forms of conversation. However, it is important to understand that fluid conversation is not some pure form of polar opposition to repetition
>
> (Stacey 2007, pp. 283–4).

This gives expression to the idea that no special kind of language is necessary for the emergence of new knowledge. Rather, the fluidity, spontaneity, and 'good enough holding of anxiety' of the conversational interaction itself (Stacey 2007, p. 285) seem important in encouraging potentially transforming themes. The deliberate utilization of the clients' everyday language in SFBT and the conversational focus on small details, as will be seen from the case study below, show how this emergence of knowledge is encouraged without ever referring to it in such terms.

Solution-focused brief therapists' interest in initiating change through small and often provisional steps is also consistent with complexity theorists' appreciation of modest depictions of social realities (Cilliers 2005). Modest proposals acknowledge and accept the limitations of our understandings of and control over the complex processes of life. They also orient to the unpredictability and transformative potential that are built into complex interactional processes. McKergow and Korman (2009) explain that the interactional emergence of modest proposals in SFBT occurs 'inbetween'—neither inside (stemming from inner drivers, urges, motivations or other mentalistic explanatory mechanisms) nor outside (determined by external systems, narratives or other mechanisms).

The intersecting assumptions and concerns of SFBT and complexity theory suggest how complexity theory and affirmative postmodernism might be used to put new language to therapists' and clients' practices. Complexity theory is a standpoint for organizing discursive analysts' studies of SFBT sessions as interactional events. For example, the concept of complexity is a possible point of departure for examining the claim that change in SFBT involves a language game shift from problems talk to solutions talk. This claim justifies therapists' recurring use of particular questions and other techniques in interacting with clients. It also glosses the complexity of these different, but not fully separate, orientations to language and social reality. Specifically, complexity theory sensitizes us to the diversity of potential meanings that are available within particular interactional events. They also implicitly challenge therapists and researchers to attend to the presence of both types of meanings in therapy interactions, including how therapists' recurring use of so-called solutions-focused techniques might undermine the development of potentially useful insights about clients' problem talk.

Complexity theory extends analyses of therapy sessions as interactional events by stressing the unpredictable and improvisational aspects of social interaction, particularly how small shifts in conversation may have transformative implications for conversationalists' understandings of what has already been said and what needs to be said next. This is one way in which inferences and meanings emerge in self-organizing interactions. It also points to how Derrida's (2004) analysis of traces might be applied to ongoing therapy interactions. The interactions include traces of other events and interactions but also orient to what has already occurred within the present interactional event and perhaps to what the conversationalists assume is likely to be said later in the interactions. This has been described by solution-focused practitioners as 'possibilities from past, present and future' (Jackson and McKergow 2007).

Complexity theory also has implications for rhetorical studies of solution-focused interactions. Perhaps most significant are the possible implications of complexity theorists' emphasis on description as a process of change. They explain that while we cannot fully grasp or represent complex processes, it is still useful to develop partial and selective descriptions (modest proposals) that may provide insights into otherwise unnoticed aspects of the processes. As socially constructed realities in therapy, such descriptions are potentially transformative because they invite clients to imaginatively experience change as an alternative reality for their lives. The modest proposals emergent in clients' descriptions of their possible new lives may be self-justifying, because they may be interpreted by clients as good reasons for embracing change.

For us, the most important implication of complexity theory for narrative analysis of SFBT involves the seemingly underdeveloped nature of narrative construction in these interactions. We have stated that narratives emergent in SFBT are best characterized as storylines rather than as full-fledged restoryings of clients' lives. Viewed as aspects of complex processes, the storylines are modest proposals. They are organizing themes that clients and therapists might use to create comprehensive stories that assign coherence to clients' lives. It is significant, then, that such elaboration occurs so seldom in SFBT interactions. It appears that clients may 'try out' these provisionally constructed storylines in between therapy sessions, allowing a fit to develop between their life experiences, and the reworked storylines in the same way as a new pair of shoes might feel a little strange at first and become more comfortable with repeated wear—which is not to say the shoes did not fit in the first place. Analysts might draw upon Burke's (1969) dramatistic framework in exploring this aspect of SFBT.

We see narrative emergence in SFBT working within the open and indeterminate processes of complex systems. Whether intended or not, the construction of storylines is a way of forestalling premature understandings that might make other potentially useful and transformative constructions unavailable to clients as they decide how to go on. This practice fits with the idea that we discover the unknowable future by engaging it. The practice also fits with affirmative postmodernists' definition of changes as continuing effort.

While complexity theory complements aspects of discourse analytic perspectives, it is also a framework for asking questions about their limitations. We believe that an important limitation of most conversational, rhetorical, and narrative approaches to social interaction is their overwhelming concern for the present. This focus might be interpreted in several ways. For example, it might be understood as suggesting that past practices are useful predictors of the future, a claim that is often but not always true. Another interpretation is that discursive analysts' emphasis on the past is an implicit acknowledgement that the future is unknowable. This claim is also often but not always true. Complexity theory reminds us of a third truth, which is that the future emerges within past and present interactions. It is an emergent narrative because the future is an ever present possibility in the past and present, an open set of emerging and continually transforming narratives always under construction. Complexity theory is a rubric for engaging this possibility in solution-focused interactions. Complexity theory represents one form of mindfulness about the future possibilities that pervade our lives and depictions of social reality. Adam (1995, p. 174) explains that such mindfulness involves:

> explicit cognizance of the future, not the prediction of the future, a regard for the future which takes responsibility for potential outcomes of present actions and incorporates this into present plans and decisions.

We continue our emergent narrative in the next section by discussing a case example,

A case example

This is the second meeting of the therapist and client. The client is a middle-aged white woman whose initial complaints emphasized her uncertainties about her employment status and dissatisfaction with aspects of her work relationships. She also voiced concerns about some aspects of her family life. The session is divided into the interview, which a therapy team observes from an adjoining room, a break when the therapist joins her team to construct a parting message, and the delivery of the parting message to the client. The therapist framed the parting message as a report and request from the team. The message is a selective depiction of the clients' answers in the interview that rhetorically justifies a modest solution-oriented storyline of client agency, competence, and success in creating noteworthy changes in her life.

Specifically, the therapist stated that the team was impressed with the client's clarity in describing what she wants to be different and what she has already done to improve her life. They also stress the client's personal strengths and her flexibility in managing problems in the past. The therapist continued by stating, 'The thing that most impressed us is that you've already figured out how not to be everyone's answer, and you started doing that. You call them small ways but we thought that they were pretty big ways'. She concludes by explaining that the team is confused and wants to know more about how and when the client delegates tasks to others at work and home, and a request that the client take some time before her next therapy session to 'think about that process, how you figure out how and when to do it and stuff like that'.

The parting message draws on aspects of the interview but it does not describe its contingencies, particularly how the client and therapist negotiated the focus of their therapy conversation. In looking closely at their negotiations we see how SFBT is an emergent micro-political process in which therapists and clients work at building practical orientations to clients' circumstances. It is also significant that solution-focused brief therapists, who have a clear interest in focusing the interactions on solutions talk, only rarely make this interest a condition for continuing therapy. Rather, they use questions and assessments to signal their interest in solution-oriented talk. The therapists display their assessments of clients' answers as promising by inviting elaboration, whereas they respond to client answers deemed unpromising by asking new questions that call for new lines of talk or by waiting for a more promising line to emerge in clients' depictions of themselves and their lives.

We see such negotiation at the outset of this session when the therapist asks, 'So, what's better since last time?' This optimistic question announces the therapist's interest in talking about solutions but the client responds by describing several recent incidents that suggest that her job is at risk. The client's account includes an instance of reported speech in which she quotes a brief interaction with a co-worker about their supervisors' discussion of possibly finding a replacement for the client. The therapist then asks how the incidents have been helpful to the client who replies that they have not been helpful. The therapist follows with, 'Ok. Let me ask you another question then. What would be most helpful for us to talk about here today that would help kind of get things going in the right direction as far as what, what do you want to accomplish here?'. The therapist's initial question explicitly invites the client to change the topic under discussion, while the 'Ok' may be heard as a marker indicating that the prior topic is completed and as a justification for a raising new topic.

The therapist's subsequent questions continue to express her interest in talking about change. But the client responds by stating that her boss says that she is 'suffering from a major depression', and she wonders if they should be talking about why she is suffering this illness. The client's answers foster further negotiation about the topical focus of the interview. This line of interaction fills the first 20% of the session with the therapist continuing to respond to the client's expressions of concern for the causes of her seeming depression with questions that address the therapist's 'need to know just a little bit to be able to take the next step'. The interaction takes a significant turn in the following exchange that began when the client stated that she once thought that she understood 'what makes me work the way I am,' but not anymore. The designation of [] represents overlapping talk and ↑ represents rising intonation. These and other markings are intended to convey the measured—even thoughtful—pace of the interaction, and how the therapist used her voice to highlight some client statements.

Therapist:	Ok, when you thought you did [pause]
Client:	[Hmhm, ok]
Therapist:	have a clear understanding. Ok, what kinds of things were you?
Client:	Well, I always thought of myself (pause) as a (pause) pretty strong person. Um, (pause) could handle (pause) pretty much anything that came my way.
Therapist:	Uh, huh.
Client:	(pause) Um, (pause) I had moments (pause) but I hid, I hid those moments from people. So, [no one knew]
Therapist:	[You had moments] of?
Client:	Well, (pause) they were, (pause) uh, I was not as strong as I thought I was, but I hid them away so no one would know. (pause) No one would see me blah. (pause) Um, (pause)
Therapist:	How did you get yourself through those moments to get back (pause) to the (pause) strong person that could (pause) do whatever she wanted?
Client:	Just turn it off?
Therapist:	It worked? ↑
Client:	Yeah. (pause)
Therapist:	Ok, (pause) simple as that? ↑
Client:	Yeah. (pause)
Therapist:	Ok. (pause)
Client:	[I don't know.]
Therapist:	[So, you're an expert] at it. (pause)
Client:	(laughs) I guess, (pause) I don't know, (pause) I can't just, (pause) I mean (sighs), I can go, like people are just baffled, I hear at work, that I, (pause) that anything being wrong with me like this.

We next discuss some of the complex discursive processes at work in this interaction.

Solution-building as discursive processes

This therapy session shows how therapists and clients do interactional work to construct and justify the sorts of optimistic storylines that solution-focused brief therapists call solution-building. It illustrates one way that solution-focused brief therapists and clients negotiate entrance into the solutions language game. We see this shift in the therapist's responses in the exchange, which begin with a request that the client elaborate on her prior answer. The therapist's 'Uh huh' response is significant because it fills the therapist's interactional turn without explicitly calling for any particular response from the client. Later, the therapist asks more pointed questions, such as 'How did you get yourself through those moments to get back (pause) to the (pause) strong person that could (pause) do whatever she wanted?'. This question might be analysed as an extreme case formulation, one that casts the client as not just strong but as someone who 'could do whatever she wanted'.

This and subsequent therapist questions build a context for the further reformulation of the client as an expert at getting back to being a strong person. The therapist's claim overrides the client's simultaneous statement of 'I don't know', thereby sustaining their focus on the client's agency. Of course, the client is also a significant actor in the interaction. Perhaps her most important contributions are in providing answers that advance the therapist's interest in socially constructing the client as an agent of change. The therapist's questions generally focus on positive aspects of the client's experience–in keeping with the findings of Tomori and Bavelas (2007) who noted this as a key distinction between solution-focused and client-centered therapies (McGee et al. 2005).

This exchange initiated a lengthy interaction about the client's desire to delegate many of her responsibilities at work and home, which might be seen as culminating in the therapist's parting message. This is not to say, however, that their interactional work was done. Rather their work changed as they negotiated what a solution might look like, how the client might take the next step toward change, and even how their shared interaction should proceed. For example, the client responded to the miracle question by stating, 'Can we go about it in another way? I really have trouble with this miracle thing'. The therapist agreed to this condition and asked a different question. We also see interactional work in the therapist's response at the end of the interview to the client's restatement of her concern about her job situation. This client move might be treated as a request to talk about problems and the therapist's response as a way of 'finessing' (i.e. not granting while also not explicitly rejecting) the request. Initially, the therapist responded to the client's statement with 'Yeah' and replied to the client's elaboration of it with 'Hmhm' and 'Ok'. She also congratulated the client on not letting an administrator at work intimidate her and then announces, 'Ok, ok, that's all. . . . I'll be back in 5 minutes'.

Solution-building as complex processes

Viewed from a complexity perspective, this session illustrates the value of multiple descriptions. The meaning and salient aspects of the interaction vary depending on observer concerns and descriptive practices. It might, for example, be interpreted as evidence of how work and family systems intersect and organize clients' lives. Even when solution-focused brief therapists choose to ignore this aspect of solution-building, their therapy practices have implications for clients' social systems. This is so because, as we see in this session, one aspect of SFBT involves encouraging changes in how clients relate to others at work and in their families. Alternatively, the session might be interpreted politically and rhetorically as a struggle over who controls the interaction and the meanings (storylines) that are honoured within it. This view challenges solution-focused brief therapists' depiction of therapy as a client-therapist collaboration concerned with moving from problems talk to solutions talk. These interpretations and descriptions of SFBT point to the myriad of issues that might be raised to expand conversations about solution-building as complex processes, while avoiding claims to having captured the essence or full reality of the processes.

A complexity perspective also reminds us to notice how therapists orient to the future possibilities in the clients' talk about their worries, while maintaining the 'good enough holding of anxiety' referred to by Stacey (2007). For example, the therapist's question about how talking about the client's work problems might be useful in helping her move on invites the client to reflect on the future possibilities in her past and present experiences. Mindfulness about the future is particularly evident in the therapist's responses to the client's statement that she was once a 'pretty strong person' who 'could handle pretty much anything'. Further, the therapist's parting message casts the future as unknown but possibly discoverable through a process of figuring out how and when the client delegates tasks 'and stuff like that'.

This session also points to the blurred boundaries between therapy interactions and the encompassing environments of clients' lives. For example, the client's work environment is introduced early in the session through the client's portrayal of her worries about her employment status and of a co-worker's depiction of her as possibly depressed. The client's statement is more than a simple report, however. It is an account that was constructed and made to fit within the therapy interaction. The account oriented to both the client's perceptions of her work world and assumptions about what is relevant in therapy. The boundary between therapy and the client's work environment is further blurred as the therapist and client talk about how the client has managed to delegate tasks and effectively handle other problems in the past, as well as the actions that she might take to gain greater control over her life. Finally, the parting message further obscures the therapy environment boundary by asking the client to continue to participate in therapy by observing and thinking about her life outside of therapy.

All of the complex processes discussed here point to how SFBT interactions are self-organizing activities. The therapist and client construct the past, present, and future as they interactionally respond to each other in predictable and unanticipated ways. It is a concrete instance of narrative emergence in SFBT. The interaction is improvised to the extent that they provisionally 'try out' different orientations to therapy, clients' problems and solution-building, sometimes seeming to settle on a solution-oriented line of talk but, as we see at the end of the session, not necessarily abandoning concern for problems. We also see how traces of prior talk may emerge at virtually any time in SFBT interactions. This brings us back to the affinity between SFBT and affirmative postmodernism. Solution-building is a continuing work project that may take uneven (nonlinear) forms that are not adequately appreciated within accounts of SFBT as movement from one language game to another. Taking the process as one where narratives emerge, are changed and transformed, are 'tried out', adapted, and even discarded provides us with a new view of this practice.

Conclusion

We have discussed a possible future path for talking about SFBT as a discursive therapy. Our overriding concern has been with showing how the limitations of treating SFBT as an interactional event may be overcome by adopting a complexity perspective. The complexity perspective treats the discourse of SFBT as a constellation of complex processes of self-organizing that we call narrative emergence. We see this line of thought and talk as a source for new insights into how solution-focused discourse operates within the larger politics of life in the contemporary world. It is a site for re-examining conventional wisdom about SFBT and for developing new questions that might transform discourse analysts' observations of and theories about it. We conclude by suggesting how therapists and researchers might use complexity theory to enlarge their conceptualizations of SFBT.

Possible futures

Complexity theorists emphasize that complex systems are open systems because the boundaries separating the systems from their environments are blurred and easily crossed. We believe that this observation has important implications for understanding the relationship between clients' experiences in therapy and their lives outside of therapy. Connections between these domains of experience are partly observable in therapy sessions when clients and therapists talk about how particular people, relationships, and activities in clients' non-therapy lives might be used to foster change. Solution-focused brief therapists also acknowledge this connection when they talk about the between session changes that clients report in therapy sessions.

But, interestingly, solution-focused brief therapists and researchers know very little about how clients actually address their problems outside of therapy. The literature provides no adequate answers to such important questions as, 'What aspects of clients' therapy experiences do they use in managing their non-therapy lives, how do clients identify resources for change in their non-therapy lives, and what other discourses do clients use in orienting to their life circumstances?' We believe that an important reason why these and related questions are not explored is because solution-focused brief therapists and researchers too often define the term 'therapy conversation' as an interactional event that begins and ends with therapist-client interactions. Complexity theory is a strategy for redefining the idea of therapy conversation.

Viewed from a complexity perspective, solution-focused interactions are embedded in the environments of clients' lives. While it is impossible for therapists and researchers to fully describe these complex environments, they can observe traces of them in clients' social interactions in diverse settings. As Cilliers (1998) stresses, complex systems are best understood by developing a wide variety of descriptions that represent a range of standpoints for seeing what can only be partially seen. This approach to SFBT directs attention to how clients interpret, adapt, and use their therapy experiences to engage the politics of their lives. It is a rationale for expanding the concept of therapy conversation to include clients' solution-building activities outside of therapy rooms and for accentuating the affirmative postmodern belief that therapy may facilitate—but does not cause—change.

Conceptualizing SFBT conversations as complex processes of self-organizing also opens new opportunities for talking differently about what goes on in therapy interactions. One issue involves ethics. A useful starting point for engaging this issue from a complexity standpoint is Griffin's (2002) analysis of how ethical understandings emerge as meanings constructed in human actions and interactions (see Andersen 2001; Anderson 2001; Donovan 2003; Gergen 2001; Ray 2001; Swim et al. 2001;

and Strong and Sutherland 2007, for related approaches to ethics in therapy). This orientation to ethics stands in contrast to the commonplace Western view of them as rules and values that exist independent from particular social contexts and interactions. These external and often abstract rules and values are then compared and contrasted with actual events in life as part of assessing whether people have acted ethically. Griffin contrasts the typical Western view of ethics with a complexity approach that treats ethics as a consciousness that people apply, clarify, and extend in social interactions concerned with managing the practical problems of life. He states that

> moral advance ... consists not in adapting individuals to the fixed realities of a moral universe, but in constantly reconstructing and recreating the world as the individuals evolve
>
> (Griffin 2002, p. 182).

Griffin's discussion of ethics as emergent aspects of complex processes has some important implications for thinking about solution-building activities. It reminds us to ask, 'How do clients and therapists express ethical consciousness in their mutual deliberations and how do they give practical meaning to that consciousness as they identify, assess and select clients' options in changing their lives?' Therapists and researchers might also learn about how clients express their ethical consciousness in social interactions with family members, friends, and neighbours about clients' problems, experiences in therapy and options for taking their next steps in life. As Cilliers (2005) points out:

> Ethical considerations are not to be entertained as something supplementing our dealings with social systems. They are always already part of what we do. One could attempt to deny that and operate as if one can deal with complexity in an objective way – as if we can calculate everything – and thereby avoid the normative dimension. But this denial of the ethical becomes an avoidance of responsibility and is, of course, ethical in itself, albeit a negative (and much too prevalent) ethics
>
> (Cilliers 2005, p. 264).

Another line of development involves the unavoidable uncertainties of life that necessitate making choices under less than optimal circumstances (Shaw 2002). We see this process unfold in SFBT as clients and therapists explore the possibilities for change, despite having incomplete information about the practical impact that any proposed action might have on clients' lives. Similar uncertainties and choices are implicated in discussions about clients' personal agency and ability to effectively change the trajectories of their lives. Complexity theorists treat such conditions as paradoxes to which people adapt in going on with their lives (Letiche 2008). Perhaps the most important paradox for therapists and clients involves the necessity of acting 'as if' they can shape the future, while knowing that this assumption is, to varying degrees, unfounded.

Parting message

The path to the future that we have sketched here leads to a host of anticipatable and unknown issues. Put differently, this essay is designed to foster narrative emergence. It is a beginning point for developing new narratives about SFBT and new understandings of how SFBT is itself a story under construction (Miller and de Shazer 1998).

Complexity theorists teach that it is in pursuing the unknown that we construct the future and, thereby, come to know it. But we are also keenly aware that the path that we have sketched here is only one of many future possibilities. Thus, we invite others to develop their own discursive paths into the future.

Acknowledgement

We wish to thank Theresa Zakutansky for her help with this paper.

References

Adam, B. (1995). *Timewatch: The social analysis of time*. Polity Press, Cambridge.

Andersen, T. (2001). Ethics before ontology: A few words. *Journal of Systemic Therapies,* **20**, 11–13.

Anderson, H. (2001). Ethics and uncertainty: Brief unfinished thoughts. *Journal of Systemic Therapies,* **20**, 3–6.

Bavellas, J. B., McGee, D., Phillips, B., and Routledge, R. (2000). Microanalysis of communication in psychotherapy. *Human Systems,* **11**, 47–66.

Burke, K. (1969). *A grammar of motives*. University of California Press, Berkeley, CA.

Cilliers, P. (1998). *Complexity and postmodernism: Understanding complex systems*. Routledge, London.

Cilliers, P. (2005). Complexity, deconstruction and relativism. *Theory, Culture & Society,* **22**, 255–67.

de Shazer, S. (1982). *Patterns of brief family therapy: An ecosystemic approach*. The Guilford Press, New York.

de Shazer, S. (1988). *Clues: Investigating solutions in brief therapy*. W.W. Norton & Company, New York.

de Shazer, S. (1991). *Putting difference to work*. W.W. Norton & Company, New York.

Derrida, J. (2004). *Positions*. Continuum, London.

Donovan, M. (2003). Family therapy beyond postmodernism: Some considerations on the ethic orientation of contemporary practice. *Journal of Family Therapy,* **25**, 285–306.

Elkaim, M. (1981). Non-equilibrium, chance and change in family therapy. *Journal of marital and family therapy,* **7**, 291–7.

Emerson, R. M. (1981). On last resorts. *American Journal of Sociology,* **87**, 1–22.

Frank, A. W. (1995). *The Wounded Storyteller: Body, Illness and Ethics*. University of Chicago Press, Chicago, IL.

Gale, J. E. (1991). *Conversation analysis of therapeutic discourse*. Ablex, Norwood, NJ.

Gale, J. and Newfield, N. (1992). A conversation analysis of a solution-focused marital herapy session. *Journal of Marital and Family Therapy,* **18**, 153–65.

Gell-Mann, M. (1994). *The quark and the jaguar: Adventures in the simple and the complex*. W.H. Freeman, London.

Gergen, K. J. (2001). Relational process for ethical outcomes. *Journal of Systemic Therapies,* **20**, 7–10.

Gill, J. H. (1996). *Wittgenstein and metaphor*. Humanities Press International, Atlantic Highlands, NJ.

Goodman, N. (1978). *Ways of worldmaking*. Hackett Publishing Co., Indianapolis, IN.

Griffin, D. (2002). *The emergence of leadership*. Routledge, London.

Heritage, J. (1984). *Garfinkel and ethnomethodology.* Polity Press, Cambridge.

Heritage, J. (1984). A change-of-state token and aspects of its sequential placement. In J. M. Atkinson and J. Heritage (Eds.) *Structures of social action: Studies in conversation analysis*, pp. 299–345, Cambridge University Press, Cambridge

Jackson, P. Z. and McKergow, M. (2007). *The solutions focus: Making coaching and change SIMPLE.* Nicholas Brealey Publishing, London.

Jantsch, E. (1980). *The self organizing universe: Scientific and human implications of the emerging paradigm of evolution.* Pergamon Press, New York.

Järvinen, M. and Miller, G. (2010). Methadone maintenance as last resort: A social phenomenology of a drug policy. *Sociological forum,* **25**, 804–23.

Langellier, K. M. and Peterson, E. E. (2004). *Storytelling in daily life: Performing narrative.* Temple University Press, Philadelphia, PA.

Letiche, H. (2008). *Making healthcare care: Managing via simple guiding principles.* Information Age Publishing, Inc., Charlotte, NC.

Levinson, S. C. (1983). *Pragmatics.* Cambridge University Press, Cambridge.

Lewin, R. (1992). *Complexity: Life on the edge of chaos.* Macmillan, New York.

Lyotard, J.F. (1989). *The postmodern condition: A report on knowledge.* University of Minnesota Press, Minneapolis, MN.

MacMartin, C. (2008). Resisting optimistic questions in narrative and solution-focused therapies. In A. Peräylä., C. Antaki, S. Vehiläinen, and I. Leudar (Eds.) *Conversation analysis and psychotherapy*, pp. 80–99. Cambridge University Press, Cambridge.

Mattingly, C. and Fleming, M. H. (1994). *Clinical reasoning: Forms of inquiry in a therapeutic practice.* F.A. Davis Company, Philadelphia, PA.

Maynard, D. W. (1991). The perspective-display series in the delivery and receipt of diagnostic news. In D. Boden, and D. H. Zimmerman (Eds.) *Talk and social structure: Studies in ethnomethdology and conversation analysis,* pp. 331–58. University of California Press, Berkeley, CA.

McGee, D., Vento, A. D., and Bavelas, J. B. (2005). An interactional model of questions as therapeutic interventions. *Journal of Marital and Family Therapy,* **31**, 371–84.

McKergow, M. (1996). Complexity science and management—What's in it for business? *Long Range Planning* **29**, 721–7.

McKergow, M. and Korman, H. (2009). Inbetween—neither inside nor outside: The radical simplicity of solution-focused brief therapy. *Journal of Systemic Therapies,* **28**, 39–49.

Merry, U. (1995). *Coping With uncertainty: Insights from the new sciences of chaos, self-organization, and complexity.* Praeger, Westport, CT.

Miller, G. (1986). Depicting family troubles: A micro-political analysis of the therapeutic interview. *Journal of Strategic and Systemic Therapies,* **5**, 1–13.

Miller, G. (1997). *Becoming miracle workers: Language and meaning in brief therapy.* Transaction Publishers, New Brunswick, NJ.

Miller, G. (2001). Changing the subject: Self-construction in brief therapy. In J.F. Gubrium and J.A. Holstein (Eds.) *Institutional selves: Troubled identities in a postmodern world,* pp. 64–83. Oxford University Press, Oxford.

Miller, G. and de Shazer, S. (1991). Beyond complaints: A foundation for brief therapy. In L. Reiter and C. Ahlers (Eds.) *Systemic thinking and therapeutic process,* pp. 117–35. Springer-Verlag, Heidlberg. [English translation: Miller, G. and de Shazer, S. (2009). Beyond complaints: A foundation for brief therapy. InterAction 1, pp. 78–102.]

Miller, G., de Shazer, S., and DeJong, P. (2001). Therapy Interviewing. In J. F. Gubrium and J. A. Holstein (Eds.) *Handbook of interviewing*, pp. 385–410. Newbury Park, CA: Sage Publications.

Ormerod, P. (1998). *Butterfly economics.* Faber & Faber, London.

Pitkin, H. F. (1972). *Wittgenstein and justice: On the significance of Ludwig Wittgenstein for social and political thought.* University of California Press, Berkeley, CA.

Pomerantz, A. (1986). Extreme case formulations: A way of legitimizing claims. *Human Studies,* **9**, 219–29.

Ray, F. K. (2001). Ethics in therapy: Moving from the mind to the heart. *Journal of Systemic Therapies,* **20**, 25–36.

Richardson, K. A., Cilliers, P., and Lissack, M. (2001). Complexity science: A 'gray' science for the 'stuff in between'. *Emergence,* **3**, 6–18.

Rosenau, P. M. (1992). *Post-modernism and the social sciences: Insights, inroads, and intrusions.* Princeton University Press, Princeton, NJ.

Roth, P. A. (1987). How narratives explain. *Social research,* **56**, 449–78.

Roy-Chowdhury, S. (2006). How is the therapeutic relationship talked into being. *Journal of Family Therapy,* **28**, 153–74.

Sacks, H. (1992). *Lectures on conversation: Volumes I & II.* Blackwell, Oxford.

Shaw, P. (2002). *Changing conversations in organizations.* Routledge, London.

Shotter, J. (1993). *Conversational realities: Constructing life through language.* Sage Publications, London.

Stacey, R. (2007). *Strategic management and organisational dynamics: the challenge of complexity.* 5th ed., Englewood Cliffs, NJ: Prentice-Hall, Pitman Publishing, London.

Stacey, R., Griffin, D., and Shaw, P. (2000). *Complexity and management: Fad or radical challenge to systems thinking?* Routledge, London.

Stein, D. L. (1989). *Lectures in the science of complexity.* Addison Wesley, Reading, MA.

Strong, T. and Lock, A. (2005). Discursive therapy? *Janus Head,* **8**, 585–93.

Strong, T. and Sutherland, O. (2007). Conversational ethics in psychological dialogues: Discursive and collaborative considerations. *Canadian Psychology,* **48**, 94–104.

Swim, S., George, S. A. S., and Wulff, D. P. (2001). Process ethics: A collaborative partnership. *Journal of Systemic Therapies,* **20**, 14–24.

Throgmorton, J. A. (1996). *Planning as persuasive storytelling: The rhetorical construction of Chicago's electric future.* University of Chicago Press, Chicago, IL.

Tomori, C. and Bavelas, J. B. (2007). Using microanalysis of communication to compare solution-focused and client-centred therapies. *Journal of Family Psychotherapy,* **18**, 25–43.

Waldrop, M. M. (1992). *Complexity: The emerging science at the edge of order and chaos.* Simon & Schuster, New York.

White, H. (1978). *Tropics of discourse: Essays in cultural criticism.* Johns Hopkins University Press, Baltimore, MD.

Wittgenstein, L. (1958). *Philosophical investigations.* Macmilan Publishing Co., Inc., New York.

Chapter 10

Activity and performance (and their discourses) in social therapeutic method

Lois Holzman and Fred Newman

As collaborators on the development of social therapy, Fred Newman and Lois Holzman bring different things to the task. Newman was trained as a philosopher, originated social therapy and practises it, and is a playwright and director. Holzman was trained as a developmental psychologist and psycholinguist, and practises as a teacher, trainer, and researcher. Both of us write on social therapy theory/practice, sometimes together and at other times separately. When we write together, we sometimes speak in one voice and at other times in two (or perhaps more). For this chapter we decided to preserve our two voices. After a brief historical and conceptual overview of our approach, the chapter is organized as three discourses on *social therapy as performance*. In Discourse 1, we together introduce that topic in relation to the practice of social therapy, the teaching of it, and directing plays. Discourse 2 was written by Holzman who takes a developmental psychologist (Vygotskian) perspective. Discourse 3, written by Newman, is a concise philosophical-political characterization of social therapy's performance modality.

Overview

Social therapy (or the broader practice/theory of social therapeutics) is an approach to human development and learning at the leading edge of the critical and postmodernist movements in psychology. It challenges, in practice and theory, many of psychology's and psychiatry's presuppositions about persons; therapy, the therapeutic relationship and therapeutic discourse; illness, cure, and treatment; emotions and cognition; and mind, body, and brain. This orientation locates social therapy within the diverse grouping of non-medical model approaches that identify as discursive, collaborative, and/or social constructionist.

Social therapy was introduced in the 1970s by philosopher and lay therapist Fred Newman. Since then it has continuously been developed by Newman and developmental psychologist Lois Holzman into a practical human development methodology (social therapeutics) with broad application in the myriad of settings that children, youth, and adults create and inhabit. As a psychotherapy, it is a positive, relational approach with special focus on emotional development and group creativity. While philosophically informed, social therapy is a practically oriented method in which human beings are related to as creators of their culture and ensemble performers of their lives (Holzman and Mendez 2003; Newman and Holzman 1996/2006).

Developed outside of academia at the East Side Institute for Group and Short Term Psychotherapy in New York, social therapy has been practised since the mid-1970s in social therapy centres, clinics, schools, hospitals, and social service organizations in the USA and, increasingly, abroad. As a method for social-emotional growth and learning, the social therapeutic approach has impacted on education in school and outside of school, and youth development (Feldman and Silverman 2004; Holzman 1997, 2006, 2009; Lobman 2005, 2010; Sabo 2007); on training and practice in medicine and healthcare (Massad 2003); and on organizational development and executive leadership (Holzman 2009; Salit 2003).

While several intellectual traditions have informed the social therapeutic approach as it has evolved since the late 1970s, the conceptual frameworks of Karl Marx, Lev Vygotsky, and Ludwig Wittgenstein have been most influential. Their writings have helped us to understand both the potential for ordinary people to effect radical social change and the subjective constraints that need to be engaged so as to actualize this potential. Social therapy has evolved as an unorthodox synthesis of these three seminal thinkers.

Marx

In the works of Karl Marx, one finds a radically social humanism and methodology, especially in his early writings (for example, *Economic and Philosophical Manuscripts* and *The German Ideology*). More than his political economy, it is this that has influenced and inspired the development of social therapy (Newman 2000b; Newman and Holzman 2003). For Marx, human beings are first and foremost social beings. He posited that both human activity and human mind are social, not just in their origins but in their content. Methodologically, the transformation of the world and of ourselves as human beings is one and the same task: 'The coincidence of the changing of circumstances and of human activity or self-changing can be conceived and rationally understood only as *revolutionary practice*' [revolutionary, practical-critical activity] (Marx and Engels 1974, p. 121). It is this capacity that makes individual and species development possible.

Vygotsky

Vygotsky brought Marx's insights to bear on the practical question of how human beings learn and develop (Vygotsky 1978, 1987). It is human activity (qualitative and transformative) and not behaviour change (particularistic and cumulative) that is the unique feature of human individual, cultural, and species development (Newman and Holzman 1993). Human beings do not merely respond to stimuli, acquire societally determined and useful skills, and adapt to the determining environment. The uniqueness of human social life is that we ourselves transform the determining circumstances.

Vygotsky's departure from traditional psychology's understanding of development—that it is not an individual accomplishment but a *sociocultural activity*—helped us to see more clearly how our therapeutic and educational practices worked.

His writings on cognitive development, play, and language in early childhood have great relevance to emotional growth at all ages. Children learn and develop, according to Vygotsky through being related to as beyond themselves, and being supported to play or perform, 'a head taller' than they are. We take Vygotsky to be a forerunner to a new *psychology of becoming*, in which people experience the social nature of their existence and the power of collective creative activity in the process of making new tools for growth (Holzman 2009, 2010; Newman and Holzman 1993).

Wittgenstein

Ludwig Wittgenstein challenged the foundations of philosophy, psychology, and linguistics (1953, 1965). His was a radically new method of doing philosophy—without foundations, theses, premises, generalizations, or abstractions. Especially important to how social therapy relates to emotional life is how Wittgenstein exposed the 'pathology' embedded in language and in accepted conceptions of language, thoughts, and emotions. His work can be seen not only as therapy for philosophers (as some have noted, e.g. Baker 1992; van der Merwe and Voestermans 1995) but also for ordinary people. For, by virtue of the complicated network of social, communicative institutions that have evolved since human beings invented language, versions of philosophical pathologies permeate everyday life and create intellectual-emotional muddles. In *Unscientific Psychology: A Cultural-Performatory Approach to Understanding Human Life* (1996/2006), we put it this way:

> His self-appointed task was to cure philosophy of its illness. (Ours, as we will try to show, is closer to curing 'illness' of its philosophy.) We are all sick people, says Wittgenstein. No small part of what makes us sick is *how* we think (related in complicated ways to what we think and, even more fundamentally, to *that* we think or *whether* we think), especially how (that or whether) we think about thinking and other so-called mental processes and/or objects—something which we (the authors) think we (members of our culture) do much more than many of us like to think! It gets us into intellectual-emotional muddles, confusions, traps, narrow spaces; it torments and bewilders us; it gives us 'mental cramps.' We seek causes, correspondences, rules, parallels, generalities, theories, interpretations, explanations for our thoughts, words and verbal deeds (often, even when we are not trying to or trying not to). But what if, Wittgenstein asks, there are none?
>
> (Newman and Holzman 1996/2006, p. 174).

Indeed. Nearly all therapies, whether Freudian, neo-Freudian, or cognitive-behavioural, begin with the assumption that certain kinds of physical acts of the individual have a causal connection to certain kinds of mental acts of the individual. Social therapy does not. Instead, inspired by Vygotsky, but developed well beyond his writings (which were not therapeutic), social therapy works with the notion that there is not so much a connection but a *non-causal connectedness* between so-called mental acts and physical activity. Vygotsky's word for this (translated from Russian into English) is 'completion' (Vygotsky 1987). His radical challenge to both pictorial and pragmatic views of language, and the understandings of the thought–language relationship that follow from these views, was that thoughts are completed—not expressed—in speaking (and other actions).

> The structure of speech is not simply the mirror image of the structure of thought. It cannot, therefore, be placed on thought like clothes off a rack. Speech does not merely serve as the expression of developed thought. Thought is restructured as it is transformed into speech. It is not expressed but completed in the word
>
> (Vygotsky 1987, p. 251).

This non-expressionist conception of thinking/speaking as a dialectal unity (a non-causal connectedness) is, theoretically, in the best sense of the word, at the very core of social therapy. Causal connection, or what is known in the philosophy of science as deductive connection, is what social therapy has tried to move beyond in finding a foundation for a genuinely humanistic therapy.

Discourse 1 (by Holzman and Newman)

While social therapy can be counted among the discursive therapies, it is historically (and discursively) rooted in an activity theoretic and a performance ontology. Marx's understanding of activity and dialectics has been important in the development of social therapy since its beginnings over three decades ago, followed closely by Vygotsky's application of these aspects of Marx to psychology (especially human development and learning and the role of play in both). Performance, and more generally the language of the theatre, began to occupy a prominent place in our work a bit later, about 20 years ago. The creativity that is entailed in both activity (and its discourse) and performance (and its discourse)—as radically humanistic methodologies—has a particular intellectual and political appeal to us that 'discourse' and 'talk' talk do not. (Both of us have studied language, discourse, talk, communication, conversation, etc. fairly extensively—Holzman within the discipline of linguistics/psycholinguistics and Newman within the discipline of philosophy of language/science.)

With that said, social therapy is the social–cultural–historical activity of groupings of people collectively creating environments in which they can and do perform therapy. They create both the environment and the performance simultaneously. Therapeutic talk, in social therapy as in all discursive therapies, begins as individuals telling their stories. The work of social therapy is to transform the culturally and institutionally overdetermined psychological and truth-referential environment-and-talk into a 'theatre without a stage' upon which the therapy group, qua group, creates a play (in this case, their therapy play).

Why? Because we are interested in human development and engage in activities that we believe help people to grow and transform qualitatively. Theatre and therapy can be developmental/transformative because both are opportunities for people to experience life in new ways, in ways other than those we have been socialized to—i.e. without a problem-solution or conflict resolution paradigm, but rather seeing life's uncertainty and unknowability.

Newman is a playwright who has written over 30 plays and directed many of them, as well as those of the late avant-garde East German playwright Heiner Müller. As therapist and theatre person, he has a particular take on the social therapy play (which is, perhaps, applicable more generally to the theatricality of therapy and the therapeutics of theatre).

Let's hear from him:

> I try to create plays at which my ideal audience member walks out of the play and says, 'What in the hell was that?' I've been doing group therapy for 35–40 years now and, as far as I can tell, that's what the people whom I work with walk out of every session saying. Because every session is a play. It's a play that we create together. Sometimes people walk out and say, 'Oh I got it,' and then someone else from the group usually helps me by saying, 'What are you talking about? What do you mean you got it? If you got, you don't get it.'
>
> That human process of not just questioning ourselves, but of *not knowing*—of allowing ourselves to stop thinking that we know what's going on, and instead simply have the kind of social experience that is poetic and growthful and developmental—makes us more human.

What is a poetic and growthful and developmental social experience? Over the years we have come to identify it in simple (to say, not to do) terms—it is the activity of creating something new out of what exists. This is not, we suspect, very controversial. Where it becomes so, in our experience, is in the nature of 'what exists' and what is usable to create with. In therapy, what exists is what people bring to each session, which is typically their problems, pain, hurt, victimization, depression, insecurity, fears, and so on (inseparable from their ways of talking and their stories about them). The social therapeutic task is to create something out of all this ugly stuff, to transform it—not narratively but performatorily. The difference is, we believe, big. Social therapists are not working with clients to make the ugliness go away or to create a prettier or better story of their lives. They are, instead, working with clients to give their ugliness/their stories to the group as material with which to create the therapy (play).

Newman and I have discussed this distinction relative to theories of language and therapeutic approaches (see Holzman 2009; Newman 2000a; Newman and Holzman 1996/2006, 1999). Here we use some of our experiences to highlight the performatory nature of therapeutic creativity as we understand it in our work.

First, Newman's experience directing Heiner Müller's *Hamletmachine* sparks some comparisons with doing social therapy:

> In the play Müller writes of 'lugging his overweight brain'—a beautiful, if ghastly, poetic image. Postmodernism, the overly intellectualised effort to move beyond modernism, is surely lugging modernism's overweight brain. And indeed, so is Müller, the brilliant poet, lugging his overweight brain. Müller is one of the great brains of the 20th century, yet from the vantage point of lugging, it is merely overweight. His brain is a cancer and it killed him long before his death. The work that I try to do hopes to revive him not simply by doing his plays, but by doing something with his plays. To me, theatre is as least as much a way to help people grow as therapy is. I'm trying to get Heiner Müller to grow because I think his work is brilliant in the spirit of deconstruction that calls out to destroy everything. That touches me and I think that's marvelous. My own vision, in psychology as well as in theater, is to take what's being destroyed, what's being smashed into a million pieces, and create something with it. So Müller is someone whom I feel very close to because he makes it possible for there to be something for me to work with. He destroys everything. My concern is to build with all the garbage, with all the crap. That's my theatrical, poetic vision—to take the garbage of the world and not make it look good, not put a lot of fancy smelling stuff on it or shape it up, not to do what's done on Broadway where

crap is made to look beautiful and therefore mislead people and mis-teach people politically. What I try to do is political theater that shows that we have to learn how to create with the crap that we have inherited. Because this is our working material. And no mental act, in my opinion, can turn crap into anything but crap, though we can create with it as the material.

That's what therapy is all about. That's what people bring into therapy after all, and it is what we expect them to bring in. They bring in that which has been destroyed, which they call by various names, but fundamentally they call it 'my life'. They bring in their pain, their destroyed lives, their destroyed visions. They bring these lives into a therapy room and they share them with other people in the group in what I think is a wonderful act of love. And then we take that terrible, ugly stuff, which is for all of us in varying degrees who and what we are, and the work I try to do is to help people create something out of that. 'Let's build something with that'. And that's a play. That's as much a play as anything I put on the stage. Social therapy groups are fantastically interesting plays—week after week a different play. The only difference is that we don't sell tickets to watch them and we don't do a video of them. But they're plays.

As a trainer and teacher, I (Holzman) work social therapeutically to create something new out of what exists. Often the topic and substance of what I'm training people in or teaching is social therapy, which means that people are involved in learning social therapeutics—the method—social therapeutically. The class or workshop (the group) has to create the learning environment by using 'what exists' (the material, their histories, responses, understandings, and so on) in order to learn (about) the method. They are creating, in Vygotsky's words, 'simultaneously the tool and the result' (Newman and Holzman 1993; Vygotsky 1978).

This raises some similar and some different issues from the therapy activity. The desire to 'get it' is similar—and in an educational setting to be asked to suspend this goal can be particularly frustrating for some. An individualistic bias/strategy is operative as well. Going into therapy, the working assumption is that the way to get help is to talk about oneself; in the case of students entering classes and seminars, they are consumed with what they themselves will get out of it. Unlike in therapy, where people expect to talk about how they are feeling, educational settings are generally constructed as emotion-free zones. One's fears of not knowing or looking stupid, competitive feelings towards others, the frustration and anxiety that accompany boredom and lack of concentration—all these and more are not usually related to as material that can be made use of in learning. All of us have been very well socialized to see therapy and education as they have been constructed through their institutional and popular discourse, which makes these working hypotheses completely understandable, and challenges to them quite a provocation.

Creating development 'out of garbage' was difficult to contemplate for a group of educators and psychologists whose country had gone through an intensely violent civil war during the 1990s. In my work with them, they told painful personal stories of death, destruction, bewilderment, loss of meaning, and paralysis. It seemed from the telling that they had repeated these stories very often. At the same time, when I invited them to perform their lives 'on stage' they were fully and playfully creative and improvisational. Without the stage, they spoke from their scripts. The challenge was, could they create *with* their scripts; could they perform off the stage as well; could we play with their stories together and in doing so transform the pain they were talking *about* into a performed conversation, whose meaning (and meaningfulness to all) was in its creating and not in any aboutness; could we create something new with the 'garbage' of the world? Raising these questions used and built with the material they had already given to the learning environment. Through this activity, we discovered together that as a group they were not willing to transform their activity from 'telling the truth' about their lives into performing their lives conversationally. The group consensus was that garbage is garbage; you cannot create with it. Many of them felt that all they now had of their own was their pain and loss and they were not about to give it up. They would tell their story but not share it. They would narrate but not perform.

It is tempting to see this shift from talking to performing conversation in terms of scripted and improvisational performance—don't! In therapy sessions, classrooms, and training workshops, we all have our roles and our lines. The social therapeutic work is to collectively take these roles and lines and in some nuanced way create something new. Again, Newman's way of understanding theatre helps make this point:

> Actors get their roles in the play. Now they know what their lines are, just as we know what our lines are in life. And the actors say those lines. But that's not the creative part of the play. The creative part of the play is what the ensemble does. The creative part is the relational part. It's how people say things to each another and exactly how people move when they say them. That's improvisational and there is tremendous variation in it. The creative and developmental element in theatre is finding a way—after you've discovered your role—to abandon your role. Learn your role well. Accept it. Internalise it. Now forget about it. You've got to go beyond it if you want to create something. Move beyond it to create. In therapy as well. We work hard to learn who is there in the therapy room in order to create something together that is bigger than any of us and what we brought in. That is a strong similarity between roles, scripts and improvisation in terms of what goes on developmentally in theatre and therapy.

Discourse 2 (by Holzman)

Developmental psychology tends to relate to culture in one of two ways. Within the broad mainstream of the discipline, culture is considered to be a factor in human development, that is, something that influences the developmental process. Within constructionist and cultural–historical psychology, development *is* cultural, in that what it means for children to develop is that they adopt ('appropriate') the culture that they are born in to. My own perspective is that human development consists of both the appropriating and the creating of culture, and that their dialectic interplay is what is most interesting and relevant to understand. That is one way I see the social therapeutic activity of transforming narrative into performance.

Vygotsky's writings on development, learning, and play, and language and thought have shaped this way of seeing (no doubt, working with social therapy has equally, if not more, shaped how I understand his writings—the simultaneous shapings being an instance of appropriating and creating culture). These processes are, for Vygotsky, cultural–historical and *collectively produced*, accomplished through 'a collective form of working together' (Vygotsky 2004, p. 202). Vygotsky's zone of proximal development (zpd) is for me the prime example (Holzman 1997, 2009, 2010). Young children and their caregivers together create the zone by their activity (playfully and creatively imitating and completing each other's speech, movements, and actions). Before school age, children's learning is seamless with their everyday activities, which are nearly all playful. Not only do they spend a lot of time playing in the sense of what adults identify as children's play (free play, pretend play), but with caretakers and older children they also play speaking and reading and making dinner and getting dressed, etc.

This kind of play (and, thereby, learning in early childhood) is performatory, that is, non-didactic, non-cognitively based, and non-individuated. Fifteen-month-olds who do not yet know the language of their family perform as speakers of it; two-year-olds who are not literate perform as readers; three-year-olds who know nothing of perspective or representation perform as artists. The performatory zpd supports them doing things they don't yet know how to do; it activates what Vygotsky referred to as 'the child's potential to move from what he is able to do to what he is not' (Vygotsky 1987, p. 212). In the performatory zpd children develop because they are both who they are and beyond, or other than, who they are at the same time. This is akin to Vygotsky's notion that play is developmental for children because it is when they act as if 'a head taller' (Vygotsky 1978, p. 102). Perhaps the collective form of working together in early childhood is better identified as a collective form of playing together. It is a playing together in which culture (i.e. the 'stage' and the performance) is created and simultaneously appropriated.

With respect to language, this means that speaking as performance (performed conversation) precedes and makes possible speaking as narrative (talking about things). (While psychologists have noted that narrative is a rather late development in childhood, as far as I know they have not explored the performatory nature of pre-narrative speech.)

And once narrative begins, it pretty much takes over in most people's lives. This is the social–cultural–historical 'presenting problem' for social therapy. Adults speak narratively. To grow emotionally, they need to learn how to do speaking as performance. The group needs to create a performatory zpd in which they, with the support of the therapist, can do what is beyond and not known to them (as young children do): take their ways of speaking and listening to each other—their narratives and stories and accountings—and use them to create a new kind of conversation, a conversation that is not merely spoken, but performed. The process of this transformation (creating the therapy play) creates in the group new ways to understand and relate to talk and to emotionality. It is emotional growth by virtue of the group growing.

Discourse 3 (by Newman)

In 'Where is the magic in cognitive therapy? (a philo-/psychological investigation),' a chapter in *Against and for CBT* (Newman 2009), I wrote what might be the most complex sentence I ever intentionally created. I called it Sentence NAD: (Not a definition) and it goes like this:

> Within a performatory (as opposed to a cognitive) modality (community), we (social therapy/social therapists) seek to help create a pointless dialectical (a mixture of Plato's and Marx's) group conversation (a conversation oriented toward discovery/creation) in

order to generate a new game (a Wittgensteinian game) which completes (in a Vygotskian sense) the thinking, and is itself (by magic, a.k.a. art) a performance (though more activity than an action) (p. 229).

I didn't have the chance to unpack the sentence in that chapter, but will do so now.

Within a performatory (as opposed to a cognitive) modality (community)...

Much as very traditional psychoanalysis attempts to overcome this hard fact, *all* therapy is done in a historical spatio-temporal environment. Classical social therapy is carried out in a self-consciously organized community which could be identified as a synthesis of a 1970s-style therapeutic community, a 1960s-style alternative school community, an activist progressive political community, and an avant-garde political theatre community begun in the late 1960s (in the midst of the mini-upheaval that now bears the label 'the Sixties').

It is now, some 40 years later, of substantial size, located in various places throughout the world (plus cyberspace) with thousands of people with varying degrees of interest in one or many of its varied forms. All of those involved are hardly the same. It is not a cult. Indeed, it is not even remotely cultic. Most members of the community have no idea what other members of the community are doing. It has been designed to be (and succeeds in being) methodologically and structurally *disconnected*; it is what we call a *practice of method* (Hood [Holzman] and Newman 1979).

That our critics persist in calling it a cult shows their need and indeed international society's need to comprehend something by way of connectedness.

...we (social therapy/social therapists) seek to help create a pointless dialectical (a mixture of Plato's and Marx's) group conversation (a conversation oriented toward discovery/creation)...

The classical social therapy group is roughly made up of 25 people (the more diverse, the better) who gather weekly with a therapist/leader/facilitator and an assistant. Most of the members have 'been through' or are still going through individual therapy, in some cases at one of the social therapy centres.

The group is asked to form themselves as a therapeutic environment which could help the members with their emotional problems. In almost all cases, this soft directive is misheard and seen as an opportunity for individual members to get individual therapeutic help (a relatively traditional form of traditional group therapy).

The early stages of group social therapy (perhaps years) is devoted to conversation intended to clarify this distinction. But the group (made up of individuals, after all) never quite abandons its individualistic drive. So even after years of working together, individuals in the group will attempt to come to group 'seeking help' with *their own* problem at home, at work, with a lover, etc. As the group develops a longer history it will tend all the sooner to have a group recognition that they have gone off in the 'wrong' direction. The group then returns, though often begrudgingly (and characteristically via the therapist), to collectively building an environment for helping individuals.

How is the above description pointless activity, or equivalently, how does the group do this?

This is unknown. But pointless conversation is recommended. Pointless in that the group's engagement in conversation, the activity of conversing, is what creates the group. What the group talks *about* makes little difference. *How* the group talks about it makes a great deal of difference.

Do emotional concerns tend to dominate, as opposed to, let's say, quantum physics? Yes. Unless the group happens to be made up of all and only quantum physicists (which is rare—indeed, it has never happened). But typically emotional issues will dominate. But when and if individual members slip and slide toward individual problem solving, the social therapist will politely (sometimes not so politely) reconvene the group as a group attempting to create an environment for helping people with their emotional problems.

Such is the performatory dialectic of the classical social therapy group. It is the dialectic of classical Marxist theory and workers seeking higher wages, the dialectic of art theory and making art, the dialectic of theory and practice.

> . . . in order to generate a new game (a Wittgensteinian game) . . .

Wittgenstein's notion of a 'language game,' which could just as easily be called a 'life game,' is, properly understood, central to fully appreciating postmodernism (at least in its psychological expression) for it gives performatory dominance to the ever-present activity/abstraction dialectic. Within our legitimate culture everything said is related to as both something said and something said about something. Philosophers of language have searched for exceptions but in ordinary language usage this paradigm (the denotative) dominates and with this dominating paradigm comes the corollary that what is said is more what it is *about* than it is the activity of saying. Wittgenstein's notion of the language game challenges this long-standing paradigm at its very heart and soul.

> . . . which completes (in a Vygotskian sense) the thinking…

Vygotsky, who died of tuberculosis in his thirties in the 1930s, was a brilliant Soviet psychologist with a keen and revolutionary interest in educational development. Social therapy has considered the applicability of his ideas to *emotional* development. Amongst the many things we have discovered in Vygotsky's writings is his recognition of and sensibility to the classical mind/body problem. Moreover, he offers a solution to it in his insistence that what the mind creates is indiscernible, separate from what the listener 'completes' in her or his hearing. Hence, there is nothing to be connected, for discourse is essentially social.

> . . . and is itself (by magic, a.k.a. art)…

Art, even in classical terms has (we believe) always been seen as the 'connectedness' of the 'disconnected'. Science, as well, especially in late modernist times, has also come to be seen as the 'connectedness' of the 'disconnected', e.g. quantum physics.

> . . . a performance (though more an activity than an action)

Aristotle and many of his late modernist followers seem more focused on *an action* as a particular expression of a particular thought process. Social therapy focuses more on the activity (of either the individual or the group) than on the particularistic action.

Endview

The origin and evolution of social therapy over the decades has been humanitarian and, thereby, political. The philosophical conundrum it has dealt with—'What is going on in therapy that makes talking about one's inner life helpful when there is no such thing as an inner life?'—has contributed immeasurably to whatever effectiveness it has had in ameliorating privatized emotional pain and activating the human capacity to create development. We have come to understand that talking about one's inner life is therapeutic because and to the extent that it is a socially completive activity and not a transmittal of private states of mind, a performance and not a representation, a non-causal connection, a completion that is as ongoing as people choose to make it.

One of the formal functions of the social therapist is to say, 'I think we have to stop.' We think we have to stop.

References

Baker, G. P. (1992). Some remarks on 'language' and 'grammar. *Grazer Philosophische Studien*, **42**, 107–31.

Feldman, N. and Silverman, B. (2004). The let's talk about it model: Engaging young people as partners in creating their own mental health program. In K. E. Robinson (Ed.) *Advances in school-based mental health, best practices and program models*, pp. 12.2—12.21. Civic Research Institute, New Jersey, NJ.

Holzman, L. (1997). *Schools for growth: Radical alternatives to current educational models*. Erlbaum, Mahwah, NJ.

Holzman, L. (2006). Activating postmodernism. *Theory & psychology*, **16**(1), 109–23.

Holzman, L. (2009). *Vygotsky at work and play*. Routledge, London and New York.

Holzman, L. (2010). Without creating zpds there is no creativity. In C. Connery, V. John-Steiner and A. Marjanovic-Shane (Eds.) *Vygotsky and creativity: A cultural-historical approach to play, meaning-making and the arts*, pp. 28–39. Peter Lang Publishers, New York.

Holzman, L. and Mendez, R. (2003). *Psychological Investigations: A Clinician's Guide to Social Therapy*. Brunner-Routledge, New York.

Hood [Holzman], L. and Newman, F. (1979). *The practice of method: An introduction to the foundations of social therapy*. Practice Press, New York.

Lobman, C. (2005). 'Yes and': The uses of improvisation for early childhood professional development, *Journal of early childhood teacher education*, **26**(3), 305–19.

Lobman, C. (2010). Creating developmental moments: Teaching and learning as creative activities. In C. Connery, A. Marjanovic-Shane, and V. John-Steiner (Eds) *Vygotsky and creativity: A cultural-historical approach to play, meaning-making, and the arts*, pp. 199–214. Peter Lang Publishing, New York.

Marx, K. and Engels, F. (1974). *The German Ideology*. International Publishers, New York.

Massad, S. (2003). Performance of doctoring: A philosophical and methodological approach to medical conversation, *Advances in mind-body medicine*, **19**, 6–13.

Newman, F. (2000a). Does a story need a theory? (Understanding the methodology of narrative therapy). In D. Fee (Ed), *Pathology and the postmodern: Mental illness in discourse and experience*, pp. 248–62. Sage, Thousand Oaks, CA.

Newman, F. (2000b). The performance of revolution (More thoughts on the postmodernization of Marxism). In L. Holzman and J. Morss (Eds) *Postmodern psychologies, societal practice and political life*, pp. 165–76. Routledge, New York.

Newman, F. (2009). Where is the magic in cognitive therapy? (A philo/psychological investigation). In R. House and D. Loewenthal (Eds) *Against and for CBT: Towards a constructive dialogue?*, pp. 218–32. PCCS Books, Ross-on-Wye.

Newman, F. and Holzman, L. (1993). *Lev Vygotsky: Revolutionary scientist.* Routledge, London.

Newman, F. and Holzman, L. (1996/2006). *Unscientific psychology: A cultural-performatory approach to understanding human life.* Praeger and iUniverse, Westport, CT.

Newman, F. and Holzman, L. (1997). *The end of knowing: A new developmental way of learning.* Routledge, London.

Newman, F. and Holzman, L. (1999). Beyond narrative to performed conversation ('In the beginning' comes much later). *Journal of Constructivist Psychology,* **12**, 23–40.

Newman, F. and Holzman, L. (2003). All power to the developing! *Annual Review of Critical Psychology,* **3**, 8–23.

Salit, C.R. (2003). The coach as theatre director, *Journal of excellence,* **8**. 20–41.

Sabo, K. (2007). *Youth participatory evaluation: Strategies for engaging young people.* Wiley, New York.

van der Merwe, W. L. and Voestermans, P. P. (1995). Wittgenstein's legacy and the challenge to psychology. *Theory & psychology,* **5**, 27–48.

Vygotsky, L.S. (1978). *Mind in society.* Harvard University Press, Cambridge, MA.

Vygotsky, L. S. (1987). *The collected works of L. S. Vygotsky.* Vol. 1. Plenum, New York.

Vygotsky, L.S. (2004). The collective as a factor in the development of the abnormal child. In R.W. Rieber and D. K. Robinson (Eds) *The essential Vygotsky*, pp. 201–19. Kluwer Academic/Plenum Publishers, New York.

Wittgenstein, L. (1953). *Philosophical investigations.* Blackwell, Oxford.

Wittgenstein, L. (1965). *The blue and brown books.* Harper Torchbooks, New York.

Chapter 11

Developing a 'just therapy': context and the ascription of meaning

Charles Waldegrave

Context and meaning

The ways in which meanings are ascribed often indicate both the nature of the relationship and the understandings that can be expected to ensue. If, for example, a school teacher says to a young pupil that they need to complete a task or there will be consequences, then it is reasonably clear that the teacher is drawing upon his or her senior status to direct the pupil. When a member of the police force says the same thing to another adult it carries an authoritative nuance that is quite different from the nuance of a woman speaking to her partner, or an employee addressing his or her boss. Human beings are very sensitive to meaning. They perceive the nature and value of relationships through the meanings they understand emanate from the other.

'Just therapy' grew out of a seed that sought to distinguish the branches of meaning in therapeutic encounters. It grew in a soil of disenfranchised people, who though vulnerable and searching for help, were often subject to established and prescribed trunks of assessment and direction. These therapeutic prescriptions carried with them the claims of professionalism to neutrality and higher knowledge, and in so doing, often bypassed the fundamental core of meaning that had developed among the people they were designed for. Although cultural boundaries and expectations differed, the fields were ploughed as though every paddock was the same. Gender differences and socioeconomic status distinctions played a minor role when compared with the universality of the chosen therapeutic direction.

The 'just therapy' approach, by contrast, privileges the notion of *context* as being critical to a person's or family's health and well-being rather than universal approaches (Waldegrave et al. 2003a). 'Context' refers to the impact and ongoing influence of the lived experience of people from their earliest, given relationships to their mature choices and expressions of culture, gender, and to a lesser extent socioeconomic positioning. Although genetic inheritance is a major determinant of individual functioning, people learn to value certain ways of acting in the world over others through the primary expressions of care they receive that in turn impart culture, socioeconomic status, and gendered cues. These cues take on specific meanings, and words with associated emotions and body cues amplify those meanings.

People learn to interact and communicate through explanations and modelling from the intimate group they are born into or placed in. Their sense of security, predictability, and order stems from this contextual mixture of cultured and gendered experience of belonging, and is also influenced by the socioeconomic position through which it is expressed (Erikson 1950; Gerhardt 2004; Quintana et al. 2006). They learn the behaviours that are considered to be acceptable and those that are shameful. Socioeconomic status in modern democracies is more fluid than it used to be, and changes for some people during the course of their lifetime.

Think for a moment of the notion of family, and recall what families pass on directly through their guidance and instruction, and indirectly through their demeanour and interactions with others. Families can vary from two people living in the same house to large extended families living in different households and one-parent-led households. Families provide a structure for intimacy, a safe place to be nurtured, grow, and learn (Cozolino 2006; Shonkoff and Phillips 2000; Waldegrave and Waldegrave 2009). It has to be said, unfortunately, that although safety is the norm in all our cultures, it is not always guaranteed.

From families we learn the basis of gender identification and role expectations. We are taught the finer points of social interaction that involve values and expectations such as reciprocity, mutuality, sensitivity, boundaries, and the plethora of unwritten rules of communication (Posner and Rothbart 2007; Schore 2003). Families are the foundational purveyors of cultural mores, gendered expectations, and broad socioeconomic standing. They provide a critical entry point to society and a preparation for broader social interaction with other families who have similar underlying values. The collectivity of these, in a region over time, inherits and passes on what we refer to as culture.

Within cultures particular meanings are accorded to certain events and physical entities. We may wear certain clothing, acknowledge certain types of people, and express particular rituals. Each of these actions has ordinary or sacred meaning in a particular culture. A monetary gift or a formal acknowledgement in front of peers, a glass of wine or a tea ceremony, a diamond in Europe or a fine mat in the Pacific, a cross in Christendom or a crescent in Islam, gatherings of women or activities with children, each take on special significance.

Our sense of belonging is very closely tied to our participation in all these processes, most of which we have had very little choice over until late adolescence and adulthood. Whatever our sense of self-determination may be, much of it was shaped by the generations before us and our interactions in the culture or cultures in which we were brought up. Our heritage creates meaning and accords status. It creates a space among others, where we are recognized and where certain expectations are justified by those around us.

This sense of belonging runs very deep for human beings. It provides the basis for primary loyalties, social networks, and social behaviour. This is not static, of course, each generation is influenced by developments and change. Nevertheless, it is the persistence of the significance of this identity through generations, and its power to explain and create meaning for people, that suggests it would be very wise to respect and honour it (Love 2000; Sue and Sue 1990; Tamasese et al. 2005).

This persistence of multigenerational identity raises serious questions about modern notions of subordinating particular cultural and gendered ways of doing things to a more commodified, globalized, and universalized approach. This is not to suggest that there is no place for globalization or common practices and laws across cultures. There is much to be gained, for example, from common laws and practices, the free flow of people and ideas and international trade. It is rather to suggest that the 'melting pot' idea of universalizing therapy and institutions has taken an excessively one-dimensional approach, within and between countries, that has seriously marginalized large groups of people in inequitable ways.

Cultural, gender, and socioeconomic influences of meaning

The 'just therapy' approach is termed 'just' for two reasons. Firstly, 'just' refers to equity and justice. The work has grown up around the notion that many of the physical health, mental health, and relationship problems people have are the consequences of power difference and injustice. There is certainly a substantial body of literature that associates cultural marginalization, gender inequities, and low-income households with physical and mental ill health (Benzeval et al. 1995; Kawachi and Berkman 2003; Kawachi and Kennedy 2002; Mackenbach 2006; Marmot 2010; Ministry of Social Development 2009; National Equality Panel 2010; National Health Committee 1998; Waldegrave et al. 2003b; Wilkinson and Pickett 2009).

Secondly, the approach attempts to identify the essential elements of therapeutic work. It is just (or simply) therapy, devoid of the commonly accepted excesses and limitations of some professional approaches and Western cultural bias. It is a demystifying approach that enables a wider range of practitioners, including those with skills and community experience or cultural knowledge. The term 'just therapy' does not suggest a dilution of therapeutic knowledge and competence, but rather a distillation of therapeutic practices.

It was developed by a group of people at the Family Centre, Lower Hutt, Wellington, New Zealand who wanted to push out the boundaries of therapeutic practice and apply a fresh critique. We wanted to address the profound experiences of social pain that were not being adequately responded to by caseworkers, because of a narrower clinical focus. The group were women and men. We were Māori, Samoan, and Pakeha (European). Some were very highly educated and well qualified. Others had barely finished the compulsory requirements of the New Zealand education system. Some were community development workers. Some were family therapists. Most were both.

There were a plurality of starting points and a plurality of knowledge and experience. Firstly, there was the vast body of international social science knowledge. Secondly, and of no less importance, were the traditions of healing and the processes of healthy relationships in the three cultures from which we came, Māori, Samoan, and Pakeha. Thirdly, were the separate gendered experiences of the women and men. Fourthly, there was a shared commitment to social justice. And fifthly, an open belief in a universal spirituality that acknowledged the sacredness of people's stories, particularly in their exposure of pain: a view of spirituality that was not institutionalized in form, but spirituality that was essentially about relationships. These five aspects were the pivotal points of collectivity in our early reflections, sharing, and debate.

Early on the Centre realized that many families who came to them with problems that included psychosomatic illnesses, violence, depression, addiction, delinquency, marital stress, psychotic illnesses, parenting problems, relationship stress, and so on, after some questioning, located the onset of their problem with events that were external to the family. These were events like unemployment, bad housing, homelessness, racist, sexist, or heterosexist experiences, and the like. They were extremely depressing ongoing experiences that eventually led parents and children into a state of stress and/or depression that opened them up to physical and mental illnesses.

At first, the Centre endeavoured to address the symptomatic illnesses, treating those problems as though they were the result of internal family dysfunction. As family therapists, it was thought the problems being seen were the symptoms of family relationship difficulties. After years of listening attentively to the stories of these people, however, the Centre learned that for many clients, their problems were actually the symptoms of poverty, of unjust economic planning, of racism, sexism, and heterosexism.

We learned that when people came to us depressed and in bad housing, and we treated their clinical or social problems (symptoms) within the conventional clinical or social work boundaries, we were simply making them feel a little better in poverty. Usually we were able to quite effectively help move them out of depression, but then simply sent them back to the conditions that created the problems in the first place. Unintentionally, but nevertheless very effectively, we recognized we were adjusting people to poverty. Significantly we realized that this is what most therapists and social workers do when working with poor or marginalized families.

Further, by implication we also recognized we were encouraging in the families the belief that they, rather than the unjust structures, were the authors of their problems and failures. Like so many other therapists, we did this despite our knowledge of structured unemployment in most post-industrial countries, despite our knowledge of the physical and psychological pathologies associated with inadequate housing; despite our knowledge of the same pathologies associated with ongoing racist experience; and despite our knowledge of the patriarchal determinants of physical and sexual abuse.

Liberating meaning

Psychology, social work, and the other helping professions have been taught within a largely positivist and modernist framework. The claims to a superior professional body of knowledge often centre on the social science claims to notions of independence, neutrality, objectivity, and verifiability (Habermas 1971; Weiten 1995). Medical metaphors with notions of diagnosis and cure, and biological metaphors with a systemic focus are often used. The term 'social science' is itself a metaphor modelled on the physical sciences. These all combine to create practitioners who search in varying degrees for objective diagnoses, objective causes, objective explanations, and objective cures.

These processes have built a status of superiority for the social sciences over other forms of knowledge, such as gender, cultural and socioeconomic knowledge. Over time this has created many problems, because the social sciences have grown up in environments that involve a range of assumptions.

Prior to the last quarter of the 20th century, reasonably well-resourced white men devised most of the theory and taught most of the practice. Books written in Western Europe or North America by such people were sold throughout the world. Thus the cultural assumptions of a healthy family, for example, grew out of an environment where individual self-worth, choice, and secularism in science were seen as primary values. They were then picked up and taught in cultures whose primary values centred around communal identity, genealogical ties, and spirituality. To be professionally qualified, one had to adopt the dominant assumptions in training and practice. In Western Europe and North America, these assumptions are still dominant and African American, First Nations people and Asian cultures in Europe are expected to absorb them as part of their professional growth and development.

There were gender blind spots as well. It wasn't so very long ago that sexual and violent abuse were looked upon by psychologists, and other therapists, in clinical terms within the old medical, biological, and social science metaphors, characteristic of the more patriarchal assumptions of the times. Causes were sought, and symptoms were treated, but the abuse itself was often ignored or considered outside the clinical arena.

This began to change substantially in the 1970s and 1980s when women politicized the issue. Articulate feminists (Bograd 1984; Goldner 1985; Kamsler 1990; Pizzey 1982) challenged the helping professions and policy-makers to identify violence, expose its damage, and devise policies and therapies that would hold offenders accountable and create safety. Judith Herman (1992) went further, placing domestic violence alongside other forms of terror beyond an individual experience into a broader political frame. She argued that psychological trauma can be understood only in a social context.

Psychologists, social workers, doctors, nurses, and therapists can no longer act as they did before. Policy and law makers have been required to address the broader structural issues around violence and safety. The movement for change that was spearheaded by feminists soon drew support from other women and some groups of men.

The term 'abuse' and the meanings we now give it have changed our practice, our explanations, and even the law. Most people are now trained to recognize violence when it occurs and to ensure that those victimized by it are properly supported and freed from self-blame. Perpetrators are usually exposed and encouraged to take responsibility. Men's and women's groups have sprung up to teach non-violence, refuges and safe houses now exist in most cities and towns, and large community educational drives including television advertising take place to highlight the horrors of domestic violence.

The problem of violence has not been solved, of course, but it has been exposed and it is being addressed. Safety is understood today to be a primary issue when dealing with gender equity. It is written into most professional codes of ethics. It is recognized by most of the helping professions as needing to be addressed immediately when it arises and it has become a priority in policing.

We have learned that violence is endemic in our societies and it is going to require much more effort to extinguish such deeply embedded cultural responses. Nevertheless, the courage of those who began the big push to expose the injustice has achieved an incredible amount. In fact, they offer an example of what can be accomplished in other areas when sufficiently large and motivated groups of people are determined to turn an injustice around.

This was not discovered scientifically, it was the result of a critical analysis accompanied by a political movement that created new awareness by drawing attention to the meanings given to these events. In a critical postmodern sense, the old practice was deconstructed and all its assumptions exposed. The chosen word 'abuse' floated a new meaning that highlighted women's experience and placed responsibility on the perpetrators. None of this emerged out of the so called objectivity of psychology or the social sciences. A political movement identified the injustice and insisted that the practice be changed.

This example serves to expose one of the dubious assumptions in the development of social science knowledge. There are many others. The just therapy approach questions assumptions that lock people into disadvantage or injustice. In that same critical postmodern sense, the meaning behind assumptions are sought, where appropriate they are exposed and new meanings are created which liberate and inspire resolution and hope.

Cultural knowledge offers another good example. All cultures carry with them history, beliefs, and ways of doing things. Cultures particularly carry meanings. We experience practically all the most intimate events in our life, within a culture or cultures. Within our families or intimate groupings, we learn the rules and the accepted ways of doing things. Public life is also determined by the meanings created by cultures. There is nothing more basic to our identity and sense of belonging than our culture (Durie 2004; Ross 2009; Tamasese and Waldegrave 1993).

Most of the psychological theories, however, have been developed in Western Europe, and white North America. These Western cultures tend to favour notions of individual self-determination over extended family or collective notions of self-determination. They primarily focus, for example, on individuals within disadvantaged ethnic communities succeeding rather than the community as a group succeeding. As a consequence most theories of counselling, psychotherapy, and clinical psychology posit individual self-worth, in one form or another, as the primary goal of therapy (Owusu-Bempah and Howitt 2000; Sampson 1993; Sue and Sue 1990). That is because destiny, responsibility, legitimacy, and even human rights are essentially individual concepts in most Western cultures. It follows that concepts of self, individual assertiveness, and fulfilment are central to most of these therapies.

However, for many of the cultural communities within Western countries, and for most cultures internationally, collective notions of family and groups of families' well-being are favoured over individual ones. If, for example, you come from a communal or extended family culture to some form of therapy because of traumatic experiences you may have endured, questions that encourage individual family members to expose their personal feelings with no regard to the family's cultural sense of order, may be inappropriate and even alienating. Likewise notions of self-assertion, common in many Western therapies, may be experienced as confusing and unhelpful. Among individually-based cultures, such questions can be quite appropriate. Outside these cultures, however, the questions are often experienced as intrusive and rude. They can crudely crash through the sensitivities in communal-based and extended family cultures. They can rupture cooperative sensitivities among people, and destroy the essential framework for meaning that should be drawn upon for healing.

It is important not to exaggerate notions of individualism as being dichotomous with collective concepts. The welfare state in most English-speaking democracies expresses strong notions of collective responsibility, but not as strong as those of most continental European countries (Esping-Andersen 1996). Most Western cultures also have collective notions of family, but shared obligations and resources among extended family members tend to be weaker than in other cultures. Nevertheless, individualistic concepts are often powerfully embedded in the assumptions, constructs, and policies in Western countries.

This does not mean that individualistic concepts are better or worse than collective or family concepts. Rather, it is to suggest that they are different. There should be room for both. There should even be room for contradictions, as some will hold, for example, a strong collective sense of family and at the same time be resolute about their commitment to their individual self-determination. The homage to the primacy of the individual has deep philosophical roots in the West as a whole (Tawney 1926; Weber 1905), with particular potency in the English-speaking world. It is so much a part of the culture that the notion has since been frequently purveyed uncritically through social science literature (Bellah et al. 1985; Maslow 1970).

Surely good social work and clinical practice should enhance people's sense of identity and belonging, but unfortunately the practices of applied social science have developed with Western cultural assumptions that so often render them ineffective with most non-white groups. This explains why so many marginalized cultural groups fail to communicate with the social professions who are paid to help them.

Spirituality offers another important aspect that stands out. Social scientists often boast that their discipline is a secular science. They are suspicious of notions like love or transcendence because they cannot measure or verify them. Families in non-Western cultures frequently associate healing with spiritual practices and traditions. At the Family Centre, Māori and Pacific Island people when working with people from their culture often share dreams, prayers and numinous experiences that are important to the life of the family and the issues of health and wholeness. When violations are being talked about, there is often a need for spiritual rituals of protection. Those important aspects are considered sacred, and yet they are frequently disregarded by social workers and psychologists. As such the social or clinical work is often perceived as being culturally unsafe for the client family.

The mainstream assumptions, which are usually considered by their proponents to be somehow more professional and objective, are deconstructed in these examples. Tragically, they illustrate a colonial mentality that ensures that the health and welfare resources seldom reach the marginalized cultural groups, on their own terms. It is little wonder these communities continue their disadvantaged profiles.

Alternative knowledge and plurality for those whose values are different is often minimized or ignored. In this manner, the distinctiveness of cultural, gender and socioeconomic meaning is made in a sense invisible, and is not recognized (Taylor 1994). Services for families and family policies are devised within this ideological context. Health and therapeutic services assume a primarily individualistic approach, and policy settings cater to the same values as though they were objective and robust. The 'experiences of belonging' of those who are not part of the mainstream are usually denied. Their critical contexts of meaning are largely, although not entirely, overlooked. The assumptions of the dominant culture, gender and socioeconomic position generally prevail, and those who are dissimilar are expected to adjust to the mainstream, or to translate the processes into their own cultural milieu.

A strange world of universalized therapeutic and policy prescriptions emerges in such a context. In a therapeutic setting, for example, families, whose traditions of meaning and ways of doing things may be centuries old, are often co-opted into the world and constructions of the therapist or counsellor. The metaphors of the families' culture are usually absent. So too are their rituals. And this happens when the families are in very vulnerable states, which is why they are seeking therapeutic help in the first place.

The consequences of this universalized approach, as it works its way through our social and economic systems, are all too apparent. Within countries like the United Kingdom (Office for National Statistics 2005), the United States, Canada, Australia, and New Zealand (Ministry of Social Development 2009), they manifest themselves in the statistical measurement of outcomes. The social, educational, health and economic results for many immigrant and indigenous people, for example, are consistently poorer than for the mainstream. This strongly suggests that most immigrant and indigenous cultures approach learning, socialization, and economic activity from different perspectives than the mainstream, and educational and other systems disadvantage them, while favouring those more in tune with the mainstream.

Effective clinical practice and social work needs to be developed by people from those cultures. All cultures have people who have the confidence of their community and know the emphases and meanings that enable health and well-being. In a just therapy, resources are moved from ineffective mainstream outlets to cultural groups to develop their own paradigms that give dignity and add colour and variety to the field. Where these become effective and gain the support of their communities, they then need to be recognized as a new and valid practice to be equally funded by government and private health and welfare funders. Furthermore, this process also enhances employment opportunities in communities that often have higher unemployment rates.

Public policy settings and therapeutic responses

As was noted earlier in this chapter, there is now a substantial body of literature that associates cultural marginalization, gender inequities, and low income households with physical and mental ill health. The studies consistently show a distinct relationship between inequalities in society and physical and mental ill health. Poorer people die earlier, consistently have the poorest health and the highest hospitalization rates (Benzeval et al. 1995; Kawachi and Berkman 2003; Kawachi and Kennedy 2002; Mackenbach 2006; Marmot 2010; Ministry of Social Development 2009; National Health Committee 1998; Wilkinson and Pickett 2009). Furthermore, when there is an overall improvement in a country's population health status, the health inequalities do not decrease.

The evidence is so overwhelming that a number of major government enquiries have been set up over the last decade and a half to study the evidence and recommend new directions for national health services to address health status from the perspective of inequalities. The famous Acheson *Independent Inquiry into Inequalities in Health Report* in the United Kingdom (1998), *The Social, Cultural and Economic Determinants of Health in New Zealand: Action to Improve Health* (1998) and the Marmot Review, *Fair Society, Healthy Lives* (2010) also in the UK, are three such examples.

Given the substantive evidence of the relationship between inequality and physical and mental ill health, it is reasonable to suggest that many of the problems that families present in therapy result from poverty, inadequate housing, unjust economic planning, unemployment, racism, and so on. As such, where this is the case, they can be conceived as the symptoms of inequality. From this perspective, these symptoms, which are usually construed in mental health or social categories, should not be considered as simply personal, intra-psychic or intra-family disorders when they arise in association with broader structural problems in society. They can be more accurately viewed primarily as the symptoms of those structural social problems. The tighter clinical categories are secondary, and only useful if viewed in relation to the primary focus.

This suggests a notion that many, though obviously not all, of the mental health and relationship problems people have are the consequences of power differences and injustice. Such a notion only infrequently features in clinical literature or as a major theme in therapeutic conferences. If it did, however, there would be considerably more exploration and analysis around public policy ethics and social justice themes as they relate to family context and less exclusive focus on the boundaried space of individuals, couples or families.

Central to the 'just therapy' approach is the view that therapists, be they psychologists, social workers, counsellors, psychiatrists, or nurses, etc, have a critical role in post-industrial and largely secular states. They are the predominant professional group who listen to the pain of individuals and families. They work in the institutions that address pain in these societies, like the health, welfare and justice services. They work in the non-government (NGOs) and community organizations that provide family support and services around abuse, poverty, housing, general counselling, mental and physical ill health, and so on. They also work privately, but are often contracted into the work of these larger organizations.

Therapists, as a professional group, are the most informed 'experts' of the collectively grounded levels of hurt, sadness, and pain in modern countries. Those who live in deep pain are, of course, the primary 'experts' in the sadness and hurt they and their communities experience, but therapists are the professional helpers who continually witness that pain with many individuals and families and across a variety of communities week after week. As such, they carry a substantial responsibility to identify, quantify and describe the severity and causes of it. This is ethically essential if they are committed to honouring their client group. They have a responsibility to publish and publicise the causes and outcomes of people's pain in order that they may be addressed in the public debate and impact on policy. Good public policy in this sense can address issues of well-being and inclusion in informed and effective ways and actually prevent the need for therapy.

Therapists in this view, can be healthily seen as the 'thermometers of pain' in modern countries. Instead of withholding their knowledge in clinical vacuums, they can quantify, describe and identify causality for all to see. Where issues around housing, poverty or race become dominant in caseloads, for example, their descriptions can inform the public by adding reality and depth, and providing a more helpful basis for intelligent public discussion. A good example of this can be seen in the public work many fine therapists have carried out highlighting the levels of abuse occurring in many countries, the causes of that abuse and the policies and laws required to stop it. A parallel level of action and commitment is required in a range of other pain causing factors therapists identify.

There is a further need for therapists to engage directly with disadvantaged communities, which requires them to take the critical context beyond the family into account. Those most in need of the health and welfare resources in most societies and communities are those who experience the most trauma, the greatest stress, and as a consequence the most ill health. They are usually those on low incomes, people in cultures that have been marginalized in the societies in which they live, and most frequently women. Unfortunately, therapeutic resources are spread rather thinly for this group because they are outside the mainstream and have less money.

Gender equity and the feminization of poverty

During the course of the last five decades, gender roles, expectations, and understanding have undergone enormous change. The patriarchal inequalities that were accelerated over the period of the industrial revolution and continued right through into the post-war welfare states were glaringly exposed by feminist critique in the 1960s, 1970s, and since, in which almost every aspect of gender inequality was assessed (Friedan 1963; Gilligan 1982; Greer 1970; hooks 1999). The results of that assessment have fuelled the challenges that took place then and have continued since.

Traditional notions of family and gender roles have been transformed as a result. This is not to suggest that the old patriarchal structures have completely crumbled, but their foundations have been substantially shaken and their assumptions are continuously challenged. At the same time, the shapes of families have changed markedly. In New Zealand, for example, 90% of families with dependent children in 1976 were living in two-parent households and 10% were in one-parent households. Thirty years later in 2006 (the last census), 71% were living in two-parent households and 29% in one-parent households (Ministry of Social Development 2009). This is not to suggest that two-parent households are devalued, or that the demographic change is simply due to feminism, but the change is significant. The labour market has also changed, with higher female participation rates and women represented much more in senior and managerial positions.

There was a period recently in New Zealand when women occupied each of the positions of Prime Minister, Governor General, Attorney General, Chief Justice, and CEO of our largest company. While this is not typical, it is indicative of substantial changes in leadership and influence. Many of these changes are welcome, but they do not always find their balance. The changes in many households are often superimposed on a patriarchal structure, where women work in the labour market but continue to be the primary carers for children and responsible for domestic tasks (Hochschild 2003). While some couples find a new and equitable balance, deep resentments can occur when gender arrangements do not adjust to the new situation. The stresses that modern families experience can stem from inequities in the home.

They can also spring from inequities in society. Not the least of these is the post-industrial phenomenon often referred to as the feminization of poverty. In post-industrialized countries, sole-parent woman-led households are usually the poorest (Jones 2005; Ministry of Social Development 2009). Furthermore, in recent years they have become an increasing proportion of all households with children. Not all single parents are living on low incomes, but analysis by the New Zealand Poverty Measurement Project demonstrated as early as 1993 that over 70% of single-parent households lived below the poverty threshold (Stephens et al. 1995), and they continue to dominate the poverty statistics.

Contemporary globalized market societies seem to consider the two-income family as their societal norm. If there is only one income earner, they have to be earning a high income or work extremely long hours to be financially comfortable. This imposes an extraordinary strain on most sole parents, because alongside their working life they can be the only parent for their children and they are also responsible for household domestic tasks. Their costs are only marginally less than those for two-parent families. In most cases, they require houses with the same number of bedrooms as two-parent families with the same number of children. Children require the same amount of transport, food, clothing, and other costs. It is no wonder, then, that a large proportion of sole parent families have few resources and low living standards. It is also not surprising that many of these households are much more susceptible to mental and physical sickness.

Very few countries have been able to devise policy responses that adequately overcome the disadvantages single-parent households' experience. They usually lack money and support to relieve their ongoing parental roles, and workplaces can be insensitive to the flexibility they require when children are sick or they are simply exhausted. They are often stigmatized by others for being single parents. When they arrive at counselling centres or other service providers, it is very important to recognize and address the contextual factors in their lives and avoid working on the symptoms of their distress out of context.

From the perspective of 'just therapy', the challenge for therapists and policy-makers is to develop policies that facilitate the social inclusion and participation of single parents, while working with the demands they face from their multiple roles. These can include education and training, pathways into the workforce, the development of informal social networks, and well-funded holidays and activities for children. Sole-parent families need recreation, activities they can afford, and opportunities to build relationships.

Applying the 'just' context in the therapeutic process

There can be many ways a 'just therapy' can be practised or applied. At root the relevant cultural, gender, and/or socioeconomic context plays a major role in framing the therapeutic conversation. Where it is possible, people who live and participate within a particular cultural community are usually seen by someone from that community. From the outset, the rituals of welcome and respect, appropriate to that culture, are introduced as the therapist or counsellor enters the conceptual world of the client or client family. This enables the family to speak and act freely without having to translate their perceptions and experience into the language and concepts of the dominant social group in their region or country. Sometimes cultural consultants, who may not be trained in the social sciences but clearly have a role in their community, will work alongside a more mainstream therapist. This enables the skills and metaphors of the culture to play their appropriate part in the therapeutic process.

The questioning is respectful in the sense that the therapist is often receiving deeply personal information about clients' vulnerabilities and they indicate that they honour the trust accorded. 'Who' and 'what' questions are preferred over 'why' questions, because they encourage unselfconscious narrative without requiring justification. The therapist's role is to facilitate the telling of events around the presenting problem and other associated events, in order to discern the meanings family members give to them. People often construct negative meanings around their or other members of their family's circumstances and the task of the therapist is to help deconstruct the negativity and encourage the family to develop positive and sustainable ways of living together.

It is beneficial, for example, when questioning low-income household members to sensitively address their stories around accessing necessities. The adequacy of household income, the quality of housing, and access to good healthcare are critical contexts. Families in these situations struggle and are often highly motivated to share coping strategies and survival skills. These, in turn, offer genuine stories for the therapist to admire, honour and in a sense to be in awe of.

Poor families are often viewed in derogatory ways by others in their society and a sense of defeat sometimes sets in that can lead to serious depression and other mental health problems. The construction of meaning centres on pathological notions of failure. The professionals will often speak of 'dysfunctional' and 'multi-problem families' and the families can come to view themselves in a negative light. This consistently negative view, combined with the sense of social failure and lower status conferred by mainstream society, can quickly become self-fulfilling.

However, many of these people have suffered extreme disadvantage and developed many survival skills. It is critical to the 'just therapy' approach to recognize where their strength lies and to honour it. It is usually found in their resilience under the sort of stress middle-income households are seldom required to endure. Families who are forced to live in overcrowded houses, for example, often live under extreme stress as are others whose right to sustainable adequate housing is threatened. There is nothing more basic to a family and family health than a house. Without adequate, safe and secure housing all families are at risk of mental and/or physical sickness.

The meaning therapists assign to poor families' housing problems determines whether or not the problem will be located internally or in its socioeconomic context. If the former route is taken, then feelings of inadequacy and self-blame will be encouraged. If the latter contextual route is chosen, then the focus will move towards understanding the socioeconomic context and developing smart survival strategies. It is important to challenge the failure meanings that so many poor families take on board as a result of their constrained circumstances and the reactions of others to them.

A 'just therapy' endeavours to untangle the malign threads of meaning and weave new patterns of resolution and hope. Having explored their stories of resilience, resistance, and survival, therapists and counsellors would commend such people for surviving the housing crisis with their family still intact. They would recognize their ability to survive the crisis not of their making, but the failure of policy makers and planners, as courageous, committed and extraordinarily competent.

In this positive context, they are able to address the symptomatic presenting problems in context, enabling families to identify the broader structural issues that have been imposed on them. Therapists can then help them recognize their strengths as the stepping stones to either survive without self-blame or to develop smart strategies to move to a more secure social place. In doing so, they are creating new and preferable meanings that recognize the socioeconomic realities and encourage the recognition of powerful inner strengths within the client/s.

This same process of deconstructing pathological meaning and creating meaning that inspires hope and resolution is just as relevant in other areas of need. The victim/survivors of sexual abuse and physical violence, for example, frequently blame themselves for contributing to the abuse and over time develop negative images of themselves as flawed and unworthy of real success in life. However, their ability to have survived the ordeals that were imposed on them and the achievements in their lives since can become the basis for helping them discard the sense of guilt and begin to value their ability to survive under duress and achieve.

In this process, the use of metaphors is central to the 'just therapy' approach. The Māori and Samoan cultures in which it grew up are rich in metaphor. Metaphors provide a vehicle for softer and less direct forms of communication than the tenets of most western therapies. They enable people to stop and reflect, while at the same time save face if they are embarrassed.

The analogy of weaving is often employed as a 'just' way of describing case or therapeutic work. Although the symbolism of weaving is international, it is particularly appropriate, because it evokes the activity of many Māori and Pacific women. People come for therapy and counselling with problem-centred webs of meaning, and the task of the caseworker is to weave new threads of meaning and possibility that give new colour and new textures. The weaving should loosen the tight and rigid problem-centred pattern, enrich the colour and enable resolution and hope.

Another metaphor that is often used in 'just therapy' is that of spirituality. Spirituality here is not referring to Christian institutionalism, but to something more akin to the sacredness of life or 'soul' as in soul music. In this view, the therapeutic conversation is a sacred encounter, because people come in great pain and share their story. The story is like a gift, a very personal offering given in great vulnerability. It has a spiritual quality. It is not a scientific pathology that requires removal, nor is it an ill-informed understanding of the story that requires correction. It is rather a person's articulation of events, and the meaning given to those events, which have become problematic. The therapist honours and respects the story, and then in return gives a reflection that offers alternative liberating meanings that inspire resolution and hope.

Finally, there are three primary concepts that characterize the 'just therapy' approach. When assessing the quality of such work, it is measured against the inter-relationship of three concepts. The first is *belonging*. This refers to the essence of identity, to who we are, our cultured and gendered histories, and our ancestry. The second is *sacredness*. This refers to the deepest respect for humanity, its qualities, and the environment. The third is *liberation*. It refers to freedom, wholeness, and justice. It is the inter-dependence of these concepts that is important, not one without another. Not all stories of belonging are liberating, for example, and some experiences of liberation are not sacred. It is the harmony between all three concepts that authentically characterizes a just therapy.

References

Acheson, Sir, D. (1998). *Independent inquiry into inequalities in health*. Stationery Office, Norwich. http://www.archive.official-documents.co.uk/document/doh/ih/contents.htm

Bellah, R., Madsen, R., Sullivan, W., Swidler, A., and Tipton, S. (1985). *Habits of the heart: Individualism and commitment in American life* (2nd ed., 1995). University of California Press, Berkeley, CA.

Benzeval, M., Judge, K., and Whitehead, M. (Eds.) (1995). *Tackling inequalities in health: An agenda for action*. King's Fund, London.

Bograd, M. (1984). Family systems approach to wife battering: A feminist critique. *American Journal of Orthopsychiatry*, **54**(4), 558–68.

Cozolino, L. (2006). *The neuroscience of human relationships*. W. W. Norton and Co, New York.

Durie, M. (2004). M ori. In C. R. Ember and M. Ember (Eds.) *Encyclopedia of medical anthropology: Health and illness in the world's culture*, pp. 815–22. Kluwer Academic/Plenum, New York.

Erikson, E. (1950). *Childhood and society*. W. W. Norton and Co, New York.

Esping-Andersen, G. (1996). *Welfare states in transition: Social security in the new global economy*. Sage, London.

Friedan, B. (1963). *The feminine mystique*. Dell Publishing, New York.

Gerhardt, S. (2004). *Why love matters: How affection shapes a baby's brain*. Routledge, East Sussex.

Gilligan, C. (1982). *In a different voice: Psychological theory and women's development*. Harvard University Press, Cambridge, MA.

Goldner, V. (1985). Feminism and family therapy. *Family Process*, **24**, 31–47.

Greer, G. (1970). *The female eunuch*. Farrar, Straus and Giroux, New York.
Habermas, J. (1971). *Knowledge and human interest* (J. J. Shapiro, Trans.). Beacon Press, Boston, MA.
Herman, J. (1992). *Trauma and recovery*. Basic Books, New York.
Hochschild, A. (2003). *The second shift*. Viking Penguin, New York.
hooks, b. (1999). *Ain't I a woman: Black women and feminism*. South End Press, Cambridge, MA.
Jones, F. (2005). *The effects of taxes and benefits on household income, 2004–05, National Statistics, U.K.* http://www.statistics.gov.uk/articles/nojournal/taxesbenefits200405/Taxesbenefits20 0405.pdf. [Accesssed January 2009.]
Kamsler, A. (1990). Her story in the making: Therapy with women who were sexually abused in childhood. In C. White and M. Durrant (Eds.) *Ideas for therapy with sexual abuse*, pp. 9–36. Dulwich Centre Publications, Adelaide.
Kawachi, I., and Berkman, L.F. (2003). *Neighbourhoods and health*. Oxford University Press, New York.
Kawachi, I. and Kennedy, B. (2002). *The health of nations*. The New Press, New York.
Love, C. (2000). Family group conferencing: Cultural origins, sharing and appropriation– A Maori reflection. In G. Burford and J. Hudson (eds.) *Family group conferencing: New directions in community-centered child and family practice*, pp. 15–30. Aldine de Gruyter, New York.
Mackenbach, J. (2006). *Health inequalities: Europe in profile*. An independent, expert report commissioned by the UK Presidency of the EU (February 2006).
Marmot, Sir M. (Chair of the Independent Review Commission) (2010). *Fair society, healthy lives: The Marmot Review. Strategic review of health inequalities in England post-2010*. The Marmot Review, Department of Health. London. http://www.ucl.ac.uk/gheg/marmotreview/FairSocietyHealthyLives
Maslow, A. (1970). *Motivation and personality* (2nd ed.). Harper & Row, New York.
Ministry of Social Development (2009). *The social report 2009*. Ministry of Social Development, Wellington. http://www.socialreport.msd.govt.nz/
National Equality Panel (2010). *An anatomy of economic inequality in the UK: Report of the National Equality Panel*. Government Equalities Office London. http://sticerd.lse.ac.uk/dps/case/cr/CASEreport60.pdf
National Health Committee (1998). *The social, cultural and economic determinants of health in New Zealand: Action to improve health*. Ministry of Health, Wellington.
Office for National Statistics (2005). *National statistics: Focus on ethnicity & identity*. http://www.statistics.gov.uk/downloads/theme_compendia/foe2004/Ethnicity.pdf. [Accessed January 2009.]
Owusu-Bempah, K. and Howitt, D. (2000). *Psychology beyond western perspectives*. British Psychological Society, Leicester.
Pizzey, E. (1982). *Prone to violence*. Hamblyn Paperbacks, Middlesex.
Posner, M.I., and Rothbart, M.K. (2007). *Educating the human brain*. American Psychological Association Washington DC.
Quintana, S., Aboud, F., Chao, R., et al. (2006). Race, ethnicity, and culture in child development: Contemporary research and future directions. *Child Development*, 77(5), 1129–41.
Ross, M. (Ed.) (2009). *Culture and belonging in divided societies: contestation and symbolic landscapes*. University of Pennsylvania Press, Philadelphia, PA.

Sampson, E. (1993). *Celebrating the other: A dialogic account of human nature.* Harvester-Wheatsheaf, New York.

Schore, A. (2003). *Affect dysregulation and disorders of the self.* Norton, New York.

Shonkoff, J. and Phillips, D. (Eds). (2000). *From neurons to neighborhoods: The science of early childhood development.* National Academy Press, Washington DC.

Stephens, R., Waldegrave, C. and Frater, P. (1995). Measuring poverty in New Zealand. *Social Policy Journal of New Zealand,* **5**, 88–112.

Sue, D.W., and Sue, D. (1990). *Counselling the culturally different: Theory and practice.* Wiley, New York.

Tamasese, K. and Waldegrave, C. (1993). Cultural and gender accountability in the 'just therapy' approach. *Journal of Feminist Family Therapy,* **5**(2), 29–45.

Tamasese, K., Peteru, C., Waldegrave, C., and Bush, A. (2005). Ole Taeao Afua, The New Morning: A qualitative investigation into Samoan perspectives on mental health and culturally appropriate services. *Australian and New Zealand Journal of Psychiatry,* **39**(4), 300–9.

Tawney, R.H. (1926). *Religion and the rise of capitalism* (1938 ed.). Pelican Books, West Drayton.

Taylor, C. (1994). *Multiculturalism: Examining the politics of recognition*, Princeton University Press, Princeton, NJ.

Waldegrave, C. and Waldegrave, K. (2009). *Healthy families, young minds and developing brains: Enabling all children to reach their potential.* Wellington: Families Commisssion. Available from: http://www.nzfamilies.org.nz/sites/default/files/downloads/RF-Healthy-Families.pdf

Waldegrave, C., Tamasese, K., Tuhaka, F. and Campbell, W (2003a). *Just therapy–a journey: A collection of papers from the Just Therapy Team, New Zealand.* Dulwich Centre Publications, Adelaide.

Waldegrave, C., Stephens, R. and King, P. (2003b). Assessing the progress on poverty reduction. *Social Policy Journal of New Zealand,* **20**, 197–222.

Weber, M. (1905). *The protestant ethic and the spirit of capitalism.* Blackwell Publishing, Oxford.

Weiten, W. (1995). *Psychology: Themes and variations* (3rd Ed.). Brooks, Pacific Grove, California.

Wilkinson, R. and Pickett, K. (2009). *The spirit level: Why more equal societies almost always do better.* Allen Lane, London.

Chapter 12

Māori expressions of healing in 'just therapy'

Maria Maniapoto

The aim of this chapter is to contextualize the underlying philosophical approaches to 'just therapy'. It discusses the cultural and philosophical perspectives of working with Māori families at the Family Centre. The views of the writer are subjective and contextualized from the experiences and realities of working with Māori families at the Family Centre. They are the views of a Māori woman staff member at the Family Centre. There are two critical points in relation to this perspective:

1) Indigenous culture plays a critical role in the way in which we provide services to our community; and
2) Incorporating indigenous views, perspectives, culture, etc. into our work practice are taken for granted.

The context

People who come to the Family Centre often come from low socioeconomic backgrounds, many have low educational qualifications, and/or many belong to a marginalized minority. Given that Māori are disproportionally overrepresented in these areas, they are among the highest users of health and mental health services in New Zealand. Consequently, many of our clients are Māori who seek to address a wide range of issues, most of which have resulted in some form of family dysfunction or breakdown. We are not a mental health service, but we are dedicated to improving the health and well-being outcomes of those who are affected by the impacts of mental health, sociocultural, and economic disorders.

Commonly, our clients have sought help from a number of different agencies over an extended period. Sometimes they have little confidence that our service will help because previous engagement in counselling or therapy has made little difference. If people have no confidence then they may never believe that they can restore harmony in their lives or find a way to live without pain and distress. Therefore, it is important that we build confidence and lift their expectations so that hope can be restored. Each family's situation has developed within a specific context, and we have to find the most appropriate framework to analyse that context, so that the family can seek some resolution.

We navigate through the personal stories, histories, life accounts, and experiences to gain a better understanding of the nature and origins of the issues. As people tell their stories, we soon identify the unique set of factors and circumstances that have caused many of the issues. This process is slow and it can be challenging to maintain a positive connection with people who have lost hope. However, if we fail to identify the true source of the issues or problems, then we may not be able to seek a long-term resolution.

The most common issues people present with are the result of domestic violence, family relationship disruption, and various experiences of economic, social, and cultural adversity. These issues are given high-priority service by our health and social service agencies, as they pose high-risk factors to the health and well-being of the entire population. Traditionally, the primary function of these agencies has been to treat the symptoms of the disorder. That is, the doctor will fix the broken limbs, the drug and alcohol addictions service will treat the addict, the truancy officer will make sure the student returns to school, etc. However, once the limb has healed there is a good chance that it might break repeatedly if the source that caused the break is not identified and dealt with appropriately. Similarly, when we talk to someone about family violence, we try not to let the issue of abuse dominate our discussions or else we end up providing a legal protection service. Instead, we try to find smart ways to stop the abuse immediately while seeking to understand the more complex reasons of why an abused partner continues to be abused, or why an abusive parent continues to abuse his or her children. Our practice has evolved as we have come to understand that it is inadequate to simply try to help someone manage anger without understanding the true nature of that anger. After ensuring the family is safe, we tend to focus on identifying the factors that produce or initiate the anger and work with them.

One issue I have observed amongst some of our Māori clients and families is that they lack a strong identity with Māori culture. That is, they do not exhibit a strong sense of belonging to Māori people or culture or they do not interpret their world in relation to the Māori world. A strong cultural identity is important, as it enables individuals to understand themselves in relationship with others (Sawrikar and Hunt 2005). Tangaere (1997) suggests a number of factors that must be present in order to achieve a strong Māori cultural identity. An individual must have ancestral links to the Māori world and this is achieved through ones genealogy (*whakapapa*). Through one's whakapapa an individual will possess a divine spirit (*mana atua*). As children they are nurtured, loved, and cared for by their *whanau* (family), *hapu* (sub-tribe), and *iwi* (main tribe), their roots are identified with the land and the child is able to develop a sense of belonging (*mana whenua*). Through the Māori language, the child is able to understand the world around them (*te ao turoa*). With all these values, the Māori child is able to develop a strong positive identity. These values carry with them the dignity and traditions of the past that they need in order for them to feel strong and comfortable with their Māori identity. Pere (1988) believes that when Māori people lack exposure to or understanding of these concepts, they are unable to form a strong identity as a Māori. Pere also states that a child should be totally immersed in the context of his or her own cultural values. In the Māori world, these values are the essence of *tikanga*[1] Māori.

---

[1] The Māori word *tikanga* has a wide range of meanings—culture, custom, ethic, etiquette, fashion, formality, lore, manner, meaning, mechanism, method, protocol, style. Generally taken to

Tangaere's model of Māori cultural identity development may help us to understand why some of our whanau and clients have not achieved a strong identity with the Māori world. Perhaps their ancestral links to the Māori world were severed through generations of cultural dislocation, loss of language, and land displacement. Aotearoa/New Zealand is a culturally diverse country where people affiliate with many cultures. It is also a colonized country where it is well known that historically little importance was accorded to Māori culture, language, and worldviews. Maurial (1999) explains that Māori and indigenous knowledge was labelled as inferior to Western knowledge within the Western world and its institutions, including schools. In Aotearoa/New Zealand, this conflict began when the first Europeans encountered Māori civilizations. We often witness the magnitude of this conflict when we hear the stories of shame, loss, and pain. Our first priority is to accord primary status to Māori worldviews, practices, beliefs, and ways of knowing. We bring the components that construct a strong cultural identity to the forefront so that being Māori is a given. We acknowledge that Māori history includes colonial history and that must be viewed in balance with contemporary realities. We also acknowledge that while history may stay the same, culture on the other hand is constantly changing and moving. Therefore we must find ways to balance traditional knowledge, concepts, and views in relation to local and current social, cultural, and political environments.

Te ao Māori in therapeutic practice

To begin with, it is necessary to understand *te reo Māori* (the Māori language), at the very minimum hold a conversation, but one must have enough knowledge of the language to be able to interpret the Māori world. For example, a word I frequently hear is *whakam*ā. Whakamā can generally be defined as embarrassment, indignity, shame, or shyness. In the context of these discussions, the word whakamā is used to reflect a sense of shame or embarrassment of one's actions. People often say that they feel whakamā that they 'beat up their misses', or because their drug or alcohol problem has caused the breakdown of their family. When used in this context, you could say that the word whakamā is a negative word. With good knowledge of the nuances of te reo Māori, we can extend a range of meanings to one word. For example, 'Ma te whakamā e patu' is a Māori saying which means 'Let the shame of your actions be your punishment'. However, it is not the same as saying 'Shame on you for your actions', te reo Māori is a passive language, and since we often work with very sensitive issues it is helpful to use a language which does not sound threatening or direct. On the one hand, the word whakamā is used to describe a negative feeling (shame or embarrassment). On the other hand, it takes strength and courage to accept that one's actions have brought about shame. Once this level of consciousness has been reached then restorative action can begin.

In my view, when someone holds a great sense of shame or whakamā for their actions they have a strength. This quality allows us to give new meaning to their stories

---

mean 'the Māori way of doing things', it is derived from the Māori word tika meaning 'right' or 'correct' (http://en.wikipedia.org/wiki/Tikanga_M%C4%81ori).

because if it were not for the great sense of shame, then they would not have the strength or determination to restore their well-being. These people come to us with great shame and after our first meeting, they leave knowing that they have a strong sense of character. This is a strength-based approach, which allows us to create new experiences, new understandings, and life stories, etc. Hence, we can begin to build the foundations for a stronger identity in the sessions which follow. There has been enough talking about the beatings and the drinking. We have to try to make people bring new meaning into their lives and help them to believe that new meaning can change lives.

These people often believe that they have little or no cultural identity; they also frequently feel that there has always been something missing in their lives. I tell them that their identity has always been with them, they were born with it. Just as Tangaere suggests, every Māori child has a divine spirit (*mana atua*), this spirit is inherited through ones *whakapapa* (ancestral links to the Māori world). It is just like an ember, all they need to do is to give it some air and fuel, and it will reignite. Part of my job is to help them reignite that ember and to return their cultural identity to the forefront. How they shape that identity depends entirely on what other cultural supports and resources they are able to access. They are able to strengthen their identity because their innate strength was always there. That is, somehow throughout all the turmoil and trauma in their lives, their *ahi kaa* still burns, all they need is the courage to rekindle the fire. In this example, the concept of ahi kaa is used as an analogy to describe a person's inner strength, their personal ahi kaa. It is a traditional Māori cultural concept, which in pre-European times referred to land occupation. Its literal meaning is 'site of burning fires'. It signified the presence of continuous land occupation. If a *hapu* or *iwi* did not maintain their ahi kaa then they extinguished their rights to control the land. This would also give opportunity for other hapu or iwi to establish their ahi kaa on that particular piece of land.[2] The use of the concept of ahi kaa provides a philosophical framework to help people re-construct a new sense of their cultural identity.

The impacts of colonization, government assimilation policies, etc. have aided in the demise of many indigenous cultures and languages. For some of our families, this means that their rights to maintain their cultural identity were extinguished while other cultures were established in its place. We are able to help some families restore their cultural identity because there is a little ahi kaa and so their ancestral links have remained intact. However, another reality we face is that some people's ahi kaa has been fully extinguished; there are no embers to rekindle. It is one thing to re-establish cultural links; it is another to try to reconnect people to something that they cannot conceive of having been there in the first place.

When families come to the Centre, we must firstly establish whose culture and language they identify with. If they identify with their tribal region, then this is usually a good indication that they identify with their culture (or at least parts of it). Then I know that they have a connection with their tribal region, culture, and maybe language. This means that it will be a little easier for us because then we can use the cultural frameworks and metaphors that we are familiar with. On the other hand, if they

---

[2] http://www.itaf.org.nz/?page_id=678

do not at least identify with their tribal region, then I am inclined to think that they may not have a strong cultural identity. The latter being the case, we can no longer assume that when Māori come to the Centre, that just because they look Māori, that they have garnered their experiences and life stories from *te ao Māori* (the Māori world). From my experience, these are the families who often present with issues which mask the deeper issues related to cultural identity. They are far more challenging to work with because they do not identify with the cultural markers, or they find it difficult to think in metaphorical terms because everything in their lives is 'rational', black and white, westernized.

Working with these families prompted me to question my beliefs that all Māori had the same cultural aspirations if only because we share a common history, heritage, culture, language. I inherited this attitude from my mother. My mother was raised at a time and in a place where cultural, gender values, beliefs, and attitudes were similar, and where people spoke a similar native language. However, by the time our family settled in Wellington during the early 1970s a change could be seen in the ways which people identified themselves. My mother told me a story about the day when she was waiting for the bus to go to work. She greeted some Māori women at the bus stop, her first instincts were to greet other Māori people in the Māori language, not only did she consider that this was courteous but it was also appropriate for her to speak her own language. She was surprised at the response she received. She said their body language sent a clear message to her, which was, this is the city, and we do not speak that language here. This was probably the first indication to her that Māori cultural identities had changed.

Western culture and language have had a profound affect on Māori people of Aotearoa, and so too for other indigenous groups around the world. However, I never realized how much of an influence it had on shaping our worldviews until I began to listen carefully to people's stories. Most people have adapted to Western culture, and they are able to live comfortably in both the Māori world and the Western world. However, some people have not been able to balance adaptation with preservation, and the cost of this imbalance has come at the expense of their language and cultural identity.

Judge Joe Williams is a prominent Māori leader, and he describes how individuals may develop a cultural identity. He says that there is a core group in the Māori community who are known as the traditional core. He describes how this group live close to or within their tribal roots. They are bicultural, bilingual, but identify strongly as Māori first. This group numbers between 100,000–150,000. He describes the next group as mainly urban. They are traditional or semi-traditional; they identify strongly as Māori but they have also created new identities from within their new urban communities. Although, he says, these people are noticeably Māori. (Although, I believe that it is presumptuous to identify Māori purely on the basis of their physical traits.) These groups are closely connected to their cultural ties and adopt all the labels of *mana* Māori. This group also numbers between 100,000–150,000. Collectively, these two groups maintain Māori culture, language, heritage, etc. They are the substance of the Māori world. If someone, who identifies with either of these two groups was to seek help from our service they might be the ones who ask for a Māori worker.

The third group is what Williams describes as 'unconnected'. He says that this group, do not hold strong ties with their kin, they may or may not identify as Māori. They probably do not care that much because they are quite happy with themselves and their identity. It is not surprising that this group numbers more than both the first and second groups put together. The fourth group represents at least 170,000. This is the group that is of mixed ethnic descent (Williams 2000).

In sum, Judge Williams' description of cultural identity highlights why we must acknowledge cultural diversity within groups. We must take into consideration how some of our people have grown up with a different sense of cultural identity and heritage. Sometimes, using cultural frameworks or metaphors is challenging when people identify with the Western world and they have garnered their experiences and life stories from a westernized culture, which we know in many ways does not support a Māori perspective. Whatever the forces were which shaped these conditions, it shifted the way in which people interpret their life experiences and how they form their worldviews. I believe that this has had a profound affect on our people's ability to cope with traumatic events in their lives.

Māori expressions of healing in 'just therapy'

When Māori families come to therapy it is the beginning of their spiritual journey to find healing. This is one of the dimensions in family therapy. Spirituality to Māori is essentially about relationships and within these relationships key aspects of Māori culture are expressed. In order to begin to understand what spirituality means for Māori and why it is so important, we must begin by looking at some key principles and values.

Key principles

In order to help people re-establish their cultural identities, I believe it is critical that they gain an understanding of the Māori world. Inevitably, we will begin working with the principle of *whakapapa*. Whakapapa has been described as the framework that links everything in the Māori world. In other words, it provides a structure for us to get to know oneself. For Māori, whakapapa is the source of all knowledge, all things animate and inanimate have a whakapapa. For the purposes of this chapter, this concept can be loosely defined as meaning genealogical knowledge. Te Maire Tau describes it as the fabric that held the knowledge of the world together, a theoretical basis for understanding the origins and interrelatedness between Māori people and their view of the world. In other words, in the Māori world, everything has a whakapapa, people, all living creatures and even issues have a whakapapa (Tau, 2001).

Belonging: the context of whakapapa

I attended a psychotherapy conference in New Zealand. The theme of the conference was: 'Imagining the Other: Initial contact in the Psychotherapy Relationship'. Prior to the conference I attended a meeting to discuss the conference theme. I did not realize that my understanding of the theme 'Imagining the Other' was a bit different to the rest of the people at the meeting. When it was my turn to say something I started talking about my ancestors and people close to me who had passed away. I just assumed that 'other' was not someone from a different culture but rather someone who had passed away. I thought that the conference theme was about *imagining dead people*. Despite my confusion, people seemed very interested in my perspective about 'the other'. As I proceeded to share my views, one of the psychotherapists at the meeting mentioned his first encounter with a Māori client. He described how the client entered his office, and as the client sat down, he turned to the therapist and asked if it was okay if his nan and koro (grandparents) could stay. The therapist replied, 'Of course, tell them to come in' (to the office). The client replied, 'Oh they are already sitting down'. The therapist could see no one else in the room. The therapist said that this was the first time he had encountered this situation. I do not know how the therapist reacted, but I do remember thinking he must have thought this client was hallucinating. This made me feel a bit nervous as I was sitting in a room full of psychotherapists talking about 'the others'. I do not mean to imply that I have 'psychic' abilities to communicate with the others; but it is not unusual for Māori people to have strong spiritual feelings. I began to wonder what happens in these situations where therapists or mental health professionals do not understand our worldview. Imagine what it is like for new immigrants, indigenous and marginalized groups who live in a very Eurocentric world and do not dress the same way and have different languages, cultural beliefs, attitudes, and rituals to those of the dominant group in society. How does the therapist engage with their client during the initial phase of contact? For me this was an important question because it is during this initial phase of contact where the context of whakapapa begins to emerge.

After listening to the discussions at the conference, I began to see that some people were struggling with this notion of 'imagining the other'. I think it is difficult for some people to 'imagine the other' when one does not know oneself, when one does not know ones whakapapa. Similarly, the first exercise in the 'just therapy' course we teach online asks students to talk about their cultural identity, the significance of their name, etc. All too often many students struggle to express their identity, cultural or otherwise, it is also a surprise to me that many people do not know where their name comes from.

Recently, I was talking to a Māori woman who has shared many of her life stories with me. She was an abused child, an abused spouse, most of her children have been removed from her care by Family Social Services, and she has had a long history of alcohol and drug addiction, etc. One day we were talking about her childhood and I asked her what the biggest challenges were for her when she was growing up. She said that it was feeling as though she did not have a sense of belonging. She wandered around most of her life, feeling as though she didn't fit in anywhere and her biggest dream when she was a child was to have a family like the Brady Bunch.[3] She and I belong to a culture where knowing who you are and where you come from is central to knowing oneself. Our whakapapa has everything to do with knowing where we come from and knowing where we belong.

---

[3] The Brady Bunch is an American television sitcom which revolves around a large blended family. The show originally aired from 26 September 1969, to 8 March 1974, on ABC television.

My friend had no connection with her whakapapa, hence she has walked around aimlessly for most of her life trying to find a sense of belonging. This is why it is important when we meet with Māori families in therapy that we are able to make those connections. Sometimes, people are not comfortable with that connection and they may prefer to go to someone who they do not know, but in the Māori world, every living thing and every thing non-living share a common descent from the same ancestral primal origin. Whether we know it or not, we are all connected through this common descent. At the conference, there was much debate about this. Non-Māori (Pakeha/European) therapists find this difficult to understand. For them it is a professional ethical issue, because they are trained and encouraged through their professional practice not to see their own family as clients. Māori do not have the privilege of being able to choose whether they see their family. This is mostly because Aotearoa/New Zealand is a small country and it is not difficult to connect somehow, somewhere to someone. It is not a dilemma for us when our *whanau* come to see us, this is our context, it is not a burden, and it is our reality.

In my view, Māori who work with their cultural frameworks cannot remove themselves from their own, because whether they like it or not they are related to each other somehow and in our worldview, making that connection with ourselves is critical in our practice. When we work with Māori families at the Family Centre the first thing we do is acknowledge our whakapapa to establish our belongingness. We work on the basis that not only are we probably connected in someway, but we respect the sacredness of that connection. That is, we acknowledge the people who come to us and their heritage, their ancestry, their forefathers and mothers, and those who have gone before. To understand this spiritual view we have to understand something about Māori belief systems. This is vital in order for us to interpret information and practice from a Māori cultural basis. However, it is not always appropriate to use these frameworks, and Māori workers must be adept at selecting the context in which they may be used. The following examples illustrate how some of these cultural frameworks work in practice.

Cultural frameworks

When a family is having difficulty overcoming the grief of having lost a close family member or friend, I will often work in the following manner. If the family are grounded in te ao Māori, or they can identify with their cultural heritage, then I will remind them about the story of why humans are mortal. A session may begin with stories about the creation of the world and how *Papatuanuku* (earth mother) and *Ranginui* (sky father) were conceived and developed. In turn, Papatuanuku and Ranginui begat seven sons. Because Papatuanuku and Ranginui were joined together, the sons plotted to split them apart so that daylight could enter the realm between them, which is where the seven sons dwelled. Because this act resulted in there being daylight, it is said that the world of light is likened to their being born. It is also said that the pain experienced by Papatuanuku as her children moved her apart from Ranginui is similar to the pain experienced by woman during child birth (Walker 1992, p. 171). Similarly, when the family is bereft with grief their state of mind, soul, and body are in a state of darkness. In order for the family to return to a state of mind, soul, and body whereby they can once again function normally, then they must leave the state of darkness and return to *te ao marama* (the world of light). If it were not for the seven sons having parted their parents, hence allowing light into the world, then there would always be a state of darkness.

Maui-tikitiki-a-Taranga (Maui) who was known as a demi-god, was born some generations after the initial fusion between celestial and earthly elements. Maui was gifted with supernatural powers. His mother was *Taranga*, during the day, she dwelt in *Paerau*, one of the divisions of the underworld, and at night she dwelt in the earthly world. Maui's father, *Makea-tutara*, dwelt permanently at Paerau. Maui was born prematurely, and his mother thought he was stillborn so she cut off the topknot of her hair, wrapped it around Maui and set him adrift out to sea. However, the special healing powers of the sea and the spiritual powers of his mother's hair ensured his survival. He was rescued from the sea by an ancestor, *Tama-nui-ki-te-rangi*, who nursed him to good health and reared him (Walker 1992, pp. 172–3).

Maui grew to be bold, resourceful, and quick, he was very precocious and somewhat cheeky. He was always playing tricks on his ancestors but there was a limit to his trickery. There came a time when Maui dared to gain immortality for humankind. To achieve this, he had to reverse the birth process by entering *Hine-nui-te-po* (the goddess of death) through her vagina, proceeding up through her birth canal and into her womb. He was then to work his way through her body, and emerge through her mouth. However, his attempt failed and Hine-nui-te-po crushed him to death (Higgins 1995, p. 13; H. Mead 2003, p. 146). How Maui died provides us with a cultural model of why humans are mortal. Maui attempted to expand the frontiers of immortality by challenging the goddess of death. The theory provides an explanation for what is the opposite of birth and that the seed of life lays in the womb of woman, and that the way to secure immortality is to reverse the process of birth by grasping the seed of life from the womb of the goddess of death Hine-nui-te-po (S. M. Mead 1997, p. 214).

When people attend a *tangihanga* (funeral) they will hear many stories pertaining to Papatuanuku, Maui-tikitiki-a-Taranga and how he attempted to seek immortality for humans. These stories may be heard repeatedly throughout the duration of the tangihanga. They not only have spiritual and mystical connotations but they serve to comfort people during their time of bereavement. Having established why we do not physically live forever the family can now begin to come to terms with the parting of their loved one and accept the death of their relative. The point of relating this story to the grieving family is to form a philosophical framework in a primary position. It has become clear to us that many of these Māori concepts do not exist merely as somewhat insubstantial counterpoints to Western concepts; rather, they are drawn from and firmly rooted in their own unique philosophical base. Earlier I stated that it could sometimes be more challenging for us when Māori people identify with the Western world and have garnered their experiences and life stories from a westernized culture because they interpret their world from a Western perspective. In this case, the story of how Maui attempted to seek mortality for all of humankind will probably make little sense to the grieving family. In which case, the use of Māori cultural frameworks or metaphors might not be helpful.

Mana and Tapu

Sometimes people can have issues which can be attributed to some form of cultural transgression. This being the case, there are two belief systems which are important to understand, these are *mana* and *tapu*.

Mana and tapu are concepts, which like many other Māori concepts cannot be easily translated into a single English definition. Both these concepts have a range of meanings, which are often defined according to the context in which they are being used. It is beyond the scope of this chapter to provide an in-depth explanation of the meaning of these two concepts. Essentially, mana and tapu are institutions in their own right and they have a close association with each other. Mana can be associated with meanings such as authority, control, influence, prestige or power and honour (New Zealand Ministry of Justice, 2001).

There are several different categories of tapu. We will discuss two of these in this chapter. Many people associate the meanings 'forbidden' or 'restricted' to the concept of tapu. However, it is much more than that because tapu also regulates or governs behaviour. Tapu in my view can be thought of as the institution, which protects the mana of a thing, object, or person, whether it is an animate and inanimate object, thing or person. If one has no faith or belief in the institution of tapu then there is essentially no potential for power. There are also strong connotations that if a tapu is breached, then something bad will happen and you can become sick.

As I explained earlier, these concepts are complex and powerful in the minds of Māori. Sometimes the power of these concepts is underestimated, misunderstood, or misinterpreted simply because some people maybe ignorant about their significance in Māori culture. Recently, a young man told me he believed that his cousin was sick, I asked 'What is wrong with your cousin?'. He replied, 'She's got one of those Māori curses *(makutu)*'. I asked, 'Why do you think that?'. He replied, 'because she might have taken something, a Māori *taonga*' [treasure]. I thought, yes that might cause someone to become very unwell. A Māori taonga could hold a great amount of value, by value I mean *mana* not monetary value. When a great amount of mana is accorded to an object, place, or person, then taking that object is a transgression or a serious breach of cultural protocol. But something which holds a great amount of mana does not necessarily deter someone from stealing it, in fact it might make them want to steal it even more simply because of its cultural value. There has to be a deterrence, therefore the object is accorded a level of *tapu* (or sacredness). Tapu might have been placed upon this object because it held a great amount of mana. Mana and tapu are derived from the *kawai tipuna* (ancestors). Thus, any transgressions against the ancestors were in former times taken very seriously and dealt accordingly.

These are the things that our ancestors believed. In today's context, people may not understand these things but every now and then we will read in the newspaper or see on the television an event which reminds us of how these customary beliefs continue to manifest in the daily lived realities of many Māori families. Whether people believe or not, in our practice, it would be unwise to disregard the qualities of mana and tapu from the kawai tipuna and the need to maintain mana and tapu to the highest degree. The following example demonstrates this view.

> Burglar 'suffered from Māori sickness'
> *The Dominion Post* | Saturday, 10 March 2007
> A man who smashed his way into a suburban Christchurch house after threatening a woman occupant was suffering from 'Māori sickness' at the time, a minister says. The Rev Whare Kawa Kaa told Christchurch District Court judge Colin Doherty yesterday that after he diagnosed Adam Daniel Cooper's problem, and took action, the young man was cured… Mr Kaa said that the problem stemmed from Cooper's carrying a taiaha (long club) and a tokotoko (walking stick). 'It is only elders who carry these things around. The Māori sickness was upon him. That is the sacredness of carrying these things. It was like a curse had been laid upon him.' He asked Cooper's mother and father to bring the items to his house so that they could be blessed, and then he had them send the items away. 'Māori sickness was pretty strong in the time of our fathers and grandfathers. It is still happening if things are not done in the right manner.' … In 2000, Tariana Turia, who was then associate Māori affairs minister, questioned whether psychologists had the appropriate training to deal with issues such as Māori sickness (mate Māori). Victoria University's head of Māori studies, Peter Adds, said mate Māori was a fairly common condition. 'It's usually brought on when people believe they have broken a tapu and are paying the consequences.'

What has been discussed is more or less how we would conduct an assessment, it would be what psychotherapists might describe as the initial contact phase. This is not a systematic clinical diagnosis. We do not use the DSM manual to diagnose symptoms. This is an assessment based on a cultural framework, one which is based on our knowledge and understandings of Māori cultural belief systems.

Sometimes we must rely on our instincts. Our instincts come from our knowledge handed down by the *kawai tipuna* (ancestors). They are not merely subjective thoughts or ideas. This is something that can be difficult for some Western-practitioners to understand or accept because this form of rationalization is different from notions of scientific rationality. I discussed earlier how Māori are connected in many ways to their tipuna (ancestors), and for me our tipuna can be our best sources of knowledge. That is, if you know how to trust your instincts and interpret that knowledge correctly. If we are working with a family who have many issues, sometimes we have to understand that the complexities of the issues manifest more problems for us to try and understand. This is the nature of the Māori world, where there is no beginning and there is no end, where life began with death. We incorporate this worldview into our everyday lives. It is more natural for me to think this way than it is to think within a Western worldview.

This chapter has attempted to illustrate one of the primary alternative worldviews that inform our practice at the Family Centre. We are aware that medical professionals have a huge influence on people's lives. As a marginalized and oppressed people, our worldviews have not been taken seriously in the past. We are also aware that some counsellors and therapists might believe that their clients who have conversations with 'the others', or who hold deep cultural and spiritual beliefs, may suffer from delusions. This is one example that illustrates how Māori cultural knowledge has not been viewed as significant within the clinical setting. We strongly believe that culture and spirituality cannot be separated from each other and as therapists and healers we have an ethical and professional responsibility to address issues with clients within the context of their culture and spirituality.

References

Higgins, R. (1995). Te Kura Tuohu–Etahi Ahuatanga o nga Hui Tangata Mate. Dissertation submitted to University of Otago, Dunedin.

Mead, H. (2003). *Tikanga Māori–Living by Māori values*. Huia Publishers, Wellington.

Mead, S. M. (1997). *Landmarks, bridges and visions: aspects of Māori culture*. Victoria University Press, Wellington.

Maurial, M. (1999). Indigenous knowledge and schooling: A continuum between conflict and dialogue. In L. M. Semali and J. L. Kincheloe (Eds.) *What is indigenous knowledge?* pp. 59–78. Falmer Press, New York.

New Zealand Ministry of Justice (2001). *He Hinatore ki te Ao Māori. A glimpse into the Māori world—Māori perspectives on justice*. Ministry of Justice, Wellington.

Pere, R. (1988). Te wheke: Whaia te maramatanga me te aroha. In S. C Middleton (Ed.) *Women and education in Aotearoa*, pp. 6–19. Allen & Unwin, Port Nicholson Press, Wellington.

Royal Tangaere, A. (1997). Māori human development learning theory. In P. Te Whaiti, M. McCarthy, and A. Dune (Eds.) *Māori wellbeing and development*, pp. 46–59. Auckland University Press, Auckland.

Sawrikar, P. and Hunt, C. (2005). The relationship between mental health, cultural identity, and cultural values, in Non-English speaking background (NESB) Australian adolescents. *Behaviour Change*, **22**, 97–113.

Tau, T. (2001). Matauranga Māori as an epistemology. In A. Sharp & P. McHugh (Eds.) *Histories power and ideas: Uses of the past–a New Zealand commentary*, pp. 68–69. Bridget Williams Books Limited, Wellington.

Walker, R. (1992). The relevance of Māori myth and tradition. In M. King (Ed.) *Te ao hurihuri: Aspects of maoritanga*, pp. 170–182. Reed Publishing, Auckland.

Williams, J. (2000). The 2000 Papers. Available at: http://pssm.ssc.govt.nz/2000/papers/jwilliam.asp.

Chapter 13

A systematic narrative review of discursive therapies research: considering the value of circumstantial evidence

Ronald J. Chenail, Melissa DeVincentis, Harriet E. Kiviat, and Cynthia Somers

In contemporary psychotherapy practice and research, the word 'evidence' has both methodological and political qualities (Sackett et al. 1996). From a methodological perspective, evidence can be the foundational information on which people base their beliefs in the usefulness and effectiveness of an intervention. In this vein, evidence can also be seen by some to offer proof or to establish truth or falsehood in a clinical approach. Methodologically this evidence can be derived from any of a variety of sense-making activities on the part of an observer or participant or yielded from a number of investigative designs ranging from the reflections of therapists on their clinical cases to highly controlled experiments wherein researchers conduct statistical analyses of effect size differences between the measured outcomes of participants who are randomly assigned to different treatments delivered by therapists operating from procedural manuals (Heneghan and Badennoch 2006).

From a political perspective, evidence can be a privileging and marginalizing process by which producers and consumers of clinical evidence establish hierarchies valuing one type of evidence over another (Walach et al. 2006). In these scenarios, a term like 'gold standard' can be used to create favouritism for the worth of evidence generated from 'highly controlled' experimental research designs such as randomized controlled trials and, at the same time, these imposed standards can be utilized to generate less partiality for the value of evidence constructed from more naturalistic, discovery-oriented studies of therapists and clients' experiences of their clinical encounters (Walach et al. 2006).

Over the last 30 years, a sizable body of evidence has been generated about a group of innovative psychotherapies known collectively as discursive therapies have gained prominence in the mental health arena (Strong and Paré 2004). These therapies go by many names including solution-focused brief therapy (SFBT; de Shazer 1982), narrative therapy (White and Epston 1990), and collaborative therapy (Anderson and Gehart 2007), as well as more generic monikers such as discursive therapy. Therapists who utilize these approaches emphasize the social construction of problems and solutions and explore how engaging relationally in conversation with each other and can positively change the way we see and act in the world (Gergen 2009).

For many practitioners and researchers the social constructional aspects of these discursive therapies seemed to encourage the use of case study, qualitative, and reflective methodologies to conduct investigations into the exploration of outcomes, processes, and experiences (e.g. De Haene 2010). For other curious observers, discursive therapies presented an opportunity to apply research designs more readily associated with positivistic or post-positivistic worldviews (e.g. Vromans and Schweitzer 2011). These researchers conduct their research to explore questions of fidelity, efficacy, effectiveness, mechanisms of change, moderators, and mediators. One outcome we see as being unfortunate with these two groups of investigators, both interested in learning about discursive therapies, is that political differences seem to have created two separate worlds of epistemological and methodological proponents who do not seem to be in ready conversation with each other.

In deciding how we wanted to approach our review of clinical research conducted on discursive therapies, we sought to minimize the political aspects of evidence and maximize our attention to studying those accounts in which investigators, in the broadest sense of the word, attempted to make something evident, plain, or clear regarding outcome, process, or experience of a discursive theory encounter. We sought to be methodologically pluralistic in this review in order to celebrate what we envision as the diversity of designs and vitality of difference in the contemporary landscape of discourse therapy research and evidence (APA Presidential Task Force on Evidence-Based Practice 2006). By making this choice, we were able to search, select, review, and report publications in which authors made assertions regarding some aspect of discursive therapy and presented indications or signs that were plain or clear to them and which provided them with the evidential confidence they required to make their pronouncements, results, findings, or understanding public.

Method

To address our research questions, we selected a hybrid model to review qualitatively the discursive therapy research literature in a systematic manner. We call our approach 'systematic narrative review' because we want to combine the qualities of a systematic review 'that [research which] strives to comprehensively identify, appraise, and synthesize all of the relevant studies on a given topic . . . often used to test a single hypothesis, or a series of related hypotheses' and a narrative review that values 'the process of synthesising primary studies and exploring heterogeneity descriptively, rather than statistically' (Petticrew and Roberts 2006, p. 19). To this end we incorporated the rigorous and transparent procedures of a systematic review, so we could detail our data collection and appraisal process, and combined these collecting and processing steps with the qualitative and methodological plurality features of a narrative review (Collins and Fauser 2005). In doing so we could compare and contrast the stories of the research design and findings within and across the three discursive therapies we researched.

We started our systematic narrative review of the discursive therapy research literature by identifying search terms we would use to guide our inquiries. We used 'solution-focused brief therapy', 'solution-focused counselling', 'narrative therapy', 'collaborative language therapy', 'collaborative therapy', and 'reflecting teams' as our major clinical method search terms, and we also used the last names of developers and leading proponents of these models (e.g. for SFBT we used 'deShazer' and 'Berg', for narrative therapy we used 'White' and 'Epston', and for collaborative therapy we used 'Anderson' and 'Goolishian'). For research methodology, we wanted to be as inclusive as we could be regarding research, so we used terms associated with evidence-based research such as 'systematic reviews', 'narrative reviews', 'randomized controlled trial', 'cohort studies', and 'case reports', as well as qualitative research terms such as 'ethnography', 'phenomenology', 'grounded theory', and 'case study'. We also searched using general research terms such as 'effectiveness', 'efficacy', 'satisfaction', 'experience', 'process, and 'outcome'. We then conducted a number of searches using bibliographic databases such as Google Scholar, PsycInfo, Social Sciences Citation Index, Cochrane Central Register of Controlled Trials, and Cochrane Database of Systematic Reviews. In addition, as we retrieved articles via our electronic searches, we also combed these publication references to identify additional publications to review. Together these two search processes yielded a collection of over 120 individual primary research studies and reviews.

Although all four chapter authors searched and collected resources, Melissa took the lead for SFBT sources, Cynthia for narrative therapy, and Harriet for collaborative therapy. As each search identified new sources, the lead searcher would catalogue the resource for her respective area. If a searcher found an article pertaining to one of the other searcher's clinical area, those sources were shared. Ron kept the composite list of sources and distributed this growing record regularly among the group.

For our analytical approach in this systematic review, we selected a qualitative approach known as narrative review that helps reviewers to examine the results of their searches, organize the articles in terms of categories, and then summarize information regarding the studies' methods and findings in a descriptive manner (Petticrew and Roberts 2006). In the case of our study, we organized the research publications by discursive therapy model (i.e. SFBT, narrative therapy, or collaborative therapy) and then into two general methodological categories: primary research studies and review or meta-studies. Within each of these general categories we then read and re-read the articles to determine: (a) the type of research study (e.g. outcome, process, experiential), (b) design (e.g. case study, cohort study, ethnography), and (c) orientation (e.g. confirmatory, discovery-oriented, mixed) for each source collected (see Heneghan and Badennoch 2006, for a more detailed account of each of these types, designs, and orientations).

As we noted these methodological distinctions within our discursive therapy categories, we began to construct a descriptive narrative or story of each methodological grouping in terms of the results produced by these researchers and the methodologies being employed. In presenting the stories within each discursive therapy by research design, we selected a reporting order that does reflect the typical hierarchical levels of evidence found in most guides to evidence-based practice (e.g. Heneghan and Badennoch 2006, pp. 94–6). At the same time, we wanted to privilege what all of the available evidence from the various designs contributes, so we also constructed a summary narrative on the collective state of evidence for these discursive therapies to celebrate a relational or circular pattern of evidence (Walach et al. 2006). As a result, the following reports on SFBT, narrative therapy, and collaborative therapy have their own particular flow and style based upon the primary reviewers' best sense of rendering the patterns we constructed from each set of studies examined.

Findings

Solution-focused brief therapy

de Shazer et al. describe SFBT as a discursive therapy that seeks to change, through conversation, the client's conceptualization of and interaction surrounding the problem to constructing solutions (de Shazer et al. 1986 cited in Berg and DeJong, 1996, p. 377). SFBT, founded by Steve de Shazer and Insoo Kim Berg, is based on the notion that clients inherently possess the resources for change and through brief conversations clients can co-construct a different reality (Berg and DeJong 1996).

According to de Shazer and Berg (1997, p. 123), the characteristic features of SFBT include: (a) asking the 'miracle question', (b) asking the client to rate something on a scale of '0–10' or '1–10', (c) taking a break, and (d) after this intermission, complimenting the client and sometimes suggesting a homework task (frequently called an 'experiment'). Despite these specific prescriptions, de Shazer and Berg go on to say:

> If any or all are missing, then – at least for research purposes – we have to conclude that the therapist is not practicing SFBT. Of course, clinically what the therapist and client are doing might well be SFBT (and it might well be good therapy), but in a research context the model used must be apparent and clearly demonstrated. Obviously, the presence of these characteristics says nothing whatsoever about the quality of the therapy
> (de Shazer and Berg 1997, p. 123).

Gingerich and Eisengart (2000) also include goal setting and a search for exceptions as intervention techniques to be included among the seven core components used in the operational definition of SFBT along with at least one or more of these core components used as agents of change for outcome research methodology.

SFBT research

We observed SFBT research as a diverse body of inquiry that includes both qualitative and quantitative investigations, systematic reviews, and meta-analyses. To date, we located two meta-analyses, three systematic reviews, 13 randomized controlled studies, 30 comparison studies, and over 40 naturalistic inquiries into the effectiveness of SFBT based on the APA (2002) template for research efficacy and best available research evidence practices (Macdonald 2010). We also discovered SFBT to be the most researched therapeutic model of the discursive therapy family. Spearheading this effort is the Research Committee of the Solution-Focused Brief Therapy Association, which has developed a manual in order to standardize SFBT practice, making it more conducive to experimental control procedures (Connie and Metcalf 2009; Trepper et al. 2008).

Research in SFBT began with Kiser's (1988) outcome study at the Brief Family Therapy Center in Milwaukee where de Shazer and Berg practised. In this study,

Kiser examined a series of follow-up surveys at various intervals after the termination of therapy and concluded that over half the clients said they had reached their goals, with over 80% reporting that progress was made and sustained over time (as cited in DeJong and Hopwood 1996; Gingerich and Eisengart 2000; Kim 2007; Macdonald 2007). As Kim (2007) points out, this initial research into SFBT effectiveness was considered low from a control design standpoint and some would consider his measures to be somewhat skewed. Nevertheless, the initial progress reported from clients' perspectives became a catalyst for research into the effectiveness of SFBT (De Jong and Hopwood 1996).

Most of the early SFBT research consisted of surveys, follow-up interviews, and single-subject designs with no replication across settings or comparison/control groups. Thus, several critiques exist regarding SFBT research methodologies noted a lack of generalizability or questionable measures for statistically significant progress. As SFBT began to gain popularity within the human service industry, the number of well-controlled studies increased, and outcome literature began reporting moderate client success across a wide variety of problems in various settings using the core SFBT techniques (De Jong and Hopwood 1996; Cockburn et al. 1997; Lindforss and Magnusson 1997; Macdonald 2007).

SFBT has been researched with subjects including children, adults, developmental disabilities, couples, college students, prisoners, and nurses (Cruz and Littrell 1998; Franklin et al. 2008; Lee et al. 1997; Li et al. 2007; Lundblad and Hansson 2006; Seidel and Hedley 2008; Shin 2009; Smock et al. 2008 Stoddart et al. 2001; Thorslund 2007; Walker and Hayashi 2009; Wilmshurst 2002). It has also been researched relative to therapeutic topics including substance abuse issues and domestic violence. Specifically, SFBT has been shown to be effective with clients seeking therapy for substance abuse and in the field of education with reference to children with behaviour problems (Connie and Metcalf 2009; Kim and Franklin 2009; Walker and Hayashi 2009).

Gingerich and Eisengart (2000) performed the first analysis on the research using the SFBT approach with specific 'efficacy criteria' set by the APA (2002, p. 495). The APA provided guidelines for researchers to qualitatively evaluate the efficacy of interventions based upon their methodological sophistication, such as randomized controlled experiments versus quasicontrolled experiments (APA 2002, p. 1054). From these guidelines, researchers were able to identify the best available research evidence. The results of this investigation concluded that only five studies were well controlled, while the rest of the research analyzed yielded less controlled procedures. Gingerich and Eisengart (2000) found that although more experimentally controlled rigorous research that focuses on establishing efficacy needed to be conducted, preliminary evidence did exist indicating that SFBT may be effective over a 'wide variety of settings and populations' (p. 495). Therefore, because of the ubiquitous application of SFBT and the beginnings of efficacy research using this approach to therapy, SFBT research has since continued to move towards developing empirically based standards of practice and becoming an evidence-based practice (EBP).

Stams et al. (2006) and Kim (2008) conducted meta-analyses on the efficacy of solution-focused brief therapy research. Kim (2008) used computer software in order to determine if SFBT research demonstrated positive treatment effects and if these results were statistically significant. Kim (2008) grouped the 22 studies analysed into three categories (externalizing behaviour problems, internalizing behaviour problems, and family and relationship problems) and then calculated their effect size compared to the control group. Kim found that SFBT was effective and yielded statistically significant results for internalizing behaviour problems. However, results for externalizing behaviour problems and relational problems were not as significant, although overall, 'SFBT demonstrated small but positive treatment effects favoring the SFBT group on the outcome measures' (Kim 2008, p. 113).

Corcoran and Pillai (2009) conducted a systematic review of the SFBT literature from 1985–2006 using experimental and quasi-experimental designs specifically analysing subject, intervention, and methodological characteristics. They concluded that SFBT is still in the early stages of evolving into an evidence-based practice. Corcoran and Pillai also found that SFBT research practices vary among populations, settings, and problems. These differences in clinical application proved challenging to them while attempting to synthesize research in order to make statements regarding SFBT's effectiveness given experimental control.

Across these review studies, Gingerich and Eisengart (2000), Kim (2008), and Corcoran and Pillai (2009) all found that SFBT delivered little to moderate effectiveness. They suggested the need for more research with larger sample sizes and randomized controlled methodologies that have a control group before saying that SFBT is a research-supported clinical approach utilizing the best available research evidence.

In contrast to the small number of controlled studies identified in the review studies and by us, there have been many SFBT research endeavours that have employed more naturalistic designs and offer a discovery-oriented approach to finding out what works in SFBT in general and with specific populations and problems (Beyebach et al. 2000; Conoley et al. 2003; Darmody and Adams 2003). These studies show effectiveness in that the intervention helped reduce the problem for the clients yielding evidence of therapeutic progress and improvements (Macdonald 2007). For instance, this research notes improvement in individual problems based on individualized quantitative measures as well as qualitative descriptions (MacDonald 2007, 2010).

Another aspect of this more naturalistic practice-based evidence is a focus on client and therapist interaction. In this focus, the intervention is not based on using the a priori operational definition of SFBT, but rather on what will work for the client based on both the therapist's and client's perspectives. There are also a larger number of naturalistic inquiries, case studies, comparison studies, and less controlled experimental designs where clients and therapists report effectiveness with certain SFBT techniques; these studies may be considered more practice-based evidence (Macdonald 2007, 2010). Perhaps the first to determine improvement from the client perspective based on a SFBT technique was de Shazer (1985), who followed up with 28 clients who had received the formulaic first session task and found that 'twenty-three (82%) of the 28 cases had improved; 25 had solved other problems' (as cited in Macdonald 2007, p. 101).

Researchers using this practice-based design utilize more individualized SFBT interventions in order to fit the client's reality; the emphasis is on benefiting the client and restoring real-life functioning and obtain client feedback in order to 'offer systematic evaluation of outcome' (Miller et al. 2005, p. 205). Studies utilizing practice-based evidence use more individualized instrumentations to measure change, such as the scaling question or questions regarding progress towards individual's goal. They also use perhaps more unsystematic sampling procedures and naturalistic discovery-oriented design in order to measure, monitor, and obtain feedback (Sapyta et al. 2005). These investigations not only have clinical utility, but are also important to SFBT research because they can assist in determining the effectiveness of SFBT across various problems.

Narrative therapy

Narrative therapy was pioneered by Michael White and David Epson in the 1970s and 1980s. This model of therapy is based on the postmodern constructivist view that there is no absolute reality (Cowley and Springen 1995); moreover, constructivists believe that reality is continuously being constructed. According to Richert (2003), 'If there is a "catch phrase" that identifies the narrative tradition in psychotherapy, it is probably, "The person isn't the problem; the problem is the problem"' (Epston 1993b, p. 161). Narrative therapy has blossomed into a variety of treatment applications and is considered one of the most influential within the narrative therapies (Freedman and Combs 1996; White 2007).

The narrative therapeutic process involves externalizing and personifying the problem, deconstructing the dominant narrative and mapping the influence of the problem, finding the subjugated story by uncovering unique outcomes and sparkling events, and reconstructing and reinforcing a new narrative. This discursive flow is achieved by utilizing a variety of questioning techniques (e.g. deconstruction questions, opening space questions, preference questions, story development questions, meaning questions, and futuristic questions) and reinforcing approaches (e.g. therapeutic letters, therapeutic certificates, and leagues). In essence, narrative therapy is a way of understanding people's problems (Epston 1993a; Freedman and Combs 1996; Morgan 2000; White and Epston 1990).

Narrative therapy research

Denborough (2009), on behalf of The Dulwich Centre Publications that produces resources (including books, journals, and DVDs) about narrative therapy and community work with a particular focus on making narrative approaches accessible and relevant to a wide range of practitioners and contexts, noted:

> Dulwich Centre is vitally interested in the development of new methods of research that are congruent with narrative practice principles and also vigorously test/demonstrate/ examine the real effects and outcomes of narrative practices. A number of practitioners/ researchers are engaged with this task of developing research methods that are congruent with narrative approaches and meet conventional research standards (quantitative and qualitative)
>
> (Denborough 2009, Section: Discussions about narrative research).

The categories of research present in the literature on narrative therapy consisted of one review of the literature; a few controlled studies; and numerous naturalistic case studies, client reports, and therapists' self-reports.

The critical review conducted by Etchison and Kleist (2000) was the only review of evidence for narrative therapy found in the research literature. It was a non-systematic narrative review; hence, no information was offered about the methods by which published research accounts were identified, the criteria by which eventual source materials were selected, the scales or checklist by which they were subsequently appraised or any techniques of synthesis or analysis by which they were presented (Cook et al. 1997). The authors defined narrative therapy from numerous perspectives (e.g. Cowley and Springen 1995; Monk et al. 1997; White and Epston 1990), addressed the increasing popularity and attractiveness of the model, pointed out the vast source of bibliographic narrative therapy resources, gave suggestions for the paucity of research into its effectiveness, and highlighted the implications for practitioners.

Although the article was described as a review of narrative therapy, two of the four articles reviewed (i.e. Coulehan et al. 1998; Weston et al. 1998) were not congruent with the stated focus of the review (i.e. the two articles were about narratives in therapy and narrative approaches instead of narrative therapy); therefore, these 'narrative in therapy' articles were omitted from our review.

The focus of the two pertinent articles were the effectiveness of narrative therapy using a single case design (Besa 1994) and clients' experiences of narrative therapy using an ethnographic design (O'Conner et al. 1997). Families were the target population for both studies. The studies addressed parent-child conflict and what families found helpful and unhelpful in therapy, respectively. Etchison and Kleist (2000) concluded that the 'studies provided support for the use of narrative approaches to working with families; however, support for the use of narrative approaches with families is at best tentative given the small number of clinical studies' (p. 65).

We found no randomized controlled trials among the narrative therapy studies, but we did locate other studies in which less rigorous control designs were used: a quasi-experiment (Mehl-Madrona 2007), single-system research designs (e.g. Besa 1994; Vromans and Schweitzer 2011), and the audit of the outcome of therapy (Silver et al. 1998) using a control group along with benchmarking against previous pertinent studies. The focus in the Mehl-Madrona quasi-experiment was to determine the effectiveness of a daily, one-hour narrative group in a locked inpatient unit psychiatric unit. It incorporated both pre- and post-tests measures and comparison groups. The BASIS-32 (32-item Behavior and Symptom Identification Scale), a patient self-report rating scale of symptom and problem difficulty, was the outcome measure for this study. The results for the narrative group were statistically significant; thus suggesting that the narrative therapy treatment group showed greater improvement than the control groups. However, Mehl-Madrona suggested that these results be interpreted with caution and that a randomized controlled trial format was necessary.

Besa's (1994) single-system research design to assess the effectiveness of narrative therapy in reducing parent/child conflict used a three multiple baseline design for measuring the outcome of the intervention on targeted behaviours. In the words of the researcher:

> All families documented significant improvement in target behaviors . . . This study suggested that NT was effective in reducing parent/child conflict and this may, therefore,

be applicable to families experiencing parent/child conflict under conditions similar to those found in the experiment (p. 323).

In a recent study, Vromans and Schweitzer (2011) investigated depressive symptom and interpersonal relatedness outcomes for 47 adults with major depressive disorder, depressive symptoms, and interpersonal relatedness that improved following a manualized eight sessions of narrative therapy. The research design was a single-sample with repeated measures conducted at pre-therapy, post-therapy, and at a 3-month follow-up. The outcomes (treatment gains, effect size, and clinical significance) were benchmarked against outcomes from evidence-based psychotherapies such as cognitive-behavioural therapy (CBT), psychodynamic-interpersonal (PI), interpersonal therapy (IPT), and process-experiential (PE). According to the authors, this study was the first rigorous empirical investigation of narrative therapy outcome.

Although narrative therapy controlled studies are limited, the literature was replete with naturalistic case studies about the effectiveness of narrative therapy. These studies were conducted by researching clinicians who studied their own clinical work (e.g. Crocket 2004), clinical researchers who performed the research (e.g. Besa 1994; Draucker 1998), and independent researchers who studied the work of clinicians (e.g. Gardner and Poole 2009). Numerous designs inclusive of exploratory descriptive studies, ethnographic studies, case studies, and case reports in a variety of settings (e.g. university, university clinics, outpatient clinics, rehabilitation centre, walk-in clinics) were reported. Overall, effectiveness was ascertained based on clients' reports (e.g. Fraenkel et al. 2009; Young and Cooper 2008), therapists' reports (e.g. da Costa et al. 2007; Gardner and Poole 2009; Torres and Guerra 2002), standardized measurements (e.g. Matos et al. 2009; Torres and Guerra 2002), and reports with therapists and clients as co-authors (e.g. Hogan 1999). The target populations were individual, families, and group therapies.

Though limited, there have been some instances where narrative therapy has been applied to larger systems such as different cultures (e.g. Bermudez and Bermudez 2002; da Costa et al. 2007; Keeling and Nielson 2005), and organizational settings (e.g. Barry 1997; Boje et al. 2001). Keeling and Nielson (2005) reported that the findings of their study that used a narrative intervention with Asian women indicated its suitability for this population. Barry (1997) believed that narrative therapy can be usefully applied to organizational change management. This model has been used in organizational skills training and conflict mediation (Monk et al. 1997). Boje and colleagues (2001) noted that 'Narrative therapy (White and Epston 1990) is increasingly being applied to organizational studies (Barry 1997; Barry and Elmes 1997; Boje et al. 1997)'. Barry also concluded: 'The limitations of the narrative approach within organizations still await discovery' (p. 23).

Since the evidence for effectiveness was predominantly at the case studies level, the difference of the research designs allowed for further categorization within this level of evidence. The number of sessions and the method of treatment varied across the studies. Some focused on specific narrative therapy techniques (e.g. Keeling and Nielson 2005; Matos et al. 2009) while others (e.g. daCosta et al. 2007; Fraenkel et al. 2009) employed a wider range of the core interventions of the modality. Few studies reported the use of a manualized treatment (e.g. Fraenkel et al. 2009; Torres and Guerra 2002;

Vromans and Schweitzer 2011). Some studies offered a detailed method section (e.g. Gardner and Poole 2009; Vromans and Schweitzer 2011; Young and Cooper 2008), while others (e.g. Draucker 1998; Hogan 1999) gave little to no details of the research procedures. Also, therapists' qualifications and experience were only given for some studies (i.e. Vassallo 1998). Generally speaking, the studies focused to a larger extent on the therapeutic process (e.g. Kropf and Tandy 1998) and on the outcomes of narrative therapy (e.g. Ingram and Perlesz 2004). To a lesser extent, clients' experiences of narrative therapy (Keeling and Nielson 2005; O'Conner et al. 1997; Young and Cooper 2008) and therapists' experiences of narrative therapy (O'Conner et al. 2004) were explored.

The studies covered diverse clinical problems. Examples of these problems were inclusive of, but not exhaustive of depression (e.g. daCosta et al. 2007; Vromans and Schweitzer 2011; Wirtz and Harari 2000), multidimensional partner abuse (Draucker 1998), mental illness (Vassallo 1998), brain injury (e.g. Hogan 1999), body dysmorphic disorder (da Costa et al. 2007), eating disorder (e.g. Torres and Guerra 2002; Weber et al. 2006), AIDS (Rothschild et al. 2000), childhood stealing (e.g. Seymour and Epston 1989), and homelessness (Fraenkel et al. 2009). Overall, the studies supported the effectiveness of narrative therapy to treat a variety of presenting problems and disorders across different populations and contexts.

Also prevalent within the literature were numerous case studies that focused on the effectiveness of integrating narrative therapy with other models of therapy such as art (Carlson 1997), developmental theory (DeSocio 2005), and education (Augusta-Scott and Dankwort 2002). Although these approaches reported potential or positive outcomes, the research designs were at the levels of case studies and case reports. As for narrative therapy as the sole intervention, some of the proposed interventions were manualized (Kirven 2000) while others lacked a method section (Dallos, 2004). While integration was embraced by some researchers (e.g. Carlson 1997), others did not consider it particularly necessary (e.g. Guilfoyle 2009). Even among the researchers that did not support integration, there was the acknowledgement that the process was pragmatically valuable (Guilfoyle 2009).

The narrative therapy observational studies based on both therapists/researchers and participants experiences of therapy contributed significantly to the practice-based evidence. This step towards co-composing evidence of what is useful and important in therapy is seen as valuable to both evidence-based and practice-based information. As noted by Young and Cooper (2008), 'This knowledge informs and shapes our practice of narrative therapy. It contributes to our learning, teaching, and supervision practices' (p. 80). At the same time, there continues to be a dearth of highly and moderately controlled research on the efficacy of narrative therapy (Keeling and Nielson 2005; Vromans and Schweitzer 2011).

Collaborative therapy

Collaborative therapy, a philosophical stance (Anderson 2003, 2007b) developed and honed by Harlene Anderson and Harry Goolishian (Anderson 2003), grew from beginnings in Multiple Impact Therapy (MIT; Anderson 2007a), a brief, collaborative, and family focused way of working with adolescents, primarily through communicating differently with clients, their families, and other supportive individuals within their personal community (educators, coaches, clergy, etc.). Anderson (2007a) credits the collaborative approach to some basic ideas from MIT including: (a) the team's view that they learn 'together with the family' (p. 23); (b) the team's focus on listening to and including multiple voices in the process of therapy; and (c) the team's understanding that this was a very new and different way of doing therapy.

Subsequently, influences from the Mental Research Institute (MRI) began to infuse the thinking of Anderson and Goolishian (Anderson 2007a) providing a new way for clients to describe their problems (Anderson 2003). The most notable of these influences was the use of language. Mental Research Institute therapists focused on 'learning the client's language . . . words and phrases as well as [to] beliefs, values, truths, and worldviews' (p. 24). Focusing on language and the creation of meaning through language, Anderson and Goolishian veered in a new direction and called their work a 'collaborative language systems approach' to therapy, with Anderson later changing it simply to 'collaborative therapy' (Anderson 2003, p. 130).

The stance of the collaborative therapist is 'a way of being in the world that does not separate professional and personal' (Anderson 2003, p.131). Thus, collaborative therapy is more about how the therapist experiences relationships and conversations with clients, and includes the following ideas: (a) therapists and clients are conversational partners; (b) clients are the experts; (c) therapists take a not-knowing stance; (d) therapists utilize their own voices as part of the conversation (i.e. rather than hypothesize internally, they will express their ideas); (e) there is an uncertain direction or outcome of therapy; and (f) therapy resembles ordinary conversation.

Collaborative therapy research

The categories of research present in the literature on collaborative therapy consist of reviews of the literature, case studies, client reports, and therapists' self-reports. At the time of this writing, there were no controlled or moderately controlled studies available to include in this analysis. Furthermore, there is no evidence-based practice (e.g. controlled studies) research supporting the efficacy of collaborative therapy (Sundet 2011). The focus in this section will be on the naturalistic and practice-based evidence of the extant research in collaborative therapy.

We have included two narrative reviews of the literature in this chapter (see Anderson 2003, 2007b). In the first work, Anderson (2003) compared and contrasted the premises and effectiveness of collaborative work with narrative and solution-focused therapies. She noted that the significance of highlighting these three examples of postmodern therapy was the growth of therapeutic influences 'under a postmodern/social construction umbrella' (p. 127) and the search for substantiating evidential effectiveness within this framework. Furthermore, much of the literature reviewed in this article demonstrates the naturalistic, therapist-driven research resulting in practice based evidence for these models. There was no description of a methodology or a systematic account as to how she selected the literature for this chapter. However, the author did acknowledge the historical and fundamental natures of the frameworks described in her review, and appropriately credited the important contributors to the field. She included common values (e.g. non-pathological, respectful, collaborative, etc.)

and distinctions (e.g. power, therapeutic relationship, process, etc.), as well as the specific tenets of the models to allow the reader to make comparisons with greater ease. In addition, Anderson acknowledged the isomorphism between clinical work and research in collaborative therapy, indicating the phenomenon of 'therapists and clients as co-researchers in during the process of therapy, as well as at its conclusion' (p. 133). These findings suggest effectiveness of the model with various populations (e.g. child abuse, substance abuse, eating disorders, etc.). Similarly, Anderson's 2007 chapter contained a description of the collaborative model of therapy and listed anecdotal/qualitative studies supporting the effectiveness of the model and reiterating what she discovered in the previous evaluation. Additionally, there appeared to be a correlation between what the clients deemed successful with the therapists/researchers' findings. Both of the reviews (conducted by the co-developer of the model) generally applied to the global aspects of collaborative therapy although Anderson briefly characterized some specific populations where the work was determined to be effective. We discuss many of these populations in the next section of this chapter.

At least ten of the studies that we reviewed included the therapists' perspective and the voice of the client (Andrews 2007; Fernández et al. 2007; Gehart 2007; Gehart-Brooks, and Lyle 1999; Levin 2007; McDonough and Koch 2007; Messmore 2002; Penn 2007; Sparks and Muro 2009; Wagner 2007), and varied in the adherence to rigor of method. In a recent review of postmodern and evidence-based practice (EBP), Jacobs et al. (2010) suggested that postmodern therapists view client feedback as 'key evidence' (p. 190) of the usefulness of therapy. Since, client voice is paramount in collaborative therapy it is logical to utilize the format for research (Anderson and Gehart 2007).

For instance, Gehart-Brooks and Lyle (1999) researched the change in perspective over the course of therapy for both the therapist and the client. The authors clearly stated the methodology for this ethnographic study, defined the parameters of the work, and specifically detailed the procedures, and subsequent analysis of the interviews (use of a data coding software program).

Likewise, Levin (2007) fully described the 'design and process' (p. 110) of her work with battered women, specifically indicating her method for creating the proper 'constructionist and collaborative interview approach' (p. 111) and therefore setting the context for her work. Levin shared how her questions were constructed based on the responses of her interviewees. She detailed the population and the protocol used to recruit the women for her study as well as provided the implications for this study, which suggested the importance of a non-expert, not-knowing stance when working in areas that are not in the therapists' areas of expertise.

In a similar manner, Fernández et al. (2007) utilized 'consultation interviews' in their research on people suffering from eating disorders. This study was more narrative in nature than Levin's work telling a story rather than providing a more traditional research study format. Although the method of the study was clear, and a non-team member conducted the interviews of the clients subsequent to therapy, there was no indication of how the resulting client narratives were selected.

One study purporting the effectiveness of collaborative language systems with parents and children (McDonough and Koch 2007) utilized a description of collaborative therapy as the method for research and included therapist reflections and client reactions in the narrative. Subsequently, since the authors did not conduct the research until after they terminated therapy, and the results were all positive, confidence in this study is questionable.

Alternately, and garnering more credibility, was Gehart's (2007) paper on using collaborative therapy with children. In presenting the results of her work, she displayed more transparency by specifically indicating questions used within context of play with children that allow them to afford the therapist a clearer understanding of the situation and to aid in a more productive dialogue. The author's intention of creating a safe place for children and the outcomes from therapy were clear.

For the most part, the studies mentioned thus far support the effectiveness of collaborative therapy from a naturalistic design perspective relying on therapists' studying their clients' reports of what works in therapy. A number of the articles/chapters use the term collaborative therapies to include narrative and/or solution-focused practices (see, for example, Chang 1999; Fraenkel et al. 2009; Messmore 2002). Therefore, one cannot substantiate the level of effectiveness of the collaborative therapy piece itself if it was not the singular method of therapy utilized in the study. It is clear that the research has to be more methodologically transparent (e.g. specifically indicating how the research method was developed or more descriptive in the manner with which data was collected) if those outside the collaborative arena are to hold credence in the results. Interestingly, the collaborative community does not necessarily agree with this point of view (Gehart et al. 2007).

Conducting research in the same way as one does therapy is the heart of the naturalistic aspect to the research in collaborative therapy and the reason that most of the practice based evidence is anecdotal. Unfortunately, those who have a stake in the outcome conduct much of the research. Harlene Anderson is a co-creator of collaborative therapy and by conducting research independently, it appears that there could be bias in the outcome. There is also an isomorphic tendency within the collaborative community to collaborate with clients on the research as they collaborate in therapy.

According to Gehart and Lucas (2007), 'A social constructionist perspective recognizes that it is impossible for a researcher to be completely bias-free . . .' (p. 44) and they suggest that conducting research from a *not-knowing* stance may aid in reducing researcher bias. Gehart et al. (2007) support the collaborative method of doing research. They point out that researchers utilize pre-formulated questions, for example, only as a place to begin the interview and researchers/interviewers create subsequent questions through the collaborative conversation. They further suggest ways of including quantitative research methods within the collaborative stance.

Discussion

Even though we diligently queried numerous databases utilizing a long list of search terms and reviewed the references lists of the resources collected, the fact remains that we may have overlooked some studies whose methods and findings might have changed the narratives we constructed regarding discourse therapy evidence. We also decided to focus on the well-known discursive therapy models and did not review those studies whose authors referred to the therapy under investigation in generic terms such as 'discursive', 'constructivist', or 'post-modern'. Although these decisions may have reduced the size of our sample, we still located over 120 studies spanning all three major discursive therapy models and including a variety of methods and designs. This rich and diverse collection gave us a degree of confidence that the narrative we have presented herein appears to capture the depth and breadth of the current body of discursive therapy research.

We also did not include sources from what is commonly referred to as the 'grey literature' (i.e. dissertation and conference papers). We excluded these studies because we wanted to concentrate on research that would be more readily available to therapists (i.e. journals) and would have received more formalized peer review. Of course relying solely on research published in journals and books does introduce a publication bias since journal and book editors have a tendency to favour studies which present significant findings potentially creating a halo effect skewing the effectiveness of models investigated towards being more positive than the total body of extant research (Petticrew and Roberts 2006). Having said that, we did note some studies in which the researchers reported a lack of statistically significant evidence to support the effectiveness of a particular discursive therapy model thus giving us some degree of confidence that we were reviewing a variety of results countering publication bias somewhat.

In the introduction of this review, we suggested evidence has both a methodological and political character that can shape the way we look at clinical research. We can elect to support one method over another due to our backing of a particular candidate epistemology or design and thus we can privilege one type of evidence over another. In our review we attempted to be methodologically neutral and remain politically independent from any one methodological or epidemiological party. In doing so, we endeavoured to poll the extant body of discursive therapy research to see what the investigator turn-out suggests.

Our reflections on these studies lead us to observe that collectively the research on SFBT, narrative therapy, and collaborative therapy is methodologically diverse and growing. We were able to locate controlled, confirmatory studies; naturalistic, discovery-oriented studies; as well as outcome, process, and experiential studies. Across all three therapies, naturalistic, discovery-oriented methods made up the majority of studies located. In the cases of SFBT and narrative therapy we observed more controlled-style studies than what we saw with collaborative therapy, but then again, collaborative therapy is a more recent clinical approach so this observation may be as much a case of time and in another decade another set of reviews might find a different pattern among this group.

Even though we declared our intentions to be politically independent, our pronouncement still suggests a political aspect nonetheless. By favouring inclusiveness and juxtaposing evidence from controlled and naturalistic designs and social constructionistic and positivistic epistemologies we do acknowledge we are attempting to make a political statement. We hold that all evidence has value when we are attempting to examine what researchers hold evident about discursive therapies.

In discussing evidence we think it is important to recognize that there is also a legal context within which to consider the meaning of the term. In law there are many ways to characterize evidence. There are best, circumstantial, clear and convincing, competent, corroborating, and direct evidence to name a few. In a court of law, legal representatives put forth these various types of evidence in order to convince a judge or jury as to the veracity of their case and to ultimately gain a verdict or decision that favours their side. In research we know a final verdict is never reached for the jury is always out and each instance we conduct therapy constitutes another case on which a verdict needs to be resolved. Despite these circumstances, we continue work to build evidence on a case-by-case manner for or against a particular perspective regarding psychotherapies such as the discursive ones.

In our review of SFBT, narrative therapy, and collaborative therapy, we came away with an appreciation of the value of 'circumstantial' evidence in how these researchers made their cases for their understandings of outcome, process, and experience. By circumstantial evidence we mean that we could comprehend the results of these studies, be they expressed in numbers or words, as being of, pertaining to, or derived from a particular set of circumstances. From this point of view, we could better regard the evidence as being offered by certain investigators, from certain cases, at certain times and places. We could also hold, from this perspective, that research like politics is local.

Along these lines we suggest discursive therapy researchers continue to produce research that is of local value and to construct circumstantial evidence of note. We also propose that these researchers explore the evidence produced by other local researchers under different circumstances to see what patterns can be connected across outcome, process, and experiential investigations regardless the methodological or epistemological choices utilized. By systematically choosing to include circumstantial evidence from methodological variant studies in our research and practice, we hold that discursive therapist and researchers along with their clients can only benefit from such evidential diversity.

References

American Psychological Association. (2002). Criteria for evaluating treatment guidelines. *American Psychologist,* **57**(12), 1052–9.

American Psychological Association Presidential Task Force on Evidence-Based Practice. (2006). Evidence-based practice in psychology. *American Psychologist,* **61**(4), 271–85.

Anderson, H. (2003). Postmodern social construction therapies. In T. L. Sexton G. R. Weeks, and M. S. Robbins (Eds.) *Handbook of family therapy,* pp. 125–46. Brunner-Routledge, New York.

Anderson, H. (2007a). Historical influences. In H. Anderson and D. Gehart (Eds.) *Collaborative therapy: Relationships and conversations that make a difference,* pp. 21–31. Routledge, New York.

Anderson, H. (2007b). The heart and spirit of collaborative therapy: The philosophical stance- "a way of being" in relationship and conversation. In H. Anderson and D. Gehart (Eds.) *Collaborative therapy: Relationships and conversations that make a difference,* pp.43–59. Routledge, New York.

Anderson, H. and Gehart, D. (Eds.) (2007), *Collaborative therapy: Relationships and conversations that make a difference.* Routledge, New York, NY.

Andrews, J. (2007). Honoring elders through conversations about their lives. In H. Anderson and D. Gehart (Eds.) *Collaborative therapy: Relationships and conversations that make a difference*, pp. 149–66. Routledge, New York.

Augusta-Scott, T. and Dankwort, J. (2002). Partner abuse group intervention: Lessons from education and narrative therapy approaches. *Journal Interpersonal Violence*, **17**, 783–805.

Barry, D. (1997). Telling changes: From narrative family therapy to organizational change and development. *Journal of Organizational Change Management*, **10**(1), 30–46.

Barry, D. and Elmes, M. (1997). Strategy retold: Toward a narrative view of strategic discourse. *Academy of Management Review*, **22**(2), 429–52.

Berg, I. and De Jong, P. (1996). Solution-building conversations: Co-constructing a sense of competence with clients. *Families in Society: The Journal of Contemporary Human Services*, **77**(6), 376–91.

Bermudez, J. M. and Bermudez, S. (2002). Altar-making with Latino families: A narrative therapy perspective. *Journal of Family Psychotherapy*, **13**, 329–49.

Besa, D. (1994). Evaluating narrative family therapy using single-system research designs. *Research on Social Work Practice*, **4**(3), 309–25.

Beyebach, M. M., Rodriguez Sanchez, M. S., De Miguel, J. A., et al. (2000). Outcome of solution-focused therapy at a university family therapy center. *Journal of Systemic Therapies*, **19**(1), 116–28.

Boje, D.M., Rosile, G., Dennehy, B., and Summers, D. (1997). Restorying reengineering: Some deconstructions and postmodern alternatives. *Journal of Communication Research*, **24**(6), 631–68.

Boje, D. M., Alvarez, R. C., and Schooling, B. (2001). Reclaiming story in organization: Narratologies and action sciences. In R. Westwood and S. Linstead (Eds.) *The language of organization*, pp.132–75. Sage Publications, London.

Carlson, T. D. (1997). Using art in narrative therapy: Enhancing therapeutic possibilities. *The American Journal of Family Therapy*, **25**(3), 271–83.

Chang, J. (1999). Collaborative therapies with young children and their families: Developmental, pragmatic, and procedural issues. *Journal of Systemic Therapies*, **18**(2), 44–64.

Cockburn J. T., Thomas F. N., and Cockburn O. J. (1997). Solution-focused therapy and psychosocial adjustment to orthopedic rehabilitation in a work-hardening program. *Journal of Occupational Rehabilitation*, **7**, 97–106.

Collins, J. A. and Fauser, B. C. J. M. (2005). Balancing the strengths of systematic and narrative reviews. *Human Reproduction Update*, **11**(2), 103–4.

Connie, E. and Metcalf, L. (2009). *The art of solution focused therapy*. Springer Publishing Company, New York.

Conoley, C. W., Graham, J. M., Neu, T., et al. (2003). Solution-focused family therapy with three aggressive and oppositional-acting children: An n=1 empirical study. *Family Process*, **42**(3), 361–74.

Cook, D. J., Mulrow, C. D., and Haynes, R. B. (1997). Systematic reviews: Synthesis of best evidence for clinical decisions. *Annals of Internal Medicine*, **126**(5), 376–80.

Corcoran, J. and Pillai, V. (2009). A review of the research on solution-focused therapy. *British Journal of Social Work*, **39**, 234–42.

Coulehan, R., Friedlander, M. L., and Heatherington, L. (1998). Transforming narratives: A change event in constructivist family. *Family Process*, **37**, 17–33.

Cowley, G. and Springen, K. (1995). Rewriting life stories. *Newsweek*, **125**(16), 70–74.

Crocket, K. (2004). From narrative practice in counseling to narrative practice in research: A professional identity story. *The International Journal of Narrative and Community Work*, **2**, 63–67.

Cruz, J. and Littrell, J. M. (1998). Brief counseling with Hispanic American college students. *Journal of Multicultural Counseling and Development*, **26**, 227–38.

da Costa, D., Nelson, T. M., Rudes, J., and Guterman, J. T. (2007, A narrative approach to body dysmorphic disorder. *Journal of Mental Health Counseling*, **29**(1), 67–80.

Dallos, R. (2004). Attachment narrative therapy: Integrating ideas from narrative and attachment theory in systemic family therapy with eating disorders. *Journal of Family Therapy*, **26**, 40–65.

Darmody, M. and Adams, B. (2003). Outcome research on solution-focused brief therapy. *Journal of Primary Care Mental Health*, **7**, 70–5.

De Haene, L. (2010). Beyond division: Convergences between postmodern qualitative research and family therapy. *Journal of Marital and Family Therapy*, **36**(1), 1–12.

De Jong, P. and Hopwood, L. E. (1996). Outcome research on treatment conducted at the Brief Family Therapy Center, 1992–1993. In S. D. Miller, M. A. Hubble, and B. L. Duncan (Eds.) *Handbook of solution-focused brief therapy*, pp. 272–98. Jossey-Bass, San Francisco, CA.

Denborough, D. (2009). *Research, evidence, and narrative practice.* http://www.dulwichcentre.com.au/narrative-therapy-research.html. [Accessed 29 September 2010.]

de Shazer, S. (1982). *Patterns of brief family therapy.* Guilford Press, New York.

de Shazer, S. and Berg, I. (1997). What works? Remarks on research aspects of solution-focused brief therapy, *Journal of Family Therapy*, **19**, 121–4.

de Shazer, S., Berg, I., Lipchik, E., et al. (1986). Brief therapy: Focused solution development. *Family Process*, **25**, 207–22.

DeSocio, J. E. (2005). Accessing self-development through narrative approaches in child and adolescent psychotherapy. *Journal of Child and adolescent Psychiatric Nursing*, **18**(2), 53–61.

Draucker, C. B. (1998). Narrative therapy for women who have lived with violence. *Archives of Psychiatric Nursing*, **XII**(3), 162–8.

Epston, D. (1993a). Internalized other questioning with couples: The New Zealand version. In S. Gilligan and R. Price (Eds.) *Therapeutic conversations*, pp. 183–96. Norton, New York.

Epston, D. (1993b). Internalizing discourses versus externalizing discourses. In S. Gilligan and R. Price (Eds.) *Therapeutic conversations*, pp. 161–77. Norton, New York.

Etchison, M. and Kleist, D. M. (2000). Review of narrative therapy: Research and utility. *The Family Journal*, **8**(61), 61–6.

Fernández, E., Cortés, A., and Tarragona, M. (2007). You make the path as you walk: Working collaboratively with people with eating disorders. In H. Anderson and D. Gehart (Eds.) *Collaborative therapy: Relationships and conversations that make a difference*, pp.129–47. Routledge, New York.

Fraenkel, P., Hameline, T., and Shannon, M. (2009). Narrative and collaborative practices in work with families that are homeless. *Journal of Marital & Family Therapy*, **35**(3), 325–43.

Franklin, C., Streeter, C. L., Kim, J. S., and Tripodi, S. J. (2008). Effectiveness of solution-focused brief therapy in a school setting. *Children and Schools*, **30**(1), 15–26.

Freedman, J. and Combs, G. (1996). *Narrative therapy: The social construction of preferred realities*, W. W. Norton and Company, New York.

Gardner, P. J. and Poole, J. M. (2009). One story at a time: Narrative therapy, older adults, and addictions. *Journal of Gerontology*, **28**(5), 600–20.

Gehart, D. (2007). Creating space for children's voices: A collaborative and playful approach to working with children and families. In H. Anderson and D. Gehart (Eds.) *Collaborative therapy: Relationships and conversations that make a difference*, pp. 183–96. Routledge, New York.

Gehart, D. R. and Lucas. (2007). Client advocacy in marriage and family therapy: A qualitative case study. *Journal of Family Psychotherapy*, **18**(1), 39–56.

Gehart, D., Tarragona, M., and Bava, S. (2007). A collaborative approach to research and inquiry. In H. Anderson and D. Gehart (Eds.) *Collaborative therapy: Relationships and conversations that make a difference*, pp. 367–87. Routledge, New York.

Gehart-Brooks, D. R. and Lyle, R. R. (1999). Client and therapist perspectives of change in collaborative language systems: An interpretive ethnography. *Journal of Systemic Therapies*, **18**(4), 58–77.

Gergen, K. J. (2009). *Relational being: Beyond self and community*. Oxford University Press, New York.

Gingerich, W. J. and Eisengart, S. (2000). Solution-focused brief therapy: A review of the outcome research. *Family Process*, **39**(4), 477–98.

Guilfoyle, M. (2009). Theorizing relational possibilities in narrative therapy. *Journal of Systemic Therapies*, **28**(2), 19–33.

Heneghan, C. and Badenoch, D. (2006), *Evidence-based medicine toolkit*. Blackwell, Malden, MA.

Hogan, B. A. (1999). Narrative therapy in rehabilitation after brain injury: A case study. *NeuroRehabilitation*, **13**, 21–25.

Ingram, C. and Perlesz, A. (2004). The getting of wisdoms. *The International Journal of Narrative and Community Work*, **2**, 49–56.

Jacobs, S., Kissil, K., Scott, D., and Davey, M. (2010). Creating synergy in practice: Promoting complementarity between evidence-based and postmodern approaches. *Journal of Marital and Family Therapy*, **36**(2), 185–96.

Keeling, M. L. and Nielson, L. R. (2005). Indian women's experience of a narrative intervention using art and writing. *Contemporary Family Therapy*, **27**(3), 435–52.

Kim, J. S. (2007). Examining the effectiveness of solution-focused brief therapy: A meta-analysis using random effects modeling. *19th National Symposium on Doctoral Research in Social Work*, Columbus, OH.

Kim, J. S. (2008). Examining the effectiveness of solution-focused brief therapy: A meta-analysis. *Research on Social Work Practices*, **18**(2), 107–16.

Kim, J. S. and Franklin, C. (2009). Solution-focused brief therapy in schools: A review of the outcome literature. *Children and Youth Services Review*, **31**, 464–70.

Kirven, J. (2000). Building on strengths on minority adolescents in foster care: A narrative-holistic approach. *Child & Youth Care Forum*, **29**(4), 247–63.

Kiser, D. (1988). A follow-up study conducted at the Brief Family Therapy Center. Unpublished manuscript.

Kropf, N. P. and Tandy, C. (1998). Narrative therapy with older clients: The use of a "meaning-making" approach. *Clinical Gerontologist*, **18**(4), 3–16.

Lee, M. Y., Greene, G. J., Uken, A., Sebold, J., and Rheinscheld, J. (1997). Solution-focused brief group treatment: A viable modality for domestic violence offenders? *Journal of Collaborative Therapies*, **4**, 10–17.

Levin, S. B. (2007). Hearing the unheard: Advice to professionals from women who have been battered. In H. Anderson and D. Gehart (Eds.) *Collaborative therapy: Relationships and conversations that make a difference*, pp. 109–27. Routledge, New York.

Li, S., Armstrong, M. S., Chaim, G., Kelly, C., and Shenfeld, J. (2007). Group and individual couple treatment for substance abuse clients: A pilot study. *American Journal of Family Therapy*, **35**(3), 221–33.

Lindforss, L. and Magnusson, D. (1997). Solution-focused therapy in prison. *Contemporary Family Therapy*, **19**(1), 89–103.

Lundblad, A. M. and Hansson, K. (2006). Couples therapy: Effectiveness of treatment and long-term follow-up. *Journal of Family Therapy*, **28**(2), 136–52.

Macdonald, A. (2007). *Solution-focused therapy: Theory, research, & practice*. Sage, Los Angeles, CA.

Macdonald, A. (2010). *Solution-focused brief therapy evaluation list*. http://www.solutionsdoc.co.uk/ [Accessed 13 July 2010.]

Matos, M., Santos, M., Goncalves, M., and Martins, C. (2009). Innovative moments and change in narrative therapy. *Psychotherapy Research*, **19**(1), 68–80.

McDonough, M. and Koch, P. (2007). Collaborating with parents and children in private practice: Shifting and overlapping conversations. In H. Anderson and D. Gehart (Eds.) *Collaborative therapy: Relationships and conversations that make a difference*, pp.167–81. Routledge, New York.

Messmore, C. (2002). Hearing her voice: Collaborating with the client on a new story. *Journal of Systemic Therapies*, **21**(4), 1–17.

Mehl-Madrona, L. (2007). Introducing narrative practices in a locked, inpatient psychiatric unit. *The Permamente Journal*, **11**(4), 12–20.

Miller, S. D., Duncan, B. L., Sorrell, R., and Brown, G. S. (2005). The partners for change outcome management system. *Journal of Clinical Psychology*, **61**(2), 199–208.

Monk, G., Winslade, J., Crocket, K., and Epston, D. (Eds) (1997). *Narrative therapy in practice: The archaeology of hope*. Jossey-Bass, San Francisco, CA.

Morgan, A. (2000). *What is narrative therapy? An easy-to-read introduction*. Dulwich Centre Publications, Adelaide.

O'Conner, T. S. J., Davis, A., Meakes, E., Pickering, R., and Schuman, M. (2004). Narrative therapy using a reflecting team: An ethnographic study of therapists' experiences. *Contemporary Family Therapy*, **26**(1), 23–39.

O'Conner, T. S., Meakes, E., Pickering, M. R., and Schuman, M. (1997). On the right track: Client experience of narrative therapy. *Contemporary Family Therapy*, **19**(4), 479–95.

Penn, P. (2007). Listening voices. In H. Anderson and D. Gehart (Eds.) *Collaborative therapy: Relationships and conversations that make a difference*, pp. 99–107. Routledge, New York.

Petticrew, M. and Roberts, H. (2006). *Systematic reviews in the social sciences: A practical guide*. Blackwell Publishing, Malden, MA.

Richert, A. J. (2003). Living stories, telling stories, changing stories: Experiential use of the relationship in narrative therapy. *Journal of Psychotherapy Integration*, **13**(2), 188–210.

Rothschild, P., Brownlee, K., and Gallant, P. (2000). Narrative interventions for working with persons with AIDS: A case study. *Journal of Family Psychotherapy*, **11**(3), 1–13.

Sackett, D. L., Rosenberg, W. M. C., Gray, J. A. M., Haynes, R. B., and Richardson, W. S. (1996). Evidence based medicine: What it is and what it isn't. *BMJ*, **312**, 71–72.

Sapyta, J., Riemer, M., and Bickman, L. (2005). Feedback to clinicians: Theory, research, and practice. *Journal of Clinical Psychology*, **61**, 145–53.

Seidel, A. and Hedley, D. (2008). The use of solution-focused brief therapy with older adults in Mexico: A preliminary study. *American Journal of Family Therapy*, **36**(3), 242–52.

Seymour, F. W. and Epston, D. (1989). An approach to childhood stealing with evaluation of 45 cases. *Australia and New Zealand Journal of Family Therapy,* **10**, 137–43.

Shin, S. K, (2009). Effects of a solution-focused program on the reduction of aggressiveness and the improvement of social readjustment for Korean youth probationers. *Journal of Social Service Research,* **35**(3), 274–84.

Silver, E., Williams, A., Worthington, F., and Phillips, N. (1998). Family therapy and soiling: an audit of externalising and other approaches. *Journal of Family Therapy,* **20**, 412–22.

Smock, S. A., Trepper, T. S., Wetchler, J. L., McCollum, E. E., Ray, R., and Pierce, K. (2008). Solution-focused group therapy for level 1 substance abusers. *Journal of Marital and Family Therapy,* **34**(1), 107–20.

Sparks, J. A. and Muro, M. L. (2009). Client-directed wraparound: The client as connector in community collaboration. *Journal of Systemic Therapies,* **28**(3), 63–76.

Stams, G. J., Dekovic, M., Buist, K., and de Vries, L. (2006). Effectiviteit van oplossingsgerichte korte therapie; Een meta-analyse [Efficacy of solution-focused brief therapy: A meta-analysis]. *Gedragstherapie* [*Behavior Therapy*], **39**, 81–94.

Stoddart, K. P., McDonnell, J., Temple, V., and Mustate, A. (2001). Is brief better? A modified brief solution-focused therapy approach for adults with a developmental delay. *Journal of Systemic Therapies,* **20**(2), 24–41.

Strong, T. and Paré, D. (Eds) (2004). *Furthering talk: Advances in the discursive therapies*. Kluwer Academic/Plenum Publishers, New York.

Sundet, R. (2011). Collaboration: Family and therapist perspectives of helpful therapy. *Journal of Marital and Family Therapy,* **37**, 236–49.

Trepper, T. S., McCollum, E. E., De Jong, P., Korman, H., Gingerich, W., and Franklin, C. (2008). *Solution focused therapy treatment manual for working with individuals*. http://www.sfbta.org/researchDownloads.html [Accessed 29 September 2010.]

Torres, S. and Guerra, M. P. (2002). Application of narrative therapy to anorexia nervosa: A case study. *Revista Portuguesa de Psicossomatica,* **4***,* 141–56.

Thorslund, K. W. (2007). Solution-focused group therapy for patients on long-term sick leave: A comparative outcome study. *Journal of Family Psychotherapy,* **18**(3), 11–24.

Vassallo, T. (1998). Narrative group therapy with the seriously mentally ill: A case study. *Australian and New Zealand Journal of Family Therapy,* **19**(1), 15–26.

Vromans, L. P. and Schweitzer, R. D. (2011). Narrative therapy for adults with major depressive disorder: Improved symptom and interpersonal outcomes. *Psychotherapy Research*, **21**(1), 4–15.

Walach, H., Falkenberg, T., Fønnebø, V., Lewith, G., and Jonas, W. B. (2006). Circular instead of hierarchical: Methodological principles for the evaluation of complex interventions. *BMC Medical Research Methodology,* **6**(29), 1–9.

Wagner, J. (2007). Trialogues: A means to answerability and dialogue in a prison setting. In H. Anderson and D. Gehart (Eds.) *Collaborative therapy: Relationships and conversations that make a difference*, pp. 203–20. Routledge, New York.

Weston, H. E., Boxer, P., and Heatherington, L. (1998). Children's attributions about family arguments: Implications for family therapy. *Family Process,* **37**, 35–49.

Walker, L. and Hayashi, L. (2009). Pono Kaulike: Reducing violence with restorative justice and solution-focused approaches. *Federal Probation,* **73**(1), 23–27.

Weber, M., Davis, K., and McPhie, I. (2006). Narrative therapy eating disorders and groups: Enhancing outcomes in rural NSW. *Australian School Work,* **59**, 391–405.

White, M. (2007). *Maps of narrative practice*. W. W. Norton and Company, New York.

White, M. and Epston, D. (1990). *Narrative means to therapeutic ends*, W. W. Norton and Company, New York.

Wilmshurst, L. A. (2002). Treatment programs for youth with emotional and behavioural disorders: An outcome study of two alternate approaches. *Mental Health Services Research,* **4**, 85–96.

Wirtz, H. and Harari, R. (2000). Deconstructing depression: A narrative groupwork approach. *Dulwich Centre Journal,* **1/2**, 42–51.

Young, K. and Cooper, S. (2008). Toward co-composing an evidence base: The narrative therapy re-visiting project' *Journal of Systemic Therapies,* **27**(1), 67–83.

Chapter 14

Problematizing social context in evidence-based therapy evaluation practice/governance

Robbie Busch

Evidence-based evaluation and its discourse[1] has become a considerable growth industry and a concerning trend for researchers and therapists whose values and practices do not fit with its philosophy. Originating from medicine and the medical model, evidence-based practice (EBP) discourse has proliferated far beyond the precise biological demarcations of medicine into the fuzzy, intersubjective representations of the psychosocial. EBP has become a global movement, extending its authoritative policy and practice into the social and educational sciences (Torrance 2008). Even the Research Assessment Exercise (RAE) in the United Kingdom, and its variants in Hong Kong, Australia, and New Zealand has been adopted from evidence-based principles that attempt, paradoxically, to quantify quality research (Denzin and Giardina 2008; Stronach 2008). The influential American Psychological Association (APA) also appropriated EBP into its evaluation policy. EBP stipulates that psychotherapists should use the best available research, where randomized experiments are viewed as the most stringent method, along with clinical expertise and client characteristics, to help the client (APA Presidential Task Force on Evidence-Based Practice 2006). This political ideal of EBP (Tanenbaum 2003) has been often touted by clinical psychologists as a way to bridge the gap between scientific research and therapeutic practice (Kazdin 2008; Thorn 2007), and as an improvement from its predecessor in psychology, the empirically-supported treatment (EST) movement (APA Presidential Task Force on Evidence-Based Practice 2006). Others counter-argue by saying that evidence-based evaluations exclude or marginalize therapies (incl. discursively-oriented therapies) that qualitatively examine relational and contextual aspects of client experience (e.g. Task Force for the Development of Practice Recommendations for the Provision of Humanistic Psychosocial Services 2001).

In this chapter, I problematize the thinning of the social context of psychotherapy in contemporary evidence-based evaluation and end with some implications for the discursive therapies. Discursive therapists work from postfoundationalist philosophies such as postmodernism, social constructionism, and poststructuralism

---

[1] Here I conceptualize discourse as a general domain, group, or regulated social practice of a range of statements that can systematically structure human relations (Foucault, 1972).

(Anderson 1997; Drewery et al. 2000; Holzman 2003; O'Connell 2005, p. 9) and these philosophical approaches are inherently (but not exclusively) aligned with qualitative investigation. Such approaches appear to be incommensurable with the foundationalist stance of EBP. The perspective of EBP privileges the randomized controlled trial (RCT) as the gold standard, as well as measurement and standardization of human experience (Rycroft-Malone et al. 2003; Tanenbaum 2003) where clients are often quantified as, what Rose (1999) calls, calculable subjects. Clients are defined medically as patients to be treated in EBP (APA Presidential Task Force on Evidence-Based Practice 2006). However, in the discursive therapies, clients are positioned as experts of their own experiences and are part of a collaborative relationship between therapist and client (Anderson 1997; Gladding 2002). Therapists are defined as expert clinicians in EBP. In contrast, in the discursive therapies, therapists position themselves in a less expert or authority-based role by privileging the client's expertise and by being aware of dominant professional discourses that favour the authority role of the therapist (Drewery et al. 2000). Psychotherapy in EBP is framed by a medical model where the clinician administers a 'treatment' and evaluates client progress by reducing their experience into well-operationalized, calculable measures through psychometric assessment (Spring 2007). Psychotherapy in the discursive therapies is more of a qualitative endeavour, where therapy focuses on developing understanding and meaning, shared between the therapist and client, throughout the therapy.

Evidence, via a discursive perspective, is not something that is medically framed by reducing *all* research through quantifiable standards/ideals of validity and reliability (ideals expressed throughout the APA Presidential Task Force on Evidence-Based Practice 2006). Rather, evidence can be viewed as something that is constantly limited by how it is languaged, and by whom, and thus can be made questionable, in/through a political and social context:

> It is a question of who has the power to control the *definition* of evidence, of who defines the kinds of materials that *count* as evidence, of who determines what methods best produce the best forms of evidence, and of whose criteria and standards are ultimately used to evaluate quality evidence
>
> (Denzin and Giardina 2008, p. 12).

In order to understand the consequences from those who have the ability to control evaluation and those who resist its discourse, I have used the Foucaultian perspective of governmentality as an interpretative framing for this chapter. Any authoritative system that can be taken for granted can become (re)produced and reinforced as an 'ethical' practice through our own responsible autonomy (Rabinow and Rose 2003). This is the nature of governmentality in that we are free to conduct our affairs which are often shaped by a prevailing, authoritative, and governing 'mentality' (i.e. a discourse), an ethical code that may shape how we think about how we should conduct (i.e. govern) our own conduct and how we expect others to conduct themselves.[2]

---

[2] I should note that government *tries* to shape human freedom but it is not constitutive of freedom: 'The governed are free in that they are actors, i.e. it is possible for them to act and think in a variety of ways, and sometimes in ways not foreseen by authorities' (Rabinow and Rose 2003, p. 13)

Foucault's conceptualization of government is a form of activity that aims to 'shape, guide, or affect the conduct of some person or other persons' (Gordon 1991, p. 2). It involves a complex set of power relations that produce resistance or acceptance to a discourse (e.g. an authoritative system of statements) that aims to govern conduct.

So, from a governmental perspective, EBP can be thought of as an authoritative system that attempts to shape and limit how psychotherapists practice evaluation by defining what counts as evidence and what methods and evaluative criteria can be used. Psychotherapists are free to govern themselves and others in such a system/discourse of EBP policy and guidelines. The position of authority and knowledge comes not from the practitioner (and client), but instead from the policymaker for the practitioner (and client) to govern therapeutic practice (Davies, 2003; Rose, 1999).

From a social constructionist stance, there are multiple ways of speaking evaluation in that our sense of the world can be understood according to the knowledge perspective it is spoken from (Guba and Lincoln 1989; Lincoln and Guba 2004). Based on how we language and thus contextualize evaluation, we may evaluate through a quantitative, objective measurement or through a more qualitative, subjective consideration regarding concerns presented by the client in psychotherapy. It is likely that a behavioural psychologist would use objective measures such as charting the frequency of certain problem behaviours whereas a discursive therapist would use interpretative, collaborative, and socially contextual methods such as describing and understanding dialogue and discourse. Geertz's (1973) perspective of context would suggest that the behaviourist, informed by an objectivist way of knowing, would use a thin description to make sense of experience (i.e. describing the behaviour through quantifiable, calculable terms such as counting behaviour through clear operational definitions). In contrast, the discursive therapist, informed by a social constructionist way of knowing, would use thick description. That is, s/he would attempt to understand the behaviour by situating it within a broader context (Geertz 1973) such as the effects of being positioned by dominant discourse (Drewery and Winslade 1997). Both therapeutic perspectives provide different contextualizations of the client experience—one 'thin' and the other 'thick'.[3]

Discursive therapists value the qualitative importance of social context. The social constructionist stance that underpins solution-focused therapy takes the view that 'there is no objective meaning to reality and all meaning is a human creation influenced by social and cultural factors' (O'Connell 2005, p. 9). Social context is a fundamental part of social constructionism with its assumption that the self is a product of social interactions (Burr 2003). Tied up in this is language, used as a public phenomenon to make sense of the world; our knowledge of reality is formed, linguistically, as a social practice within social contexts (O'Connell 2005). Solution-focused therapy 'pays attention to the context in which the client's narrative develops' (O'Connell 2005, p. 13). Collaborative language systems therapy examines the social context of the therapeutic relationship by viewing it as a system. Its premise views therapists as non-experts and therapy as a 'language system in which the client and therapist create

---

[3] This is not say that one perspective is better than the other but that they each have different ramings of client experience.

meaning with each other' (Anderson 1997, p. 324). Social therapy focuses on the practice of dialectics, which acknowledges that although we live in a materialistic, objectifying Western culture, humans are relational and historical beings (Holzman 2003). The relational and historical context of human experience can, according to Holzman (2003), enable the rejection of objectification. Narrative therapy uses a textual analogy to examine power relations in the social context of human experience (White and Epston 1990). White and Epston also consider therapy a form of social control. The social context of psychotherapy from a discursive therapy perspective would, arguably, involve an engagement with the political, tailoring to the client-specific context, including the relationship between client and therapist, and the historical context of the client and therapist, in/through and inseparable from the textual/discursive. Since social context appears so primary to the discursive therapies it needs to be a necessary consideration in evaluation practice.

As social context can be a core part of evaluation practice for therapy, psychotherapy evaluation is immersed in its own social context, too. Psychotherapy evaluation has become a governing political ideal where public health policymakers espouse EBP as the idea 'that more science will bring about better mental health practice' (Tanenbaum 2003, p. 287). However, the evaluator cannot be value-free as 'facts' are established by his/her value system and so evaluation becomes a political act (Guba and Lincoln, 1989). Evaluation appears to be something that policy makers and researchers impose on therapists to consider.[4] Policy documents, produced by psychotherapy researchers, are made to inform and guide practitioners and researchers (e.g. American Psychological Association 2002; APA Presidential Task Force on Evidence-Based Practice 2006; Task Force on Promotion and Dissemination of Psychological Procedures 1995) who have to regulate their practice due to public healthcare policy and guidelines (Disbury 2003; Tanenbaum 2003). Therapy evaluation can thus be considered as a *governing* activity.

I aim to problematize social context in the governance of evidence-based evaluation through the reflexive examination of my own discipline: psychology. Influenced by the critical-historical and discursive perspective of governmentality (Gordon 1991; Rabinow and Rose 2003), I thematically examine a recent history of psychotherapy evaluation in psychology in relation to social context. I argue that social context has been diluted in psychotherapy evaluation in that certain practices of thin rather than thick contextualization are espoused and encouraged. I will then conclude with what implications this has for the discursive therapies.

Psychotherapy evaluation as a governing practice

The APA and its divisions' production of policy documents on evaluation can be thought of as authoritative statements that attempt to govern the conduct of psychotherapists and psychologists. Such documents include contributions from the Division

---

[4] Perhaps I am also guilty here of imposing my interpretations of psychotherapy evaluation. Although I've studied psychotherapy, I am not a therapist and I am expressing my views on evaluation to, undoubtedly, many readers who will be therapists! In the context of this research, I locate myself as both an academic and a doctoral student in psychology, so my examination of psychotherapy evaluation is limited to the domain of psychology and its discourse.

of Clinical Psychology's (Division 12) policy on empirically-validated treatments (EVTs; Task Force on Promotion and Dissemination of Psychological Procedures 1995), now termed as empirically-supported treatments (ESTs), and the APA Presidential Task Force on Evidence-Based Practice (2006) which produced policy for the establishment of EBP in psychology (EBPP). These authoritative writings enable the production of individualized governance—a rationalizing of evaluation in thinkable and practicable ways to psychotherapists so they can 'responsibly' conduct evaluation proper through prescriptive guidelines. They help 'shape, guide, or affect the conduct' (Gordon 1991, p.2) of psychotherapists and psychologists in their evaluations and/or use their use of evaluation research. So, the authoritative evaluation policy documents of the APA and its divisions can encourage or discourage psychotherapists and psychologists to include or exclude, and to value or disvalue, the importance of social context in their practice of therapy and/or evaluation.

Inspired by Foucauldian governmental and genealogical approaches (Foucault 1977, 1991; Nicholls et al. 2009; Rose 1996, 1999) as well Geertz's (1973) writings on context, I used three criteria in my governmental, thematic examination of contemporary psychotherapy evaluation: 1) find broad thematic issues of thin contextualization (or decontextualization) that appear to be the most important in psychotherapy evaluation policy of the APA and its divisions; 2) find evaluation policy statements that dilute, omit, and/or discourage thick descriptions of social context; and 3) find evaluation policy statements that advocate for or produce thick descriptions of social context. I then interpreted the policy texts as 'saying/implying something' about the governance or conduct of psychologists and psychotherapists. I came across three main thematic strands of thin contextualization in the contemporary history of psychotherapy evaluation in psychology: manualization, experimental methodolatry, and medical objectification. What follows, after a brief historical background of ESTs and EBP, is an examination of those themes of thin contextualization.

Contemporary historical context of therapy evaluation in psychology

Since the 1990s, the discourse of psychotherapy evaluation has been more or less governed by two key evidence-based evaluation movements in psychology: empirically-supported treatments (ESTs) and evidence-based practice (EBP). During the transformation of the United States managed healthcare system in the mid-1990s, the Clinical Psychology Division of the American Psychological Association (Division 12) released a task force report on psychotherapy evaluation. Division 12's Task Force on Promotion and Dissemination of Psychological Procedures (1995) produced the policy report, *Training in and Dissemination of Empirically-Validated Treatments: Report and Recommendations*. The report and its subsequent variants included criteria for 'well-established' and 'probably efficacious' treatments whereby evaluations had to use manuals, specify clearly defined clinical problems (geared towards matching specific 'treatments' for diagnostic disorders) or populations that were to be treated, and conduct such evaluations using experimental designs (Chambless and Hollon 1998; Task Force on Promotion and Dissemination of Psychological Procedures 1995).

The Task Force was created in 1992 at a time when, according to Beutler (1998), the United States was grappling with the issue of implementing a national healthcare policy. Managed healthcare which assessed therapy based on immediate cost and general access, he argued, paid little or no attention to clinical benefit. Beutler, a member of the Task Force from 1995, asserts that psychologists and psychotherapies were in danger of being excluded from national healthcare policy. Psychologists were replaced either by clinicians who practised pharmacological interventions or by practitioners who could be paid less due to their level of training. Consequently, one of the recommendations of the Task Force report was to educate and convince third party payers about empirically-validated treatments, particularly to 'convince insurance and managed care companies and governmental agencies whose decisions affect the public' (Task Force on Promotion and Dissemination of Psychological Procedures 1995, p.12). The development of EVTs came at a time when managed healthcare organizations in the United States were determining the effectiveness of psychotherapeutic interventions (Beutler, 1998).

'New managerialism' as the driving cultural ethos of this era of managed care is a possible contextual explanation for the emergence of evidence-based evaluation discourse. It is where workers are made to comply with a moral code of work conduct, produced by policy-makers, but this coercion is somewhat disguised by the emphasis on individual responsibility (Davies 2003). The emphasis on individualized accountability forces the worker to act on their own fears, guilt, and sense of responsibility, to 'stay in line' with (and 'naturalize') the moral code no matter how problematic it may be (Davies, 2003; Rose 1999). This new ethos is a genesis from a much older form of managerialism. Scientific management, or Taylorism, emerged as a paradigm from the 1920s that combined industrial psychology, sociology, and economics so that managers could scientifically study how workers could do tasks most efficiently in order to closely manage and increase their productivity (Fleischman 2000). Taylorism and evidence-based medicine are often critically compared because they both focus on changing behaviour through scientific measurement and standardization (Timmermans and Berg 2003). However, new managerialism (or by its other name, neo-liberalism) is a discourse and a 'set of practices that facilitate the governing of individuals from a distance' (Larner 2000, p. 6). Neo-liberalism, Larner argues, spawned from the political practices of Thatcherism, Reaganomics, and Rogernomics in the 1980s where state social responsibility was abdicated to individuals and private enterprise. EBP is a product of new managerialism (Davies, 2003). That is, EBP produces a way of obtaining best efficient practice from a practitioner through their individual responsibility to be 'good enough' clinicians according to the system/discourse of EBP, produced as an unproblematic, 'ethical' code of practice.

According to Beutler (1998), Division 12 elected a group of psychologists with the task of using research data to find out what interventions are of value as a response to the new managed healthcare environment. This, he maintains, was at a time when managed healthcare programmes started to shift their focus from cost to a criteria whereby treatments were required to be proven effective empirically. This ethos of new managerialism placed the onus on healthcare professionals to 'prove' the effectiveness of interventions.

So, the Division 12 Task Force report on EVTs was a strategic tool produced to persuade stakeholders in psychotherapy evaluation on the empirical research backing of psychotherapies. The Task Force were charged with the assignment to 'consider methods for educating clinical psychologists, third party payors, and the public about effective psychotherapies' (Task Force on Promotion and Dissemination of Psychological Procedures 1995, p. 3). They produced recommendations that data-based treatment approaches be published in the APA Monitor, that the APA assist in training curricula for EVTs and offer these through health management organizations and mental health centres, and that the APA work with the National Institute of Mental Health to cultivate the dissemination of results about the benefits of empirically-validated psychotherapy research. The Task Force also recommended media releases, public service announcements and media campaigns to educate the public. In addition to convincing insurance, managed care, and governmental organizations, the Task Force recommended that the 'APA needs to continue to work to make the empirically-documented benefits of psychotherapy for emotional disorders known to third party payors' (Task Force on Promotion and Dissemination of Psychological Procedures 1995, p. 12).

The Task Force's fervent promotion of EVTs resulted in a backlash from psychotherapists due to its universal and narrow evaluation criteria, as well as its incongruity with actual therapeutic settings. Bohart et al. (1998) argued that it failed to take into account the humanistic therapies, and that one criterion of EVT, manualization, may lead to a weakening of therapist skills. Garfield (1996, p. 220) noted the disparity between therapists strictly trained in manualized EVT through controlled research settings and therapist variability in clinical practice settings where therapists rely on their 'own training and experience to best meet the therapeutic needs of the individual patient'.

Consequently, the language of EVT was subdued and its concept changed to empirically-*supported* treatments. Chambless and Hollon's (1988, p. 7) rationale was 'to avoid the unfortunate connotation, to some . . . that the process of validation has been completed, and no further research is needed on a treatment'. Various divisions of the APA also set up task forces critiquing the EST movement and provided their own solutions such as the Society of Counseling Psychology (Division 17; Wampold et al. 2002, 2005), the Division of Humanistic Psychology (Division 32; Task Force for the Development of Practice Recommendations for the Provision of Humanistic Psychosocial Services 2001), and the Division of Psychotherapy (Division 29; Norcross 2001).[5]

Some 10 years after the publication of the 1995 policy report on EVTs, where empirically-supported treatments (ESTs) followed, EBP in psychology (EBPP) developed (APA Presidential Task Force on Evidence-Based Practice, 2006). EBPP was part of a wider movement in EBP, which emerged from evidence-based medicine in the 1990s (EBM; Donald 2002; Tanenbaum 2003). The rationale for EBM, and subsequently

---

[5] Although I will be using these Divisions as examples of resistance to the EST movement, I do not necessarily agree with their 'own' solutions. This is especially so with Divisions 17 and 29 who appear to model from the calculability-focused, new managerialism of EST standards rather than questioning how such a discourse enables psychotherapists to individually manage themselves and judge others according to such standards.

EBP, was to develop a structured framework for systematic clinical decision-making guided by best evidence. Academic journals were established to specifically focus on EBP (Harper et al. 2003). EBP has been increasingly accepted as a model in Western healthcare systems (Chwalisz 2003). The general idea of EBP is that the incorporation of clinical expertise and patient characteristics with established evidence makes for beneficial health decisions for the patient (Sackett et al. 1996; Sackett and Strauss 1998). Similarly, and as promoted by the APA, EBPP is 'the integration of the best available research with clinical expertise in the context of patient characteristics, culture, and preferences' (APA Presidential Task Force on Evidence-Based Practice 2006, p. 271). Architects of EBPP see it as much broader and inclusive than empirically-supported treatment policy because of its focus on the practitioner making practical therapeutic decisions on the best available evidence in the context of their expertise and the patient's characteristics (APA Presidential Task Force on Evidence-Based Practice 2006; Wyatt 2007).

However, despite the emergence of the EBPP movement, empirically-supported treatment discourse stills remains alive and abundant. This may be because the APA's Clinical Division Task Force report 'increased recognition of demonstrably effective psychological treatments among the public, policymakers, and training programs' (APA Presidential Task Force on Evidence-Based Practice 2006, p. 272). The zealous drive of ESTs is still evident in contemporary psychotherapy publications. Nathan and Gorman's (2007) *A Guide to Treatments That Work* is comprised of evaluative reviews of empirically-supported treatments and offers detailed reviews of treatments for certain mental disorders. There are discussions on balancing treatment fidelity with flexibility in ESTs (McHugh et al. 2009), making them more accessible (Smits et al. 2007), and how they can be further incorporated into the training of clinicians (Rutgers 2008). There are also websites informing the public and practitioners on empirically-supported treatments such as the Society of Clinical Psychology, Division 12 website (www.psychologicaltreatments.org) and others like Therapy Advisor (www.therapy-advisor.com; Riley et al. 2007).[6] Evidence-based evaluation in psychotherapy is a growing phenomenon with the emergence of discourse on EBP, EBPP, *and* the continuation of ESTs. This is all set in a new managerialist ethos of health management where, according to the APA Presidential Task Force on Evidence-Based Practice (2006, p. 273), 'the goals of evidence-based practice initiatives [are] to improve quality and cost-effectiveness and to enhance accountability', notably, of the individual psychologist who complies with such 'goals'.

Thin contextualizations 1: manuals versus the relationship

The EST movement in the mid-1990s stipulated that psychologists should use manualised therapies for specific clinical problems (e.g. Chambless and Hollon 1998).

---

[6] In addition, researchers have confused empirically-supported treatments with EBP even thought they are meant to be different approaches (Levant and Hasan 2008; e.g. see King and Ollendick 2006).

The original Division 12 Task Force document cited the Beck et al. (1979) volume, *The Cognitive Therapy of Depression*, marking the 'beginning of the availability of a treatment manual for a major treatment approach with a specific patient problem' (Task Force on Promotion and Dissemination of Psychological Procedures 1995, p. 4). The Division 12 Task Force argued that since then, evidence has been accumulating on the use of manuals for effective standardization of treatment and that 'such standardisation . . . through treatment manuals' diminishes 'the methodological problems caused by variable therapist outcomes and lead to more specific clinical recommendations' (Task Force on Promotion and Dissemination of Psychological Procedures 1995, p. 4). Advocates of ESTs saw manuals as necessary for the replication of a therapy (Chambless and Hollon 1998). There have also been attempts to manualize and standardize the organizational management of mental health clinics (Donohue et al. 2009). According to the Task Force on Promotion and Dissemination of Psychological Procedures (1995), a 'treatment manual is a clear description of a treatment, and this should be possible for adherents of all psychotherapy approaches to apply' (p. 6). A new managerialism of therapy delivery was set in motion.

The EST policy of psychologists and psychotherapists as 'adherents' to 'psychotherapy approaches', in using manuals as a standardization practice, may construct an artificiality in the therapeutic relationship that erodes the relational context of therapy. Bohart (2000) for example, asserts the unsuitability of manualization for solution-focused therapy, a discursive therapy, where the interaction of client and therapist responding with each other 'is the core of therapy, and not a small "detail" to be added within a manualized framework' (p. 490). The Division of Psychotherapy Task Force was against manualized and standardized therapy. The Task Force asserted that 'one-size-fits-all therapy relationships are out' and 'tailoring the therapy to the unique patient is in' (Norcross 2001, p. 353). Former president of the APA, Ronald Levant, stated that the most narrow view of manualization 'reduces the role of clinician to that of technician and allows very little deviation . . . The manuals that were personified in the Division 12 [EST] lists were really rigid manuals' (Wyatt 2007, para. 83). In a manualized time-limited dynamic therapy study, Henry et al. (1993) concluded that manualized training eroded the therapeutic relationship.

Other APA task forces have appreciated the interpersonal context of psychotherapy in evaluation. They argued that context is 'inextricably interwoven into the emergent therapy relationship' (Norcross 2001, p. 348), that therapies are 'complex amalgams of ingredients delivered in an interpersonal context' (Wampold et al. 2002, p. 209) and that therapeutic decisions are the consequence of 'multiple, interacting, and recursive considerations on the part of the patient, the therapist, and the context' (Norcross 2001, p. 354). Humanists also argued, in the Task Force for the Development of Practice Recommendations for the Provision of Humanistic Psychosocial Services (2001) document, that people live in 'relational contexts' (p. 3) and contend that the relationship is 'more powerful than any specific "technique"' (p. 15).

In the discursive therapies, social context is fundamental to customising therapy through collaborative dialogue between therapist and client (Anderson 1997; Gladding 2002). This approach is a far cry from the treatment adherent approach in

ESTs. Instead of the practitioner hierarchically imposing expert technical knowledge, they attempt to understand the client through collaborative talk (Strong 2002). Context is formed where meanings are 'negotiated and constructed in the process of communication until each party is clear that they have a grasp of what they are "talking about"' (Strong and Lock 2005, p. 585). This talk focuses on the clients' framing of their context (Strong 2002) which involves the therapist being prepared to attentively partake and collaborate in possible meanings and modes of talk that may be unfamiliar to her/him (Strong and Lock 2005). This ethnographical-esque, collaborative approach to rendering context via a co-construction of meaning forms the means for 'customizing solutions together with clients' (Strong 2002, p. 228). Such a tailored, collaborative approach to constructing context is remarkably dissimilar to administering manualized treatment protocols according to fixed diagnostic categorizations.

Evidence-based practice in psychology (EBPP) seems to place less importance on manualization (Wyatt 2007). The APA Presidential Task Force on Evidence-Based Practice (2006) mentioned that there was concern with psychologists about the selective focus on manualization. Its wider emphasis on not just best available research but also clinical expertise and patient needs acknowledged the importance of sensitivity and flexibility in therapeutic decision-making and delivery. The Task Force recognizes that the sociocultural and environmental context of the patient is important in clinical decision-making and the relationship and that 'psychotherapy is a collaborative enterprise in which patients and clinicians negotiate ways of working together that are mutually agreeable and likely to lead to positive outcomes' (APA Presidential Task Force on Evidence-Based Practice 2006, p. 280). EBPP values the therapeutic relationship in terms of the clinician as the expert knower of the doing and shifting of interaction between therapist and patient. The clinician 'fosters the patient's positive engagement in the therapeutic process, monitors the therapeutic alliance, and attends carefully to barriers to engagement and change' (APA Presidential Task Force on Evidence-Based Practice 2006, p. 277).

However, aside from clinical decision-making, EBPP has an apparent bias towards psychologists and therapists using experimental design above all other possible approaches in psychotherapy evaluation. It is believed that 'clinical trials provide optimal evidence' (Wampold et al. 2007, p. 617) and experimental designs are the most sophisticated (APA Presidential Task Force on Evidence-Based Practice 2006). This somewhat creates a paradoxical, problematic stance in EBPP; to have a therapy evaluated in a replicable, group experimental design, it would more than likely be standardized and controlled, which could (as Henry et al. 1993 found with manuals) degrade the therapeutic relationship.

Thin contextualizations 2: experimental methodolatry

A fetishism or preoccupation of using the experimental method above all other approaches in evidence-based evaluation can be termed as 'experimental methodolatry'. Methodolatry is the idolatry or worship of method. It is a practice that has a tautological function: the employment of 'good' method for the sake of good method. It is what Danziger (1994) calls a form of methodological fetishism that is a consequence of 'preoccupations with a purity of method' (p. 6) in psychology. He suggests that methodolatry is part of a social activity that is governed by mundane conditions and contexts rather than think of it as a realm of pure reason. Otherwise, he argues, we are at risk of being exposed to a 'naive and self-deluded style of scientific practice' (Danziger 1994, p. 6). Often believed as one of the most objectively pure methods, Davies (2003, p. 99) asserts that 'experiments do not remove the subjectivity of researchers; they simply work to conceal it'. Methodolatry, Chamberlain (2000, p. 286) argues, is 'characteristic of most psychology' where psychology has been preoccupied with methodology since its origins. Chamberlain notes that, throughout the history of psychology, the influences of behaviourism as a dominant paradigm, and the emphases on objectivity and measurement are reasons for the sustainment of methodolatry to its contemporary practice. Experimental methodolatry also appears to be widespread throughout evidence-based policy and practice. RCTs are promoted as the gold standard in the international health and social research enterprises, the Cochrane and Campbell Collaborations, which influence policymakers and practitioners (Denzin and Giardina 2008). Experimental methodolatry in EBP, Davies (2003, p. 100) argues, 'reveals either a naivety about research, or a hidden, managerialist agenda that has little to do with research findings and their implications for practice'.

The EST movement promoted the experimental method as the *only* method to be used by psychologists and psychotherapists where 'empirical' means 'experimental' (Chambless and Hollon 1998). According to proponents of the EST movement, 'efficacy is best demonstrated in randomized clinical trials (RCTs)' (Chambless and Hollon 1998, p. 7) where 'RCT methodology remains the best way to test new short-term, and long-term, treatments as ways to improve upon existing ESTs' (Crits-Christoph et al. 2005, p. 415). The use of 'best' indicates a moral standing in that good practitioners use experimental design as the best way to evaluate therapy.

As methodolatry involves the worship of method, there is an absence of reflection on epistemology and theoretical perspectives (Chamberlain 2000; Danziger 1994) or a reflexive questioning of the use of method and methodology. For example, well-established treatments in ESTs require interventions that are supported by 'good experimental designs' (Chambless et al. 1998, p. 4; Task Force on Promotion and Dissemination of Psychological Procedures 1995, p. 21), although the notion of what is good is unclear. Good is not defined. Yet, it is repeated four times in the criteria tables for well-established and probably efficacious treatments: 'good group design', 'good experimental designs', 'one good experiment', and 'two good experiments'. This implies that good experimental designs form a research ethic, a moral judgement in that experimental designs are in themselves good, are part of good research practice, or that good is some moral criterion but it is one that is undefined in the Task Force document. Similarly in EBPP, 'good practice and science call for the timely testing of psychological practices in a way that adequately operationalizes them using appropriate scientific methodology' (APA Presidential Task Force on Evidence-Based Practice 2006, p. 274). Such political stipulations of 'good practice' imply that psychologists must make a moral choice in determining an intervention as evidence-based where experimental and scientifically operationalizable methods are considered 'appropriate'. The Task Force on Promotion and Dissemination of Psychological Procedures (1995) encouraged psychologists and psychotherapists to survey their own training according to set empirical criteria to see if it fits particular standards to determine whether a therapy is empirically supported. The rationale for this was to not 'put psychologists in a disadvantageous position vis a vis psychiatry' (Task Force on Promotion and Dissemination of Psychological Procedures, 1995, p. 16). In an attempt to govern the conduct of psychologists and psychotherapists, the Task Force stressed that psychology training programmes '*should* increasingly move towards a concentration of effort in training students in those methods which rest on *firm empirical support*', that 'every student completing training *should* be competent in at least one intervention with *demonstrated efficacy*' (Task Force on Promotion and Dissemination of Psychological Procedures 1995, pp. 7–8, italic emphasis added). The rationale for such training was due to the rise in managed healthcare and reimbursement, contingent on empirically-supported interventions (Beutler 1998). Consequently, this motivated the Task Force to set evaluative standards, emulated from medical efficacy criteria, for psychologists so that mental health 'consumers' and 'third-party payers' were aware of them.

Borrowed from Food and Drug Administration (FDA) efficacy criteria (Beutler 1998), the paramount focus of EST evaluations is on the psychologist's moral obligation to standardize and medicalize treatment. Clients become divided into variables that aggregate a sample to determine the effectiveness of therapy. Psychologists have to demonstrate efficacy by establishing their treatment as 'superior to pill or psychological placebo or to another treatment' or as 'equivalent to an already established treatment in studies with adequate statistical power' (Task Force on Promotion and Dissemination of Psychological Procedures 1995, p. 21). With the shift to ESTs, 'superior' was defined as 'statistically significant' (Chambless et al. 1998, p. 4). If treatments are to be supported by single case design experiments, there must be a large series[7] of these studies using good experimental designs and the treatment must be compared to pill, psychological placebo, or another treatment. No matter if they are group or case design experiments, they must also be supported by two other standards: 1) the 'studies must be conducted with treatment manuals' and 2) 'characteristics of the client samples must be clearly specified' (Task Force on Promotion and Dissemination of Psychological Procedures 1995, p. 21). Client-participants in such studies have to be homogenous in that they must have the same characteristics and the same disorder. The second tier, *probably efficacious treatments* has less stringent experiment criteria such as having 'at least two good studies demonstrating effectiveness but *flawed by the heterogeneity of the client samples*' (Task Force on Promotion and Dissemination of Psychological Procedures 1995, p. 22, italic emphasis added).

The experimental methodolatry of the EST movement focuses heavily on good design for obtaining outcome at the expense of understanding the wider social context of the client. The experimental method, Levitt et al. (2005) argue, is a tautological

---

[7] Later defined as nine or greater (Chambless et al., 1998). The shift from EVTs to ESTs resulted in more definitive and specific criteria such as 'experiment' instead of 'study' and the inclusion of 'reliability' and 'validity' (see Chambless and Hollon, 1998).

process because it cannot discover anything that was not hypothesized beforehand, which makes it inapt as an approach to discover complex social processes and thus thick contexts of human experience. Burr (2003) argues that 'the experiment effectively strips the subjects' behaviour of the context that gives it its meaning and rationale, replacing this with the experimenter's own interpretations' (p. 154). Greenberg (1991, p. 5) asserts that the idolization of experimental control, statistical significance, random sampling, and generalizability indicates a reproduction of a methodological myopia where internal validity is strictly adhered to without examining the 'bigger picture' such as being 'guided by theory' and catching 'contexts, patterns, and meanings' of what is encountered.

Other APA Divisions criticized the EST movement's policy on the conduct of psychotherapy evaluation as 'context-stripping'. The Society of Counseling Psychology's (Division 17's) own Special Task Group (STG) on evaluation claimed that there were experimental practices in EST evaluations that did not match actual practice settings and so did not make outcomes generalizable to them. Some of these practices the STG claimed that did not equate the context of actual practice were 'inclusionary/exclusionary criteria that result in samples unrepresentative in practice . . . selection of effective therapists who are given specialized training and supervision . . . and a greater dose of therapy than is typically provided, at least in a managed care environment' (Wampold et al. 2005, p. 30). The STG recognized in a special issue of the *Journal of Consulting and Clinical Psychology* on ESTs (Kendall and Chambless 1998), 'not one mention of ethnicity or culture was made, thus assuming that treatments are uniformly effective across various ethnic and cultural populations' (Wampold et al. 2002, p. 206). The STG asserted that outcomes ought to be assessed locally in that evaluations should be tailored and conform to local settings. The Psychotherapy Division Task Force on Empirically-Supported Therapy Relationships was also critical of attempts to control for therapists, asserting that 'it is simply not possible to mask the person and the contribution of the therapist' (Norcross 2001, p. 346). The Society for Humanistic Psychology's Task Force for the Development of Practice Recommendations for the Provision of Humanistic Psychosocial Services (2001) also stated that experiments are difficult to apply to people in real life contexts and having a predetermined and standardized outcome measure prevents any evaluation of the complexity of the therapeutic context.

In contrast to the EST movement, the emergence of EBPP widened the notion of what is legitimate evidence-based evaluation to include non-experimental and qualitative research. The APA supports multiple kinds of evidence, although the many of the examples of 'evidence type' given seem to imply the use of quantitative methods than qualitative approaches: such examples include 'efficacy, effectiveness, cost-effectiveness, cost-benefit, epidemiological, [and] treatment utilization studies' (APA Presidential Task Force on Evidence-Based Practice 2006, p. 274). However, six of nine examples of possible 'research designs', listed in the Task Force document, could comprise of qualitative evaluations. These include 'clinical observation (including individual case studies) . . . qualitative research . . . systematic case studies . . . public health and ethnographic research . . . process-outcome studies . . . [and] studies of interventions as delivered in naturalistic settings' (APA Presidential Task Force on Evidence-Based Practice 2006, p. 274). The report also stated single case experimental designs, randomized clinical trials, and meta-analysis as possible designs to be considered. The Task Force report noted that 'qualitative research can be used to describe the subjective, lived experiences of people, including participants in psychotherapy' (APA Presidential Task Force on Evidence-Based Practice 2006, p. 274).

Although EBPP policy has allowed psychologists and psychotherapists to use multiple research approaches in psychotherapy evaluation, EBPP policy also produces a discourse of experimental methodolatry. The APA acknowledged the usefulness of both quantitative and qualitative research for compiling 'adequate studies' to be evaluated but also asserted that 'stringent tests of internal validity ... are more persuasive arguments for efficacy' American Psychological Association (2002, p. 1054). Yet, 'efficacy' and 'validity' are terms that associated with the statistical reduction of clients into variables for inferences based on measurement. This is in contrast to a more ethnographical-like approach in the discursive therapies, which involves collaborating with the client in understanding through dialogue what is meaningful and effective for her/him (Strong and Lock 2005). Such an approach does not apply, experimentalist concepts such as 'internal validity' because it is aimed at exploring thick, qualitative descriptions of client context.

The APA Presidential Task Force on Evidence-Based Practice (2006) also produces a hierarchy of evidence criteria that is biased towards the experimental method. The Task Force placed RCTs at the top of their hierarchy, arguing they 'represent a more stringent way to evaluate treatment efficacy because they are the most effective way to rule out threats to internal validity in a single experiment' (American Psychological Association 2002, p. 1054; APA Presidential Task Force on Evidence-Based Practice 2006, p. 275). Quasi-experiments and randomized controlled experiments were seen as 'sophisticated empirical methodologies'. Such idolatry of the experimental method in EBPP is made possible through a contingent relation with experimental methodolatry in evidence-based medicine where RCTs are also the gold standard (Kitson 2002).

As a form of hierarchical observation and self-surveillance (Foucault 1977), the new managerialism of EBPP enables psychologists to examine and govern their own evaluation practices and that of others to see if their evaluations employ the most 'stringent', 'effective', and 'sophisticated' designs (i.e. experimental criteria). In the wider context of EBP that EBPP emerged from, randomized controlled experiments have become the highest benchmark for across medicine and healthcare evaluation, often to the detriment or neglect of qualitative research (Kitson 2002; Rycroft-Malone et al. 2003; Tanenbaum, 2003).

This trend for experimental methodolatry does not seem to bode well for the inclusion of qualitative approaches that enable thick descriptions of social context. In EBPP, 'the validity of conclusions from research on interventions is based on a general progression from clinical observation through [to] systematic reviews of randomized clinical trials'[8] (APA Presidential Task Force on Evidence-Based Practice

---

[8] This happens while also 'recognizing gaps and limitations in the existing literature and its applicability to the specific case at hand' (APA Presidential Task Force on Evidence-Based Practice, 2006, p. 284).

2006, p. 284). Yet, this 'goal' of EBPP to get to randomized trials negates the value of qualitative research and evaluations for psychotherapy.

Thin contextualizations 3: medical objectification

Another problematic issue in the governance of psychotherapy evaluation lies with the medical objectification of social context in the empirically support treatment (EST) movement. Objectification is where human beings are transformed into 'subjects' in that they either classified scientifically as types of people according to different academic disciplines (e.g. the 'patient' with X disorder in medicine and psychiatry) or are objectified by being divided from others (e.g. the disordered versus the normal) (Foucault 1982). The subject means 'subject to someone else by control and dependence, and tied to his [sic] own identity by a conscience or self-knowledge. Both meanings suggest a form of power which subjugates and makes subject to' (Foucault 1982, p. 208).

Medical objectification creates a thin description of client's social context by reducing it into a disorder as with ESTs. EST policy encourages psychologists and psychotherapists to produce diagnostic-group descriptions of client samples in their evaluation research (Task Force on Promotion and Dissemination of Psychological Procedures 1995). EST criteria have a contingent relation with the *Diagnostic and Statistical Manual of Mental Disorders* (DSM-IV; American Psychiatric Association 1994). Chambless and Hollon (1998, p. 7) proposed evaluative criteria for establishing ESTs based on a 'specific problem or disorder' where 'participants in research trials do tend to be selected to be homogeneous with respect to the presence of a particular target problem'(Chambless and Hollon 1998, p. 15). Westen et al. (2004, p. 632) explain that empirically-supported 'treatments are typically designed for a single Axis I disorder, and patients are screened to maximize homogeneity of diagnosis'. An 'Axis I disorder' refers to the DSM-IV categorizations of mental disorders. This aggregation of homogeneous disorders can be seen as a form of hyponarrativity—a process which negates thick description of client context to focus on thin description of symptomology and functioning (Sadler, 2004). Client context can inadvertently become marginalized in therapy evaluation if clients are made into subjects through such a reduced diagnostic discourse.

The EST movement places an expectation on the psychologist to evaluate therapy in a prescriptive-like 'specific treatment for a specific disorder' framework. By 2001, around 22 adult mental disorders, eight child or adolescent mental disorders, and two personality disorders were identified as being treatable by empirically supported therapies (Chambless and Ollendick 2001). In such a framework, the psychologist administers empirically well-established treatments for disorders just as a medical officer would endeavour to prescribe drugs that have shown efficacy for treating signs and symptoms of physical disease. Indeed, EST criteria were adopted from the US Food and Drug Administration's (FDA) efficacy criteria for approving drugs (Wampold et al. 2005). Major depressive disorder may be prescribed with Beck's cognitive therapy, panic disorder may be prescribed with cognitive behavioural therapy, and so on (Chambless et al. 1998; Task Force on Promotion and Dissemination of Psychological Procedures 1995). The initial list of 25 ESTs for particular disorders from the Clinical Division's Task Force document in 1995 gained momentum and expanded into a considerably more comprehensive list of allowable prescriptions of specific treatment for specific disorder. By 2001, 145 ESTs were identified including 108 treatments for adults and 37 for children who are categorized as having different disorders, including physical pathology (Chambless and Ollendick 2001).

However, the Humanistic Psychology Division's Task Force for the Development of Practice Recommendations for the Provision of Humanistic Psychosocial Services (2001, p. 7) criticized the prescriptive 'treatment-for-disorder' approach:

> Humans are whole persons in context and therapeutic solutions must fundamentally be grounded in their life contexts. This means they must perforce be individualized, developed to meet the individual's particular life context, and cannot be chosen as treatments for decontextualized disorders.

Narrative therapists' concerns of medical objectification appear to mirror those of the Society for Humanistic Psychology Task Force. They have aimed to critically reflect and often subvert commonly-held values of the assessment and diagnosis of psychopathology in clinical psychology and psychiatry. Narrative therapists 'have been concerned to work against what we perceive as the damaging effects of many "scientific" psychological labels' (Drewery and Winslade 1997, p. 47). Narrative therapists Drewery et al. (2000) contend that due to the language of diagnostic categorization, it is uncommon to take the effects of power relations into account when examining people's problems: 'Certainly the *DSM* reads as if power does not exist in the world' (p. 248). Narrative therapy enables a contextual examination of the effects of deficit-based (i.e. diagnostic categorization) discourse in how people are positioned in their accounts of lived experience (Drewery and Winslade 1997). Such a contextual approach seems antithetical to a prescriptive method of categorizing and treating clinical problems.

Medical objectification in EBPP limits how the therapist can language the social context of the client. In contrast to EST policy, EBPP policy acknowledges encourages psychologists and psychotherapists to explore the sociocultural context of their clients when making best practice decisions (APA Presidential Task Force on Evidence-Based Practice 2006). However, as EBPP policy in the APA is an emulation of evidence-based medicine/practice, it moralizes the conduct of psychologists through medical discourse. The definition of EBPP 'closely parallels the definition of evidence-based practice adopted by the Institute of Medicine' (APA Presidential Task Force on Evidence-Based Practice 2006, p. 284) and EBPP 'is consistent with the past 20 years of work in evidence-based medicine' (APA Presidential Task Force on Evidence-Based Practice 2006, p. 284). Terms in the APA Presidential Task Force on Evidence-Based Practice (2006) policy document such as 'medical-cost offset', 'clinical utility', 'epidemiology', 'treatment utilization', 'prognosis', 'symptoms', 'syndromes', 'treatment response', and 'patient' are medical terms used for therapists to qualify the therapeutic context. Further, the term patient, used throughout the document, is preferred to be used over 'client, consumer, or person' (APA Presidential Task Force on Evidence-Based Practice 2006, pp. 273, 284). A one-size-fits-all approach of applying medical discourse to make sense of client context may not encapsulate the social complexity of human experience, especially if the 'family, organization, community, or other populations receiving psychological services' (APA Presidential Task Force on Evidence-Based Practice 2006, pp. 273, 284) are reduced to a medical object and subject ('the patient').

Although the sociocultural focus in EBPP is admirable, the use of the EBPP model to make sense of client context may decontextualise it through new managerialist reproductions of psychologists' emulations of medical discourse. Clients, already reproduced as patients, are explained in medical terms such as symptomology and comorbidity (APA Presidential Task Force on Evidence-Based Practice 2006). However, EBPP requires psychologists to be attentive to 'many other patient characteristics, such as gender, gender identity, culture, ethnicity, race, age, family context, religious beliefs, and sexual orientation' (APA Presidential Task Force on Evidence-Based Practice 2006, p. 284). Yet, these characteristics are then described as 'variables' as if they can be merely quantified. The Task Force quotes a range of cultural studies research than can inform practice but then 'medicalizes' culture by saying that it influences '*psychopathology* but also the patient's understanding of psychological and physical health and illness' (APA Presidential Task Force on Evidence-Based Practice 2006, p. 280, italic emphasis added).

Conclusion: consequences, possibilities, and questions

In a new era of medicalized managerialism, the psychologist produces 'thinned-out' descriptions of client context in psychotherapy evaluation by being expected to behave in a prescriptive fashion: manualize, favour experimental criteria, and focus on treating disorder and symptomology regard to ESTs. EBPP, which widens the possible use of methodologies for evaluation, although still favours experimental approaches as 'sophisticated', 'stringent', and 'effective', gives the psychologist more freedom to address the broader social context of the client in evaluation. Despite this, EBPP reduces social context to a medicalized context where 'good practice' involves the psychologist borrowing concepts from medical science to frame what is the 'best treatment' for the context of their patient according to 'best research' (favourably, but not exclusively, RCTs).

As social context is of primary importance to discursive therapies, the shift to a broader approach to what is empirical in EBP has some positive implications. The acknowledgement of the use of qualitative research including ethnographic research and studies of interventions delivered in naturalistic settings in EBPP allows the use of interpretivist approaches in evaluation. Since such approaches are more likely to examine thick descriptions of social context than experiments, they would be more suitable to evaluating the discursive therapies. Holzman (2003, p. 16), for example, says that social therapists are sceptical of 'so-called objectivity' and in their view of social therapy, 'objective criteria are not valid tools to evaluate it'. Narrative therapists view evaluation as a normalizing practice, and thus are critical of its judgements and their effects (White and Epston 1990). With discursive therapy, there is a collaborative emphasis where the therapist attends to the client's standpoint, their way of speaking, to contextually co-construct meaning with the client and tailor therapy accordingly (Strong 2002). This collaborative and interpretivist approach could perhaps complement the more prescriptively clinical and empirical approaches to psychotherapy evaluation. If qualitative research aims to 'describe the subjective, lived experiences of people' (APA Presidential Task Force on Evidence-Based Practice 2006, p. 274), a collaborative and interpretive approach seems more appropriate for evaluating discursive therapies than objective, standardized experimental designs that adhere to normative criteria.

However, the inclusion of qualitative research in EBPP does not necessarily equate to valuing social constructionist, discursive research, either. Qualitative research approaches can also have a positivist bent to them with a certain degree of objectivity or the belief that 'the facts speak for themselves'—e.g. grounded theory (Glaser and Straus 1967) or thematic analysis (Boyatzis 1998). The emulation of the medical scientific approach in EBP means that objectivity is privileged over interpretative approaches, as evidenced by its evidence hierarchies with experiments given the highest status and practitioner observation the lowest (e.g. Disbury 2003). There also may be a danger that thick-descriptive, qualitative approaches are misinterpreted in/through an EBP framing as opportunities to produce highly-scripted, standard practices of therapeutic micro-management/adherence. This would miss the intention of thick description as a contextual understanding, open to multiple interpretative perspectives, rather than a generalizable script to be applied homogenously. Further, Wampold (2003) warns that qualitative research is often likely to be viewed with derision among managed healthcare organizations due to the dominance of the medical model.

Nonetheless, others are more optimistic about the usefulness of qualitative research in EBP. Indeed, based on a consensus, the APA Presidential Task Force on Evidence-Based Practice (2006) report has widened the notion of 'evidence' in psychology in contrast to the EST movement. The EBPP report has opened space for additional evaluative methodologies. Now, qualitative research can be viewed as an important, complementary approach to quantitative research in EBP (Disbury 2003; Tanenbaum 2003). There are studies that have already used qualitative, discursive methodologies in psychotherapy evaluation research (e.g. Avidi 2005; Busch 2007; Frosh et al. 1996; Madill and Barkham 1997; Strong et al. 2008). In contrast to the empirically supported treatment movement, EBP 'liberates' psychologists' choice of acceptable research methodology beyond the experimental method.

Despite EBP's 'liberation' of choice, there are limits. Psychology emulates evidence-based medicine in/through EBPP, and so it *reproduces* medical discourse (e.g. patient, treatment, clinical utility) and an evidence hierarchy that prefers the experimental method. This means that possible research methodologies and therapies that favour qualitative explorations of the social context of client experience are less valued than the experimental method. Researchers' and therapists' decisions on the suitability of therapy are made within the governance of EBP discourse along with its new managerialist ethos: a wedding of an ethic of individual practitioner responsibility to a decontextualizing style of medical scientism. Therapists, according to their *clinical* expertise, must choose what is best evidence and best practice, and what is best *for* the patient, as qualified by EBP criteria. Such an emphasis on making decisions *for* the patient misses opportunities where, in the discursive therapies, there is collaborative dialogue *with* the client, and solutions are customised in that contextual process where meaning is co-constructed and focused on the client's terms of reference (see Strong 2002).

In the current context of evidence-based evaluation there are both challenges and opportunities to address social context in the governance of evaluation concerning the discursive therapies. How can we evaluate discursive therapies when therapists are encouraged to accept and reproduce experimental studies, divorced from the social context of day-to-day practice settings, to inform their practice? Further, how can we evaluate discursive therapies when researchers are encouraged to aspire to employ context-thinning experimental designs as the gold standard of evaluative practice or adopt medical discourse to describe their clients? Perhaps one possible way forward could entail a practice-based evidence (PBE) approach. In PBE, psychotherapy evaluation involves collaboration between therapist and client (Miller et al. 2004). Duncan et al. (2007, p. 41) argue for a client-directed evaluative approach that puts clients in charge of therapy, 'using their feedback to guide all decisions'. Fox (2003) argues that "'evidence' is contingent and needs to be contextualised" (p. 84) but practice-based research (PBR), leading to PBE, should also be emphasized where 'research is not a process of individual discovery but a collaborative activity' (p. 96). PBR is also transgressive and pluralist in that it constantly challenges existing structures and concepts, and rules out one true way of doing things (Fox 2003). It should be, according to Fox, more action-oriented with weight put on emancipating the client. The collaborative, socially contextual stance of PBE and PBR may suit the collaborative-focused nature of the discursive therapies where evaluation could be shared between therapist and client like in Epston's (2001) practice of co-research. Perhaps research could compare the suitability of the philosophy and principles of PBE and PBR with those of the discursive therapies in contrast to EBP, EBPP and/or ESTs. An alternative or complementary evaluative stance to EBP like PBE and PBR could also encourage more inclusive uses of therapy where discursive therapists and researchers could find some sanctuary from the standardizing governmentalities of evidence-based evaluation discourse.

The thinning of social context in evidence-based evaluation creates both problems and opportunities for the discursive therapies. Discourses of manualization, experimental methodolatry, and medical objectification operate to govern the conduct of psychotherapy in a technical, standardized, hierarchical, medicalized, and prescriptive manner that favours quantitative and statistical measurement. Discursive therapists, in contrast, use collaborative conversations with the client to try and understand and thus contextualize client experience through the client's standpoint and their language terms (Strong 2002). Such 'thick descriptive' understandings guide therapy, tailored to client context, in contrast to imposing fixed diagnostic categories or treatment protocols. The postmodern, collaborative, and non-hierarchical stance of discursive therapy could aid to complement evidence-based approaches to psychotherapy evaluation through PBE and PBR. It perhaps could even further shape current evidence-based approaches to psychotherapy evaluation. This, in turn, could help widen the possibility of what could be effective 'evidences' so as to produce a richer, more pluralistic, and socially contextual approach to psychotherapy evaluation practice.

Acknowledgements

Thank you to Emily Doyle and Murray Anderson for providing feedback.

References

American Psychiatric Association. (1994). *Diagnostic and Statistical Manual of Mental Disorders IV*. American Psychiatric Association, Washington, DC.

American Psychological Association. (2002). *Criteria for Evaluating Treatment Guidelines*. American Psychiatric Association, Washington, DC.

American Psychological Association Presidential Task Force on Evidence-Based Practice. (2006). Evidence-based practice in psychology. *American Psychologist*, **61**, 271–85.

Anderson, H. (1997). On a roller coaster: A collaborative language systems therapy approach to therapy. In S. Friedman (Ed.) *The New Language of Change: Constructive Collaboration in Psychotherapy*, pp. 323–44. Guilford Press, New York.

Avidi, E. (2005). Negotiating a pathological identity in the clinical dialogue: Discourse analysis of a family therapy. *Psychology and Psychotherapy: Theory, Research, and Practice*, **78**, 493–511.

Beck, A. T., Rush, A. J., Shaw, F. B. and Emery, G. (1979). *The Cognitive Therapy of Depression*. Guilford Press, New York.

Bohart, A. (2000). Paradigm clash: Empirically supported treatments versus empirically supported psychotherapy practice. *Psychotherapy Research*, **10**, 488–93.

Bohart, A. C., O'Hara, M. and Leitner, L. M. (1998). Empirically violated treatments: Disenfranchisement of humanistic and other psychotherapies. *Psychotherapy Research*, **8**, 141–57.

Boyatzis, R. E. (1998). *Transforming Qualitative Information: Thematic Analysis and Code Development*. Sage, Thousand Oaks, CA.

Beutler, L. E. (1998). Identifying empirically supported treatments: What if we didn't? *Journal of Consulting and Clinical Psychology*, **66**, 113–20.

Burr, V. (2003). *Social Constructionism* (2nd ed.) Routledge, London.

Busch, R. (2007). Transforming evidence: A discursive evaluation of narrative therapy case studies. *The Australian Journal of Counselling Psychology*, **7**, 8–15.

Chamberlain, K. (2000). Methodolatry and qualitative health research. *Journal of Health Psychology*, **5**, 285–96.

Chambless, D. L., Baker, M. J., Baucom, D. H., et al. (1998). Update on empirically validated therapies, II. *The Clinical Psychologist*, **51**, 3–16.

Chambless, D. L. and Hollon, S. D. (1998). Defining empirically supported therapies. *Journal of Consulting and Clinical Psychology*, **66**, 7–18.

Chambless, D. L. and Ollendick, T. H. (2001). Empirically supported psychological interventions: Controversies and evidence. *Annual Review of Psychology*, **52**, 685–716.

Crits-Christoph, P., Wilson, G. T. and Hollon, S. D. (2005). Empirically supported psychotherapies: Comment on Westen, Novonty, and Thompson-Brenner (2004). *Psychological Bulletin*, **131**, 412–17.

Chwalisz, K. (2003). Evidence-based practice: A framework for twenty-first-century scientist-practitioner training. *The Counseling Psychologist*, **31**, 497–528.

Danziger, K. (1994). Does the history of psychology have a future? *Theory and Psychology*, **4**, 467–84.

Davies, B. (2003). Death to critique and dissent? The policies and practices of new managerialism and of 'evidence-based practice'. *Gender and Education*, 15, 91–103.

Denzin, N. K. and Giardina, M. D. (2008). Introduction: The elephant in the living room, or advancing the conversation about the politics of evidence. In N.K. Denzin and M.D. Giardina.(Eds.) *Qualitative Inquiry and the Politics of Evidence*, pp. 9–51. Left Coast Press, Walnut Creek, CA.

Disbury, P. (2003). Benefits of best practice guidelines: Evaluating and applying the evidence. *New Zealand Family Practitioner*, 30, 317–23.

Donald, A. (2002). Evidence-based medicine: Key concepts. *Medscape General Medicine* [online], 4. http://www.medscape.com/viewarticle/430709 [Accessed 15 December 2005.]

Donohue, B., Allen, D. N., Romero, V., et al. (2009). Development of a standardized treatment center that utilizes evidence-based clinic operations to facilitate implementation of an evidence-based treatment. *Behavior Modification*, 33, 411–36.

Drewery, W. and Winslade, J. (1997). The theoretical story of narrative therapy. In G. Monk, J. Winslade, K. Crocket, and D. Epston.(Eds.) *Narrative Therapy in Practice: The Archaeology of Hope*, pp. 32–52. Jossey-Bass, San Francisco, CA.

Drewery, W., Winslade, J. and Monk, G. (2000). Resisting the dominating story: Towards a deeper understanding of narrative therapy. In R.A. Neimeyer and J.D. Raskin.(Eds.) *Constructions of Disorder: Meaning-making Frameworks for Psychotherapy*, pp. 243–63. American Psychological Association, Washington, DC.

Duncan, B. L., Miller, S. D., and Sparks, J. (2007). Common factors and the uncommon heroism of youth. *Psychotherapy in Australia*, 13, 34–43.

Epston, D. E. (2001). Co-research: The making of an alternative knowledge (anti-anorexia/anti-bulimia). http://www.narrativeapproaches.com/antianorexia%20folder/AAcoresearch.pdf [Accessed 28 April, 2010.]

Fleischman, R. K. (2000). Completing the triangle: Taylorism and the paradigms. *Accounting Auditing and Accountability Journal*, 13, 597–623.

Foucault, M. (1972). *The Archaeology of Knowledge and the Discourse on Language* (A.M Sheridan Smith, Trans.). Pantheon Books, New York.

Foucault, M. (1977). *Discipline and Punish: The Birth of the Prison* (A. Sheridan, Trans.). Pantheon Books, New York.

Foucault, M. (1982). Afterword: The subject and power. In H.L. Dreyfus and P. Rabinow.(Eds.) *Michel Foucault: Beyond Structuralism and Hermeneutics*, pp. 208–26. The Harvester Press, Brighton.

Foucault, M. (1991). Governmentality. In G. Burchill, C. Gordon and P. Miller.(Eds.) *The Foucault Effect*, pp.87–104. Harvester Wheatsheaf, London.

Fox, N. J. (2003). Practice-based evidence: Towards collaborative and transgressive research. *Sociology*, 37, 81–102.

Frosh, S., Burck, C., Strickland-Clark, L. and Morgan, K. (1996). Engaging with change: A process study of family therapy. *Journal of Family Therapy*, 18, 141–61.

Garfield, S. L. (1996). Some problems associated with 'validated' forms psychotherapy. *Clinical Psychology: Science and Practice*, 3, 218–29.

Geertz, C. (1973). *The Interpretation of Cultures: Selected Essays*. Basic Books, New York.

Gladding, S. T. (2002). *Family Therapy: History, Theory, and Practice*. Merrill Prentice Hall, Upper Saddle River, NJ.

Glaser, B. G. and Strauss, A. L. (1967). *The Discovery of Grounded Theory: Strategies for Qualitative Research*. Aldine, Chicago, IL.

Gordon, C. (1991). Governmental rationality: An introduction. In G. Burchell, C. Gordon and P. Miller.(Eds.) *The Foucault Effect: Studies in Governmentality*, pp. 1–51. Harvester Wheatsheaf, Hemel Hempstead.

Greenberg, L. (1991). Research on the process of change. *Psychotherapy Research*, **1**, 14–24.

Guba, E. G., and Lincoln, Y. S. (1989). *Fourth Generation Evaluation*. Sage, Newbury Park, CA.

Harper, D., Mulvey, M. R. and Robinson, M. (2003). Beyond evidence-based practice: Rethinking the relationship between research, theory and practice. In R. Bayne and I. Horton.(Eds.) *Applied Psychology: Current Issues and New Directions*, pp.158–71. Sage, London.

Henry, W. P., Strupp, H. H., Butler, S. F., Schacht, T. E. and Binder, J. L. (1993). Effects of training in time limited dynamic psychotherapy: Changes in therapist behavior. *Journal of Consulting and Clinical Psychology*, **61**, 434–40.

Holzman, L. (2003). Creating the context: An introduction. In L. Holzman and R. Mendez. (Eds.) *Psychological Investigations: A Clinician's Guide to Social Therapy*. Brunner-Routledge, New York.

King, N. J. and Ollendick, T. H. (2006). A commentary on psychosocial interventions and evidence-based practice: Time for reflection about what an 'ideal' psychosocial intervention would look like in clinical psychology? *Behaviour Change*, **23**, 157–64.

Kazdin, A. E. (2008). Evidence-based treatment and practice: New opportunities to bridge clinical research and practice, enhance the knowledge base, and improve patient care. *American Psychologist*, **63**, 146–59.

Kendall, P. C. and Chambless, D. L. (1998). Empirically supported psychological therapies. Special section of *Journal of Consulting and Clinical Psychology*, **66**, 3–167.

Kitson, A. (2002). Recognising relationships: Reflections on evidence-based practice. *Nursing Inquiry*, **9**, 179–86.

Larner, W. (2000). Neo-liberalism: Policy, ideology, governmentality. *Studies in Political Economy*, **63**, 5–25.

Levant, R. F. and Hasan, N. T. (2008). Evidence-based practice in psychology. *Professional Psychology: Research and Practice*, **39**, 658–62.

Levitt, H. M., Neimeyer, R. A. and Williams, D. C. (2005). Rules versus principles in psychotherapy: Implications of the quest for universal guidelines in the movement for empirically supported treatments. *Journal of Contemporary Psychotherapy*, **35**, 117–29.

Lincoln, Y. S. and Guba, E. G. (2004). The roots of fourth generation evaluation: Theoretical and methodological origins. In M. C. Alvin.(Ed.), *Evaluation Roots: Tracing Theorists' Views and Influences*, pp. 225–41. Thousand Oaks, Sage.

Madill, A. and Barkham, M. (1997). Discourse analysis of a theme in one successful case of brief psychodynamic-interpersonal psychotherapy. *Journal of Counseling Psychology*, **44**, 232–44.

McHugh, R. K., Murray, H. W. and Barlow, D. H. (2009). Balancing fidelity and adaptation in the dissemination of empirically-supported treatments: The promise of transdiagnostic interventions. *Behaviour Research and Therapy*, **47**, 946–53.

Miller, S. D., Duncan, B. L., and Hubble, M. A. (2004). Beyond integration: The triumph of outcome over process in clinical practice. *Psychotherapy in Australia*, **10**, 2–19.

Nathan, P. E. and Gorman, J. M. (Eds.) (2007). *A Guide to Treatments that Work*. Oxford University Press, New York.

Nicholls, D. A., Walton, J. A., and Price, K. (2009). Making breathing your business: Enterprising practices at the margins of orthodoxy. *Health: An Interdisciplinary Journal for the Social Study of Health, Illness and Medicine,* **13**, 337–60.

Norcross, J. C. (2001). Purposes, processes, and products of the task force on empirically supported therapy relationships. *Psychotherapy,* **38**, 345–56.

O'Connell, B. (2005). *Solution-Focused Therapy.* Sage, London.

Rabinow, P. and Rose, N. (2003). Introduction: Foucault today. In P. Rabinow and N. Rose. (Eds.) *The Essential Foucault: Selections from the Essential Works of Foucault 1954–1984,* pp. vii–xxxv. The New Press, New York.

Riley, W. T., Schumann, M. F., Forman-Hoffman, V. L., Mihm, P., Applegate, B. W. and Asif, O. (2007). Responses of practicing psychologists to a web site developed to promote empirically supported treatments. *Professional Psychology: Research and Practice,* **38**, 44–53.

Rose, N. (1996). *Inventing our Selves: Psychology, Power, and Personhood.* University of Cambridge Press, Cambridge.

Rose, N. (1999). *Powers of Freedom: Reframing Political Thought.* Cambridge University Press, Cambridge.

Rutgers, B. C. C. (2008). Empirically supported training approaches: The who, what, and how of disseminating psychological interventions. *Clinical Psychology: Science and Practice,* **15**, 308–12.

Rycroft-Malone, J., Seers, K., Titchen, A., Harvey, G., Kitson, A. and McCormack, B. (2003). What counts as evidence in evidence-based practice? *Nursing and Health Care Management and Policy,* **47**, 81–90.

Sackett, D. L., Rosenberg, W. M. C., Gray, J. A. M., Haynes, R. B. and Richardson, W. S. (1996). Evidence-based medicine: What it is and what it isn't. *British Medical Journal,* **312**, 71–2.

Sackett, D. L. and Strauss, S. (1998). Finding and applying evidence during clinical rounds. The 'evidence cart'. *Journal of the American Medical Association,* **280**, 1336–8.

Sadler, J. Z. (2004). *Values and Psychiatric Diagnosis.* Oxford University Press, Oxford.

Smits, A. J., Powers, M. B., Berry, A. C. and Otto, M. W. (2007). Translating empirically supported strategies into accessible interventions: The potential utility of exercise for the treatment of panic disorder. *Cognitive and Behavioral Practice,* **14**, 364–74.

Spring, B. (2007). Evidence-based practice in clinical psychology: What it is, why it matters; What you need to know. *Journal of Clinical Psychology,* **63**, 611–31.

Stronach, I. (2008). On promoting rigor in educational research: The example of the UK's Research Assessment Exercise. In N. K. Denzin and M. D. Giardina.(Eds.) *Qualitative Inquiry and the Politics of Evidence,* pp. 80–96. Left Coast Press, Walnut Creek, CA.

Strong, T. (2002). Collaborative 'expertise' after the discursive turn. *Journal of Psychotherapy Integration,* **12**, 218–32.

Strong, T., Busch, R., and Couture, S. (2008). Conversational evidence in therapeutic dialogue. *Journal of Marital and Family Therapy,* **34**, 388–405.

Strong, T. and Lock. A. (2005). Discursive therapy? *Janus Head,* **8**, 585–93.

Tanenbaum, S. (2003). Evidence-based practice in mental health: Practical weaknesses meet political strengths. *Journal of Evaluation in Clinical Practice,* **9**, 287–301.

Task Force for the Development of Practice Recommendations for the Provision of Humanistic Psychosocial Services**.** (2001). *Recommended Principles and Practices for the Provision of Humanistic Psychosocial Services: Alternative to Mandated Practice and Treatment Guidelines.* http://www.apa.org/divisions/div32/draft.html [Accessed 10 January 2005.]

Task Force on Promotion and Dissemination of Psychological Procedures. (1995). Training in and dissemination of empirically-validated psychological treatments. Report and recommendations. *The Clinical Psychologist,* **48**, 3–23.

Thorn, B. E. (2007). Evidence-based practice in psychology. *Journal of Clinical Psychology,* **63**, 607–9.

Timmermans, S. and Berg, M. (2003). *The challenge of evidence-based medicine and standardisation in health care.* Temple University Press, Philadelphia, PA.

Torrance, H. (2008). Building confidence in qualitative research: Engaging the demands of policy. In N.K. Denzin and M.D. Giardina.(Eds.) *Qualitative Inquiry and the Politics of Evidence,* pp. 55–79. Left Coast Press, Walnut Creek, CA.

Wampold, B. E. (2003). Bashing positivism and revering a medical model under the guise of evidence. *The Counseling Psychologist,* **5**, 539–45.

Wampold, B. E., Goodheart, C. D. and Levant, R. F. (2001). Clarification and elaboration on evidence-based practice in psychology. *American Psychologist,* **62**, 616–18.

Wampold, B. E., Lichtenberg, J. W., and Waehler, C. A. (2002). Principles of empirically supported interventions in counseling psychology. *The Counseling Psychologist,* **30**, 197–217.

Wampold, B. E., Lichtenberg, J. W., and Waehler, C. A. (2005). A broader perspective: Counseling psychology's emphasis on evidence. *Journal of Contemporary Psychotherapy,* **35**, 27–38.

Westen, D., Novonty, C. M., and Thomson-Brenner, H. (2004). The empirical status of empirically supported psychotherapies: Assumptions, findings, and reporting in controlled clinical trials. *Psychological Bulletin,* **130**, 631–63.

White, M. and Epston, D. (1990). *Narrative Means to Therapeutic Ends.* W. W. Norton & Co, New York.

Wyatt, R. C. (2007). An interview with Ronald Levant, EdD, ABPP. *Psychotherapy.net* [online]. Available at: http://psychotherapy.net [Accessed 3 June 2009.]

Chapter 15

The body, trauma, and narrative approaches to healing

Maureen Duffy

In many ways, the history of psychotherapy is the history of the development of camps or tribes that often have little that is pleasant to say to each other. Lewis et al. (2000) express this view and state that 'the secret identity of psychotherapy's mutative mechanism has prompted enough hot-tempered debate and factional feuding to fill a history of the Balkans' (p. 167). The rapid development of neuroscience and its application to psychotherapy is just another case in point. Neuroscience has been taken up easily by psychiatry and other medicalized practices of psychotherapy. However, neuroscience is often regarded with suspicion or even antipathy by practitioners of postmodern forms of psychotherapy who resist what they see as the totalizing and deterministic narrative of brain explanations for human behaviour.

In this chapter, I am not making a case for neuroscience as congruent with a constructionist emphasis on the constitution of personal identity and the world through language and social processes. However, I am making a case that interpersonal neuroscience has something important to contribute to constructionist perspectives given its basic premise that the brain develops and is shaped through the activity of human relationships. Another contribution neuroscience makes to constructionism, is the inclusion of the body as an important influence in social processes. In this chapter, I will focus particularly on trauma as a bodily experience that can profoundly affect the way a person is able to enter into the domain of language. I will describe how the experience of trauma impacts the brain and other parts of the body and consequently limits resourceful participation in the linguistic arena. I will then consider how narrative approaches to therapy with people who have experienced trauma, offer possibilities for connecting the stories of their traumatized bodies with healing resources unique to narrative therapies.

The ontologies from which neuroscience and the discursive traditions in psychotherapy emerge could hardly be more different in terms of their underlying assumptions about the nature of reality, what we know, how we come to know things in the world, and how we should ethically proceed. Because of these fundamental differences in beliefs about how the world is constituted, there is no question that incorporating scientific perspectives from the neurosciences into therapeutic applications grounded in discursive traditions is difficult and risky business. In this chapter, I am not at all suggesting a transcendence of those differences but simply a recognition of them.

I am, however, suggesting that communication and dialogue across ontologies and paradigms may have something useful to offer and that unless we engage more robustly in such dialogues we will not know whether such dialogue is valuable to either the social constructionist or scientific communities or both.

Mahoney (2003) suggests that the war metaphor that has been used to describe incommensurable philosophical differences between science and postmodernism, as in the 'science wars', is an unhelpful and polarizing one. He argues that 'differences—whether in belief systems, methods, or interpreted meanings—need not be dichotomised into adversarial confrontations' (p. 121). For their parts, Fortun and Bernstein (1998) maintain that 'it is better to think about the sciences as muddled rather than pure; to imagine the borders between the sciences and the worlds of language, culture, and politics as muddled rather than as clear and distinct' (p. xiii). This chapter represents an effort to engage in discourse across ontologies and paradigms and should in no way be construed as an attempt to generate consensus or resolve contradictions. While the effort may be inescapably muddled given the ontological boundary crossings involved, the goal is to create value by engaging in productive dialogue with ideas that arise from within conflicting paradigms. Another acknowledgement needs to be made at the beginning of this chapter and that is the recognition that our common language practices for describing 'mind', 'body', 'brain', and the relationships among them are also muddled at this point in time.

Interpersonal neuroscience and contingency

Modern neuroscience, rather than representing a totalizing narrative for human behaviour, presents an understanding of the construction of the self as a contingency—dependent on the interaction of the body, of which the brain is a part, with others in the world, especially important others, and with our social and cultural histories. Each element—our relationships with others, the meanings and stories of our social and cultural histories, and our bodies that include our brains and nervous systems—are all subject to change. 'Self', 'mind', 'person', 'identity', 'subjectivity', or whatever we choose to call this contingent intersection is therefore permeable and fluid, changing and reconstituting itself as the elements of body, relationships, and social and cultural histories change and evolve (Cozolino 2006; Damasio 2003; Schore 1994; Siegel 1999, 2007). This is not, however, a view of the 'self' or 'mind' as limitless in its freedom to change and evolve or unconstrained in its capacity to shift from one expressive or discursive position to another. We are embodied beings capable of shifting positions and incorporating the multiple perspectives of others—but not equally easily and largely when we are attracted to the other at some level and when we experience resonance and attunement with the ideas and emotions being expressed. It's much easier to include in our repertoire of 'self' the linguistic and practical performances of others if we like them in some way, however mundanely, whatever our ways of liking happen to be. Most of us are somewhat selective about taking particular ideas into our lives and we pay attention to the emotions those ideas arouse in us. Constructionist ideas, like any ideas that survive, spread in a sensuous way through attraction and cooption of them. Writing a particular perspective out of our 'self' repertoire is like rejecting a lover—the biochemistry of the body is very much a part of the process. The question of why we take up some ideas and reject others is as much a question of body as it is a question of the beliefs and values that we hold and perform.

Moved by the body

Including the body in constructionist dialogues does not freeze the dialogues or herald the return of a belief in a unitary self if there ever seriously was such a belief. Even the wild and radical Scottish empiricist, David Hume (1739/1978), challenged the notion of a 'core self' in his well-known statement: 'For my part, when I enter most intimately into what I call *myself*, I always stumble on some particular perception or other, of heat or cold, light or shade, love or hatred, pain or pleasure. I never catch *myself* at any time without a perception, and never can observe anything but the perception' (p. 252). We have been struggling with the idea of the 'self' for a long time.

Francisco Varela (1997) talked about how bodies are no longer unitary and noted his own liver was a transplanted one. (He has since died.) I write this chapter with cadaver bone in my wrist that has integrated into my own radius, enabling me to use my right hand to write, lift, carry, and do more or less what I want to do. It is not just that the 'self' is not unitary—between transplants, transfusions, and prosthetics—the body is hardly unitary either. Neuroscience can enter the discursive world and bring the body out from the sidelines of discursive thought and practice if the body is constituted as a permeable constraint in the same way that language, culture, and context are. Cromby and Nightingale (1999) in suggesting that the body has been benched and ignored by social constructionism state that 'bodies are the intimate place where nature and culture meet' (p. 10).

For instance, we are overwhelmingly exposed to that intimate intersection of culture and nature in the return of bodies, both living and dead, from the conflicts in Iraq and Afghanistan and the stunning impact of those returns on witnesses and observers. It is no accident that the US Pentagon had banned images of coffins carrying dead soldiers returning from conflicts in the Middle East for 19 years until the ban was lifted in April, 2009 (Seelye 2009). The images of the flag draped coffins of the dead and the images of the living soldiers returning with missing arms and legs move us to tears, to pride, to anger, to protest, to despair. But we are changed for having borne witness to them. Those bodies haunt us and we enter into relationship and conversations with the meanings that their images evoke. A recent photo collage of bedrooms of dead young soldiers left almost as shrines by their grieving family members (Gilbertson and Filkins 2010) commands the bringing to life, if only for a moment, of the bodies of the young people who will never again lie down in those beds surrounded by their teddy bears, bunny rabbits, sports memorabilia, or sexy pictures of girls. It is the absence of the presence of their bodies that we see most vividly in their empty bedrooms.

Constructing 'trauma'

The construct of 'trauma' is a highly valenced one with variable meanings ascribed to it. Colloquially, trauma is most commonly used to refer to horrific interpersonal experiences, like physical and sexual abuse, or to the experience of severe events in the natural world, like earthquakes, hurricanes, and floods, or to the experience of accidents and traumatic injuries. What all of these have in common is some degree of assault on the sense of physical and/or emotional boundaries and safety that have been constructed as the 'self'. In considering the full range of possible sources of trauma, van der Kolk (2006) states that 'most traumas occur in the context of interpersonal relationships, which involve boundary violations, loss of autonomous action, and loss of self-regulation' (p. 283), suggesting that interpersonal trauma leads to a significant reduction in resourcefulness needed to navigate in the world. From an ethical standpoint, interpersonal trauma represents a profound denial of the legitimacy of the presence of others in the world and a profaning of their hopes, dreams, and being. Interpersonal trauma, therefore, represents the dark side of relational encounters, the rendering of joint possibilities into misery and anguish as a result of abuse.

A focus on trauma in its most horrific forms, however, whether interpersonal abuse, natural disaster, or accident and injury ignore how other kinds of more mundane and everyday events and encounters in the world act on the body in ways to similar to the more horrific forms. Scaer (2005) has mounted a challenge to interpretations of trauma as the horrific only and redefines the construct in the following way:

> Trauma [is] a continuum of variably negative life events occurring over the lifespan, including events that may be accepted as 'normal' in the context of our daily experience because they are endorsed or perpetuated by our cultural institutions. More importantly, I suggest that the traumatic nature of those experiences is also determined by the *meaning* the victim attributes to them. That meaning is based on the cumulative burden of a myriad of prior negative life events, especially those experienced in the vulnerable period of early childhood (p. 2).

In Scaer's view of trauma, micro-insults and micro-injuries can be experienced traumatically and add to a person's cumulative lifetime burden of trauma.

For example, a white woman who pauses for an instant and then steps out of the elevator when an African American man enters can represent a micro-trauma for an African American man whose personal history includes multiple experiences representative of the broader social and cultural history of discrimination and prejudice. A professional employee, up from poverty, who scraped to obtain a college education and who struggled to be accepted socially into the worlds of the middle and upper middle classes, experiences the trauma of stinging rejection during an annual performance review when criticized for talking in too direct and straightforward a manner with co-workers and supervisees. The former is an example of a micro-trauma linked to a personal and cultural history of racism. The latter is an example of a micro-trauma linked to a personal and cultural history of classism that includes class-based differences in linguistic practices (Friedenberg 2008). Understood in this way, the experiences of interpersonal trauma are deeply embedded in social and cultural history and include a continuum of hurts and insults to the physical and/or emotional being of those affected.

Natural disasters resulting in large-scale human trauma are likewise culturally connected. They reflect the geography of place and politics and the profound influences on local inhabitants of the practices and priorities resulting from geographical and sociopolitical contexts. There can hardly be a more vivid example of the impact of culture on the traumatic effects of a natural disaster than the earthquakes that recently ravaged both Haiti and Chile within a seven-week period. On 12 January, 2010 a magnitude 7.0 earthquake hit about 25 km west of Haiti's capital, Port-au-Prince, leaving an estimated 230,000 people dead, 300,000 injured, and 1.5 million homeless (Bilham 2010). On 27 February, 2010 a magnitude 8.8 earthquake (500 times stronger than the magnitude 7.0 quake in Haiti) hit about 105 km northeast of Concepción, Chile's second largest city, and about 335 km southwest of Santiago, the capital of Chile. The death toll in Chile was estimated at around 700 with 1.5 million estimated to be displaced or homeless (Barrionuevo and Robbins 2010). Greater wealth, seismic preparedness in the form of strict earthquake building codes, and a substantially more active post-earthquake government helped to reduce the number of fatalities and injured in Chile relative to Haiti combined with the randomness of the Chilean epicentre which was less close to population centres than the epicentre of the Haitian earthquake. With the exception of the location of the epicentres, social and cultural factors either increased or decreased the trauma from these devastating earthquakes and the difference between the two countries during the immediate crisis aftermath period is striking evidence of the relationship between sociocultural contexts and trauma.

Trauma: an outside-in phenomenon

The experience of trauma is an outside-in phenomenon. Events in the external, social world of a traumatized individual write themselves into that person's neurophysiology and biology in ways that are enduring and challenging for the person's future. Trauma is a striking representation of an embodied social and cultural experience that leaves its mark on both the physical body of the traumatized person and on the culture from which it arises. Trauma leaves its mark on the physical body by potentially altering neurophysiology in ways that leave traumatized individuals with fewer resources for future adapting and for effectively making their ways in the world. Trauma leaves its mark on the social and cultural world from which it arises by damaging the web of trust and interdependency that sustains life and that promotes creativity and risk in the service of growth and innovation. The experience and survival of traumatic events changes both a person's neurophysiology and ways of knowing in the world. Likewise, the world itself becomes constituted as less welcoming and ever more threatening.

The sources of trauma are numerous—war, torture, dislocation, crime, imprisonment, poverty, physical and sexual abuse, neglect, motor vehicle accidents, injuries, hospitalization and medical procedures, workplace abuse, discrimination, harassment, and other forms of interpersonal abuse, and natural disasters—to name some of the more common. Interestingly, current trauma research (cf. Scaer 2005; van der Kolk et al. 2005) suggests that interpersonal abuse (whether physical or psychological) is associated with the most severe and enduring negative effects. While the trauma from having experienced a natural disaster is qualitatively different from the trauma of having experienced interpersonal physical or sexual abuse, the distinction between the two becomes blurred in the aftermath of natural disasters. Natural disasters and the dramatic reduction of basic resources for living that typically follow can lead quickly to interpersonal trauma as people compete for scarce resources of food, water, and shelter. Makeshift living conditions create opportunities for exploitation—an example being the increase in the incidence of rapes of women and girls, including girls as young as two years of age, in the tent cities created in Haiti in the aftermath of the 12 January, 2010 earthquake there (Faul 2010).

The neurophysiology of trauma

Neuroscience is important in any discussion of discourse and trauma, not least because it provides a window of understanding about the effects of trauma on comprehension and language—critical elements of discourse. The restriction of expressive language is a particular vulnerability associated with the effects of trauma on the body. A reduced capacity to narrate the story of one's trauma and survivorship limits access to a powerful cultural resource for healing.

The brain is the part of the body responsible for organizing movement and action—including actions involving moving away from or towards others. One of the difficulties in trauma is that effective action is often thwarted by the possibility of more encompassing threats to perceived survival. In the case of having to cope with an abusive supervisor, taking desired action like standing up for oneself and talking back could result in suspension or firing, increasing the likelihood of negative consequences. In the case of physical or sexual abuse, the threat of greater abuse or even death is a real possibility when thinking about fighting back, thus short-circuiting effective self-protective action. In both cases, the victim is in a double bind. Doing nothing results in serious damage to one's personal and/or physical integrity. Fighting back often risks equal or greater damage.

Changes in the brain as a result of traumatic experiencing are a part of a larger system of information exchange between the body and the outside world that include the cortico-limbic system in the brain, hormones, internal organs, and muscles. The traumatic experience itself, the information exchanges between the external and internal worlds of the person who experienced trauma, and the meanings ascribed to the trauma are fundamental to its constitution. In terms of timelines, the traumatic events and the corresponding information exchange between the outside world and the internal neurophysiological world occur almost instantaneously in time. Ascription of meaning is more likely to take place over a longer period of time.

In the brain, trauma can result in the creation of bilateral hemispheric associational networks of neurons that activate parts of the cortex and limbic system in the right hemisphere associated with the experience of affect and that deactivate parts of the cortex of the left hemisphere associated with expressive and receptive language and comprehension. The neurophysiological outcome of trauma, therefore, can be uncomfortably high affect coupled with reduced ability to process the high affect through language (van der Kolk 2006). In addition, trauma impacts procedural or sensory-motor memories (the memories of how we do things) based upon how a person attempted to escape or resolve the trauma when it was initially happening (either as an acute or chronic event). Taut and painful muscles resulting from their self-protective contraction during a motor vehicle accident or other physical injury that then become chronically painful, signify a traumatic body memory inscribed in a person's musculature. These trauma-inscribed neuronal networks in the brain and sensory-motor memories in other parts of the body are primed to light up and activate in the presence of reminders or signifiers of the original trauma. They are organism-protective responses in overdrive that haven't learned to shut down after the initial trauma and that lead to the phenomenological experience of past trauma as occurring in the present when cued or reminded (Scaer 2005; van der Kolk 2006).

The brain and rest of the body respond to incoming sensory stimuli resulting from engagement in the world with other people in ways that are not always within conscious control. When a person has experienced trauma—a perceived threat to the person's physical and/or psychological being—the brain responds in certain patterns of activity that have implications for the experience of intense emotional arousal and for the capacity to use language to express the meanings of such arousal. Brain imaging studies from people diagnosed with post-traumatic stress disorder (PTSD), for example, combat veterans and police officers, have found that when exposed to signifiers of past traumatic events, blood flow in the right hemisphere, amygdala, and insula increases while there is a corresponding decrease of blood flow in the left hemisphere, especially in parts of the frontal cortex associated with expressive language i.e. Broca's area (Hull 2002; Lindauer et al. 2004; Rauch et al. 1996).

These neurophysiological findings are interesting in themselves but are more interesting when considering their implications. Activation of the right side of the brain and limbic areas results in the internal experience of emotional arousal which is generalized throughout the body. Relative deactivation of the left side of the brain and areas governing expressive speech provides decreased access to language as a means of representing internal states. In combination, increased generalized emotional arousal throughout the body coupled with diminished capacity to provide language for the expression of such experience impairs a primary resource; namely, language, for coping with present intense feelings and past traumatic events.

This combination of increased arousal and decreased access to expressive language to symbolize and understand the arousal casts a person who has suffered traumatic experiences back into the social world with a reduced capacity for making sense of their experiences, for coping with them, and for developing strategies for moving beyond the grip of the traumatic exposure. The person who has experienced trauma has been marked by the social world and must then reengage with the same social world with fewer resources than the person had prior to the experience of trauma.

Trauma reduces rather than increases resources for effective action as a result of bodily processes outside of a person's conscious awareness and control. Van der Kolk (2006) states:

> The discovery that sensory input can automatically stimulate hormonal secretions and influence the activation of brain regions involved in attention and memory once again confronts psychology with the limitations of conscious control over our actions and emotions. This is particularly relevant for understanding and treating traumatized individuals. The fact that reminders of the past automatically activate certain neurobiological responses explains why trauma survivors are vulnerable to react with irrational—subcortically

initiated—responses that are irrelevant, and even harmful, in the present. Traumatized individuals may blow up in response to minor provocations; freeze when frustrated; or become helpless in the face of trivial challenges (pp. 277–8).

Such seemingly inexplicable responses are, in fact, not inexplicable at all. Outside of conscious awareness, the brain and other parts of the body have overwhelmed a traumatized person's capacity to pause, take a breath, and think about how they might best respond to a new situation or challenge, including how to talk about the situation. It is for these reasons that neuroscience must enter the discursive world as an important element in the conversation about how best to facilitate the replenishing of resources for dialogue and action that have been depleted as a result of traumatic experiencing.

The paradox of memory and traumatic stress

In addition to the neurophysiological cocktail of heightened arousal with reduced access to expressive language, trauma also affects the body in relation to memory. Specific autobiographical memory, in contrast with generalized memory, seems to be most affected by the experience of traumatic stress (Dalgleish et al. 2008). For example, a person who experienced traumatic stress at work may have difficulty remembering details of an encounter with a supervisor during which the supervisor assigned an unreasonable and arbitrary workload and condescendingly refused the worker any meaningful opportunity for input or dialogue. The same worker may find it much easier to make general memory-based statements about work, such as, 'I don't get treated fairly or justly by my supervisors at work' than to provide details of the specific disturbing encounter with the supervisor. Remembering in categories instead of in details takes away the flavour and texture of life. It's like seeing a blurred and fuzzy image on the photograph of a beloved child without being able to hone in on the child's scraped knee and her big eyes looking sideways out from underneath her flowered sun hat. Recalling the details of the traumatic encounter with the supervisor may have been able to help the worker support a claim for a transfer out of the department or ask for support from other co-workers or supervisors. Not having adequate access to those details reduces the range of available effective action given the intertwining of knowledge and action.

Multiple studies involving populations who have experienced trauma repeatedly support the relationship between the experience of trauma and a reduction in specific autobiographical memory. The impact of trauma on memory is associated with reduced memory specificity in a study of inpatient adolescents (de Decker et al. 2003), among women who were sexually abused as children (Henderson et al. 2002), among suicidal patients (Williams and Broadbent 1986), in those with a recent diagnosis of cancer (Kangas et al. 2005), among a group of people suffering trauma after a motor vehicle accident (Harvey et al. 1998), and in combat-related and other kinds of PTSD (McNally et al. 1994; McNally et al.1995). Reduced specificity of memory has also been identified in women with postpartum depression (Croll and Bryant 2000), and in depressed and previously depressed patients (Williams et al. 2007).

Williams et al. (2007) state that autobiographical memory is important because 'it is central to human functioning, contributing to an individual's sense of self, to his or her ability to remain oriented in the world and to pursue goals effectively in the light of past problem solving' (p. 122). They emphasize that pursuing goals includes the pursuit of vitally important interpersonal goals which are central to the ongoing story of the self. Paradoxically, the intrusive, vivid memories of previous trauma seen in many people who have experienced traumatic stress are also associated with lack of specificity in autobiographical memory (Kuyken and Brewin 1995; Wessel et al. 2002). What kind of an autobiography does a traumatized person construct about significant aspects of their life when their memory is lost in the shadow lands of categories rather than in the clarity of details?

Narrative approaches to therapy with trauma victims

Narrative approaches in trauma work can help a person give voice to the meanings, skills, and knowledges acquired as a result of traumatic experiencing and to weave such experiences into a coherent life story. The development of voice and of a narrative that incorporates their trauma helps those who have been traumatized to speak up and talk with the parts of their body that are in neurophysiological overdrive, ultimately releasing those parts from the exhausting guard duty they have been performing to protect against further harm.

This section of the chapter will focus on how narrative approaches to therapy can be utilized to help persons who have experienced trauma: (a) establish emotional resonance with a therapist who is interested in examining how one wants to live in the present and in the future and who holds as a principle that the meanings of a person's life are not fixed even when the events that engendered those meanings occurred in the past, (b) find a position of safety from which to view the meanings to which one is currently committed and to explore whether there are other meanings available to that person which may be helpful, (c) begin a conversation with one's body in the interests of improved understanding and communication of body sensations and signals, (d) incorporate the experience and meaning of their trauma into their autobiography, (e) narrate the story of their coping and survival, and (f) access wisdom derived from their experiences that they might wish to share with others.

The process of effective therapy itself is a joint somatic accomplishment in that the brains and nervous systems of both the therapist and client(s) enter into physiological connection designed to promote healing and change. Lewis et al. (2000) state:

> The mind-body clash has disguised the truth that psychotherapy *is* physiology. When a person starts therapy, he isn't beginning a pale conversation; he is stepping into a somatic state of relatedness. Evolution has sculpted mammals into their present form: they become attuned to one another's evocative signals and alter the structure of one another's nervous systems. Psychotherapy's transformative power comes from engaging and directing these ancient mechanisms. Therapy is a living embodiment of limbic processes as corporeal as digestion or respiration. Without the physiologic unity limbic operations provide, therapy would indeed be the vapid banter some people suppose it to be (p. 168).

Michael White (2004) has emphasized that narrative telling of lives allows for flexibility in generating meanings for events not previously identified as meaningful and for reconsidering existing meanings that have been applied across the timeline of past, present, and future. He says:

> The generation and regeneration of meaning also occurs across time. Our reflexive capacity provides us with new alternatives for what to make out of
> 1. the past in response to any new meanings that are assigned to our experiences of the present,
> 2. the present, in response to any new meanings that are assigned to our experiences of the past,
> 3. the future in response to any new meanings that are assigned to our experiences of the past and/or the present, and
> 4. the past and/or the present in response to any new meanings assigned to proposed or hypothetical futures (p. 35).

Given White's (2004) view of the meaning of events in time as malleable from whatever point in time one is situated, narrative approaches to therapy are of particular interest for those who have experienced trauma since one of the defining characteristics of trauma is the re-experiencing of the past as if it were in the present. An approach which allows entrance into the meaning systems of the past from the present with an understanding that change in those past meaning systems is possible is clearly attractive in trauma work.

Gabriela's story

In the following case, I will describe the story of Gabriela and the unexpected postpartum death of her daughter. I will retell her narrative of traumatic experiencing from the moment of her realization that her daughter had unexpectedly died and describe her determined efforts to find relief and help. Gabriela consulted me approximately 18 months after the birth and death of her infant daughter. Within a few minutes of entering my office and sketching the outline of the events from 18 months ago, Gabriela, overwhelmed with sorrow and anger, said plaintively and repeatedly throughout the remainder of the interview, 'I didn't touch my baby; they wouldn't let me touch my baby'.

Gabriela told me the following account of the birth and death of her infant daughter. The baby was born by Caesarean section and was taken to the nursery immediately after her birth. Gabriela's husband was with her during the birth and neither was aware that there had been any problems during the birth or with their daughter. Gabriela had had an anaesthetic so she was groggy when she woke up and the hospital staff said they would bring the baby to her once she got settled into her room.

Gabriela and her husband were in their room and heard a commotion in the hallway. Although no one said anything to them they had a feeling that the commotion was about their daughter. With help from her husband, both went out into the hallway and saw their baby being surrounded by a number of medical personnel. They became extremely upset and demanded to know what was happening. One of the medical staff told her that their baby was sick and needed to be transferred to a different hospital with a higher level neonatal intensive care unit (NICU). Gabriela asked them to stop so she could see and touch her baby and was told, 'No, the sooner we get her over to the other NICU the better and you can see her there'. Gabriela then asked if she could accompany the baby in the ambulance to which she was also told, 'No, you will have to go there yourselves, you won't be permitted in the ambulance'. Gabriela immediately got dressed and went to the other hospital with her husband. By the time they got there, their infant daughter had died.

Listening to Gabriela tell me the story of her daughter's birth and death left me feeling both sad and angry at the string of events as Gabriela had narrated them. Gabriela told me that she started screaming at the hospital staff, 'I never got to touch my baby. You didn't let me touch my baby'. Just having had the C-section she was also weak and shaky and vulnerable and had collapsed in a distraught mound on the hospital room floor. Gabriela got to touch her dead baby, but she had never had the chance to hold her baby during her baby's brief life.

Gabriela told me that she had all the support a mother in those circumstances could ask for—a loving and caring husband, family support, and an understanding boss who told her to take all the time she needed and who kept paying her even though she rarely showed up for work. It had now been 18 months and patience with Gabriela was wearing thin. A blundering but well-meaning family member had told her that she was young and could have another baby. Her boss had given her an ultimatum about her job and said she would have to decide whether she was able to keep it or not. Her husband wanted to go out occasionally and Gabriela wasn't interested, spending a lot of time in bed. She had taken antidepressants and had seen two different therapists but nothing helped, Gabriela said, so she had stopped the antidepressants and the therapy. Gabriela kept repeating 'I didn't get to touch my baby. They wouldn't let me touch my baby'. Her sorrow and anger filled the room and it felt to me as if these agonizing events had just occurred yesterday. For Gabriela, the past and the present collided in a daily cauldron of grief and anger. In her current configuration of body and narrative, Gabriela had no future. She was consigned to reliving the traumatic events from the past over and over, no different than if she had sustained a severe physical injury to a part of her frontal cortex responsible for thinking about and planning for the future.

In this section, I present a description of the focused therapeutic conversations that I had with Gabriela, influenced by the concept of the construction of limbic resonance and therapeutic attunement (Lewis et al. 2000) and the meaning-making perspectives of White (2004) and White and Epston (1990). I describe what transpired in Gabriela's life after those conversations. I will use the key points I presented above about how narrative approaches can be helpful for working with people who have experienced trauma to organize my discussion of my relationship and work with Gabriela.

Establish emotional resonance with a therapist who is interested in examining how one wants to live in the present and in the future

As she was telling me her story, I was moved by Gabriela. I listened in rapt attention to her account of what had happened after the birth of her baby daughter and the events surrounding her infant's death. I am a mother and I have given birth too and Gabriela's story engaged me at a level that connected us as women and as mothers. There were tears in my eyes as I listened to Gabriela's story and I felt my body reacting to Gabriela's anger over the events that she experienced as abject violation of her rights and needs. Gabriela's sorrow and anger came alive in my body too as I listened to her story. Emotional resonance wasn't a therapeutic goal to be achieved; it was an emotional state of connectedness between us to be experienced and acknowledged by me as Gabriela's therapist. I asked Gabriela what inclined her to continue looking for a way forward. She answered that she really didn't know other than that it was too painful continuing to feel the way she was feeling. Gabriela told me she was desperate. Her refrain 'I didn't get to touch my baby; they wouldn't let me touch my baby' was the central experience for Gabriela with its torrent of associated meanings around which I knew I would have to invite exploration of heretofore unvisited other meanings. White's (2004) notion of reflexivity as allowing for the generation of new meanings about the past from new understandings developed in the present is particularly useful for working with the effects of trauma in peoples' lives.

Find a position of safety from which to view the meanings to which one is currently committed and to explore whether there are other meanings available to that person which may be helpful

White (2004) states that 'stories about life and identity are not equal to each other in their constitutive effects. It is clearly apparent that some stories sponsor a broader range of options for action in life than do others' (p. 34). Gabriela had committed, not by conscious choice but by somatic experience, to an understanding of the events surrounding the birth and death of her infant daughter that left her with no room to manoeuvre and little or no opportunity to generate a more fluid understanding of those events. The way it had been constructed, the ending of Gabriela's story had already happened with her being denied the opportunity to touch her warm and breathing baby. It was an ending that no mother could easily bear. The safety that I was able to provide for Gabriela, was the assurance that the meanings she ascribed to her traumatic experiences, were safe with me and that I heard those meanings with all of my being.

The concept of 'touch' was the concept that ended Gabriela's story in such a heartbreaking way but in which also lay other, so far unimagined, possibilities. Any reopening of Gabriela's story needed to incorporate new understandings of 'touch' since 'touch' was the refrain that echoed through all of her descriptions of sorrow and anger. Gently, I said to Gabriela, 'You never got to touch your baby when she was alive. Can you tell me what you did to care for and protect your baby's life during your pregnancy with her?'. 'Can you tell me the ways in which you prepared for her birth and the ways in which you held her in your heart and in your body all those 9 months?'

That was it. The floodgates of Gabriela's heart opened. She knew in an instant that she had held her baby close in her heart for all those 9 long months and that she had touched her baby's life with her love, with her conscientious care for her during her pregnancy, and through her hopes and dreams for this baby's life that no one ever imagined would be as brief as a shooting star. Gabriela sobbed and sobbed. But it was the sobbing of relief and of the recognition that she could lay down her arms now.

There was no battle to continue because she, in fact, had held her baby for 9 long months in the most intimate ways physically and emotionally and in the territory of her dreams and hopes for her baby's life. In the way that White (2004) had described, together, Gabriela and I reached from the present into the past and made the acquaintance of meanings and understandings that had hidden in the background. We befriended those new understandings and brought them forward and invited them into Gabriela's now reconstituted ways of knowing.

Begin a conversation with one's body in the interests of improved understanding and communication of body sensations and signals

The body must be included in healing from trauma because through the effects of trauma on it, the body participates in organizing and shaping the restrictive narrative performed over and over again by the traumatized person. That performed narrative makes itself visible in the body through the restricted range of life options and understandings performed everyday by the person who has been traumatized. In Gabriela's case, the endless repetition and associated despair of her sorrow and anger-filled refrain, 'I didn't get to touch my baby; they didn't let me touch my baby' closed off almost all options for effective action. Her body disclosed its daily agony in multiple other ways as well. Gabriela's physical exhaustion, her spending hours upon hours in bed, her disinterest in going out, doing things, being around other people signalled her physical weakness and, simultaneously, reproduced her psychological hopelessness. Gabriela was both physically and emotionally debilitated.

We had conversations about what Gabriela thought her body needed in order to feel stronger. I asked Gabriela what signals she would receive from her body that would let her know she was feeling sad or angry or joyful. I asked her what she needed to do to become a more skilful interpreter of her body's way of communicating with her. In these early stages of becoming more resourceful, Gabriela focused mostly on movement—getting out of bed, walking around a little, going to work when she could, using her arms to hug her husband, and, in general, learning about the signals that her body was sending to her in the form of sensations from muscles, nerves, and internal organs. Siegel (2007) states that 'one role of the senses in our daily lives is to wake us up, to pull us from automaticity, to sharpen the acuity of awareness so that life is both richer and more present in the moment' (p. 77).

As she began to recognize and interpret the signals sent from the territory of her body, Gabriela found herself more active and engaged in life while also caring for herself and her body in new ways that respected its requests for rest and quiet and solitude. Listening and dialoguing with her body was a literal means of preparing the ground for more effective action in her life. By learning how to calm her body Gabriela was learning about emotional regulation even though we never used that linguistic frame per se. As Gabriela became calmer and less distressed, her access to language became easier and more rapid and, over time, she was able to access lost details of her story. Most significantly, of course, Gabriela was no longer captured by her past and her freedom was also the basis of increased movement and the initiation of effective action on behalf of herself and her husband, family, and employer.

Incorporate the experience and meaning of trauma into one's autobiography

Incorporating traumatic events into one's autobiography is a layered process. The ability to engage in mindful dialogue about the trauma, both with oneself and with others, is an early step and an ultimate joint accomplishment on the path to making sense of the traumatic experiences. The making sense process in resolving trauma is, optimally, conducted with others in contexts of emotional acceptance and resonance. Dialogue involves language and an ability to access a vocabulary that is full relative to the particular individual. Trauma that remains unresolved in language is also unresolved in neural networks of the brain. An operational definition of unresolved trauma, then, is traumatic experiencing that the person has not made sense of in their lives and about which the person is unable to tell a coherent story (Main 2000; Siegel 1999).

For Gabriela, there were several chunks of meaning that became central to her enriched autobiographical account of the trauma of her infant daughter's birth and death. The new understanding that seemed most significant to her was her realization that she had touched, held, and cherished her baby for nine long months as she joyfully anticipated her birth. Gabriela also began to think and talk about how her baby's life, as short and luminous as it was, touched her and her husband and family. In Gabriela's narrative, the concept of 'touch' was transformed into a mutual act of love, caring, and profound change, well beyond the physical skin to skin contact that was her original locked-in understanding of it. However, in thinking about how she held and carried her infant daughter throughout her pregnancy, Gabriela included an understanding of having experienced that skin to skin contact in an intimate daily way—an understanding that she had initially overlooked and now viewed sacramentally.

Gabriela also clearly saw the lack of respect and caring by the hospital staff who had ignored her and her husband's enormous anxiety and suffering. She took a stand against their apparent insensitivity but, over time, her stand softened as she took into account their focus on getting her infant daughter to the higher level NICU. This aspect of her hospital experience led her to think about how mothers and fathers in her situation could be included and given opportunities for contact with their baby such as being allowed to go in the ambulance. There are many examples of people who have suffered great traumas and who then have gone on to redirect their lives by becoming activists and reformers for a cause linked to the source of their trauma. As far as I know, this was not the case for Gabriela, but such life changes illustrate the power and far-reaching effects of meaning-making in the aftermath of trauma. Not only is the trauma incorporated autobiographically but it becomes the beginning of a new story that may indeed be life-long and life-sustaining for those who experienced the trauma and, in turn, for others.

Narrate the story of coping and survival

Few have written as eloquently about grief as has C. S. Lewis (1976) in his book, *A Grief Observed*, written after the death of his beloved wife. In writing about the experience of his own grief, he has described the visceral sensations of the body following traumatic loss. He says:

> Tonight all the hells of young grief have opened again; the mad words, the bitter resentment, the fluttering in the stomach, the nightmare unreality, the wallowed-in tears. For in grief nothing 'stays put.' One keeps on emerging from a phase but it always recurs. Round and round. Everything repeats. Am I going in circles, or dare I hope I am on a spiral? But if a spiral am I going up or down it? How often—will it be for always?—how often will the vast emptiness astonish me like a complete novelty and make me say 'I never realized my loss till this moment'? The same leg is cut off time after time. The first plunge of the knife into the flesh is felt again and again (pp. 66–7).

The past and the present are the same to the body suffering traumatic loss—they are one. It is interesting that Lewis with his access to linguistic resources beyond the imaginings of most chose the image of the experience of the body to signify the experience of his suffering.

Gabriela, with far fewer linguistic resources than C.S. Lewis, also was faced with making sense out of the experience of her suffering and the 18 months during which her central and recurring thoughts were 'I didn't get to touch my baby; they wouldn't let me touch my baby' and in which her past had utterly overwhelmed her present. As a future began to appear for the first time in almost two years on the horizon of Gabriela's vista, she began tentatively to look back. In looking back she not only saw the death of her baby and the end of the future she had imagined for herself and her family but she also saw herself and the heartbroken and exhausted person she had become after her infant daughter's death.

The conversations we had during that beginning period of looking back focused on the sources in Gabriela's life of her understandings about empathy and compassion. What had she learned about compassion and empathy and who had been her teachers? What learnings about empathy and compassion had she come to hold on to? Were there any that she particularly treasured? How would she apply those to herself and her experience of loss? How would her most compassionate and empathic self understand what she had been through? These questions and ensuing conversations formed a basis for Gabriela's narration of her own coping and survival—with empathy and compassion as a central theme. As she saw a future emerge and began to look back, other voices of family, friends, and employer were added to her story of coping and survival.

Siegel (2007) says that 'relational experiences promote the development of self-regulation in the brain' (p. 191). He is referring, of course, to attuned and self-validating relational experiences. It was important that our conversations about looking back at the pain of the past two years were organized by the frames of compassion and empathy. Gabriela had already been told more than once that she needed to move on and that she was young and could have another child. These voices of unempathic but perhaps well-meaning others represented what in the world of neuroscience are referred to as top-down cortically-driven judgements that Cozolino (2002) refers to as 'hardening of the categories'. Hardening of the categories is about preconceived representations of reality that are not attuned to the particularities of a given situation.

In Gabriela's case, these voices of others telling her to 'move on', and 'have another baby for God's sake' and the implicit but present 'you're torturing all of us' only served to continue to freeze her in her responses and further reduce her access to other options. Gabriela was frozen by top-down judgements like these but freed by empathic acceptance of her pain and immobility that then pointed to other possibilities for assigning different meanings and taking new actions.

Access wisdom derived from traumatic experiences that might be shared with others

Linley (2003) suggests in the following passage that wisdom derived from traumatic experiencing is made manifest by the evidence of a narrative acknowledging both the traumatic events of the past and the flow of life moving on:

> The development of narrative in positive adaptation to trauma is the milestone that records the distance traveled since the event: simultaneously recording the trauma, but also accepting that life has moved on, is at the core of adaptation (cf., the sense of connected detachment). Repetition of the past (cf., reenactment of the trauma) cannot be avoided without its acknowledgement; neither can reparation be made in the absence of acceptance. The development of narrative facilitates both these processes through giving voice to that which was often nameless (p. 607).

The filling in the gaps or thickening of a trauma narrative provides a social, interpersonal, and experiential account of what happened, what the effects of what happened were, and how the meanings ascribed to those effects came to be and changed over time. Wade (2007) also identifies how a person has responded to and resisted the effects of traumatic experiencing as an important perspective in the formation of a new narrative. A thick narrative signals the joint accomplishment of development of a story that is open to new meanings, possibilities, and actions. A thick narrative also represents changes in neural functioning in that the details of a thick narrative necessarily suggest autobiographical memory that has regained specificity.

From the perspective of narrative approaches to therapy, the development of trauma derived wisdom is an example of what White (2004) describes as a set of new meanings and alternatives for the future based on newly developed understandings of the present and the past. Since the effects of trauma often result in the conflation of the past and present, seeing a future filled with different possibilities is indeed quite an accomplishment. For Gabriela, her acquired wisdom and associated narrative were especially important to her in terms of her restored ability to express the deep love and appreciation that she felt for her husband, family, and her employer. Her articulation of her understanding of their frustration with her as time wore on resensitized them to the depth of her pain and suffering which, in turn, led to greater expressed mutual caring and support. Gabriela and her family created a project in which they made recordings of their feelings about the infant baby and their love and hopes for her. They gathered the symbols of that love and hope, the clothes the baby had worn in the hospital, little soft toy animals, a few family photographs, and placed them all in a carved wooden box that Gabriela's husband had made. Not only Gabriela's narrative had changed but so had the narratives of her husband, family, and employer. Gabriela's enriched narrative also included her ability to think of herself with compassion for all she had suffered and with dignity for how she had persisted in searching for an understanding of her loss that made sense to her.

Closing reflections

The experience of trauma, both of the horrific and everyday varieties, involves the body in ways that are central and undeniable. Trauma routinely reconstitutes the body by impeding a person's ability to use language while simultaneously increasing arousal and fear. This reduction of linguistic resources complicates the accessing of new meanings that may be helpful to those who have experienced trauma and to those whom they love. The effects of trauma provide vivid evidence of the inscription of the social world on the remaking of the body in trauma's aftermath. Granting the body greater discursive recognition does not involve moving away from a focus on the construction of meaning within the social world, but rather includes the body more centrally in the flow of life as the body itself becomes constituted and reconstituted as a result. Findings from neuroscience can be read as supportive of an understanding of the body as shaped in and by the world and, therefore, as a repudiation of Cartesian dualism. In many ways, it is social constructionism that is at risk of embracing an unintended dualism by not adequately accounting for the constitution of meaning as embodied discursive experience. We are neither over-weighted body masses like cartoonish homunculi nor shape-shifting mentalists without corporeality moving through the world. Trauma marks the body in ways that are both visible and invisible and profoundly affects the experience of time. Narrative approaches to therapy include a focus on both time and meaning and offer resourceful ways of working with those who have experienced trauma. Narrative approaches encourage emotional resonance with the person who has suffered trauma and are congruent with the requisites for healing that encompass mind and body together.

References

Barrionuevo, A. and Robbins, L. (2010). 1.5 million displaced after Chile quake, *The New York Times*, 28 **February**, A1.

Bilham, R. (2010). Lessons from the Haiti earthquake. *Nature,* **463**, 878–9.

Cozolino, L. (2002). *The Neuroscience of Psychotherapy: Building and Rebuilding the Human Brain*. Norton, New York.

Cozolino, L. (2006). *The Neuroscience of Human Relationships: Attachment and the Developing Social Brain*. Norton, New York.

Croll, S. and Bryant, R. A. (2000). Autobiographical memory in postnatal depression. *Cognitive Therapy & Research,* **24**, 419–26.

Cromby, J. and Nightingale, D, (1999). What's wrong with social constructionism? In D. J. Nightingale and J. Cromby (Eds.) *Social Constructionist Psychology: A Critical Analysis of Theory and Practice*, pp. 1–19. Open University Press, Buckingham.

Dalgleish, T., Rolfe, J., Golden, A.-M., Dunn, B. D., and Barnard, P. J. (2008). Reduced autobiographical memory specificity and posttraumatic stress: Exploring the contributions of impaired executive control and affect regulation. *Journal of Abnormal Psychology,* **117**(1), 236–41.

Damasio, A. (2003). *Looking for Spinoza: Joy, Sorrow, and the Feeling Brain*. Harcourt, Orlando, FL.

de Decker, A., Hermans, D., Raes, F., and Eelen, P. (2003). Autobiographical memory specificity and trauma in inpatient adolescents. *Journal of Clinical Child and Adolescent Psychology*, **32**, 22–31.

Faul, M. (2010). Women, girls rape victims in Haiti quake aftermath. *Examiner.com*, **16 March**. http://image.examiner.com/a-2530422 Women__girls_rape_victims_in_Haiti_quake_aftermath.html [Accessed 22 March 2010.]

Fortun, M. and Bernstein, H. J. (1998). *Muddling through: Pursuing Science and Truths in the 21st Century*. Counterpoint, Washington, DC.

Friedenberg, J. E. (2008). *The anatomy of an academic mobbing. The First Hector Hammerly Memorial Lecture on Academic Mobbing*. The University of Waterloo, Ontario, Canada, 11 April. http://arts.uwaterloo.ca/ kwesthue/frieden-hh.htm [Accessed 22 March 2010.]

Gilbertson, A. and Filkins, D. (2010). The shrine down the hall. *The New York Times Magazine*, 21 March, 34–47.

Harvey, A. G., Bryant, R. A., and Dang, S. T. (1998). Autobiographical memory in acute stress disorder. *Journal of Consulting and Clinical Psychology*, **66**, 500–6.

Henderson, D., Hargreaves, I., Gregory, S., and Williams, J. M. G. (2002). Autobiographical memory and emotion in a non-clinical sample of women with and without a reported history of childhood sexual abuse. *British Journal of Clinical Psychology*, **41**, 129–42.

Hull, A. M. (2002). Neuroimaging findings in post-traumatic stress disorder. *British Journal of Psychiatry*, **181**(2), 102–10.

Hume, D. (1739/1978). *A Treatise of Human Nature*. Oxford University Press, Oxford.

Kangas, M., Henry, J. L., and Bryant, R. A. (2005). A prospective study of autobiographical memory and posttraumatic stress disorder following cancer. *Journal of Consulting and Clinical Psychology*, **73**(2), 293–9.

Kuyken, W. and Brewin, C. R. (1995). Autobiographical memory functioning in depression and reports of early abuse. *Journal of Abnormal Psychology*, **104**, 585–91.

Lewis, C. S. (1976). *A grief observed*. Bantam, New York.

Lewis, T., Amini, F., and Lannon, R. (2000). *A general theory of love*. Vintage Books, New York.

Lindauer, R. J. L., Booij, J., and Habraken, J. B. A., et al. (2004). Cerebral blood flow changes during script driven imagery in police officers with posttraumatic stress disorder. *Biological Psychiatry*, **56**(11), 853–61.

Linley, P. A. (2003). Positive adaptation to trauma: Wisdom as both process and outcome. *Journal of Traumatic Stress*, **16**(6), 601–10.

McNally, R. J., Lasko, N. B., Macklin, M. L., and Pitman, R. K. (1995). Autobiographical memory disturbance in combat-related posttraumatic stress disorder. *Behaviour Research and Therapy*, **33**, 619–30.

McNally, R. J., Litz, B. T., Prassas, A., Shin, L. M., and Weathers, F. W. (1994). Emotional priming of autobiographical memory in posttraumatic stress disorder. *Cognition & Emotion*, **8**, 351–67.

Mahoney, M. J. (2003). Minding science: Constructivism and the discourse of inquiry. *Cognitive Therapy and Research*, **27**(1), 105–23.

Main, M. (2000). The Adult Attachment Interview: Fear, attention, safety, and discourse processes. *Journal of the American Psychoanalytic Association*, **48**, 1055–96.

Rauch, S. L., van der Kolk, B., A., and Fisler, R. E., et al. (1996). A symptom provocation study of posttraumatic stress disorder using positron emission tomography and script-driven imagery. *Archives of General Psychiatry,* **53**(5), 380–7.

Scaer, R. (2005). *The Trauma Spectrum: Hidden Wounds and Human Resiliency.* Norton, New York.

Schore, A. N. (1994). *Affect Regulation and the Origin of the Self: The Neurobiology of Emotional Development.* Lawrence Erlbaum, Hillsdale, NJ.

Seelye, K. Q. (2009). Coffins' arrival from war becomes an issue again. *The New York Times,* 21 February, A22

Siegel, D. J. (1999). *The developing Mind: How Relationships and the Brain Interact to Shape Who We Are.* Guilford, New York.

Siegel, D. J. (2007). *The Mindful Brain: Reflection and Attunement in the Cultivation of Well-Being.* Norton, New York.

Van der Kolk, B. A. (2006). Clinical implications of neuroscience research in PTSD. *Annals of the New York Academy of Sciences,* **1071**, 277–93.

Van der Kolk, B. A., Roth, S., Pelcovitz, D., Sunday, S., and Spinazzola, J. (2005). Disorders of extreme stress: The empirical foundation of a complex adaptation to trauma. *Journal of Traumatic Stress,* **18**(5), 389–99.

Varela, F. (Ed.) (1997). *Sleeping, Dreaming, and Dying: An Exploration of Consciousness with the Dalai Lama.* Wisdom Publications, Somerville, MA.

Wade, A. (2007). Despair, resistance, hope: Response-based therapy with victims of violence. In C. Flaskas, I. McCarthy, and J. Sheehan (Eds.) *Hope and Despair in Narrative and Family Therapy: Adversity, Forgiveness, and Reconciliation,* pp.63–74. Routledge, London.

Wessel, I., Merckelbach, H., and Dekkers, T. (2002). Autobiographical memory specificity, intrusive memory, and general memory skills in Dutch–Indonesian survivors of the World War II era. *Journal of Traumatic Stress,* **15**(3), 227–34.

White, M. (2004). Folk psychology and narrative practice. In L. E. Angus and J. McLeod (Eds.) *The Handbook of Narrative and Psychotherapy: Practice, Theory, and Research,* pp. 15–51. Sage, Thousand Oaks, CA.

White, M. and Epston, D. (1990). *Narrative means to therapeutic ends.* Norton, New York.

Williams, J. M. G., Barnhofer, T., and Crane, C., et al. (2007). Autobiographical memory specificity and emotional disorder. *Psychological Bulletin,* **133**, 122–48.

Williams, J. M. G., and Broadbent, K. (1986). Autobiographical memory in suicide attempters. *Journal of Abnormal Psychology,* **95**, 144–9.

Chapter 16

Narrative, discourse, psychotherapy—neuroscience?

John Cromby

Introduction

> *The man jumps over a high white fence and hits the ground running. Not far behind is another man, wielding a gun. Frantic, breathless, eyes popping, he runs, ducks and then hides. The chasing man, still waving the gun, searches for him.*
>
> *Now the man uses a mirror to read a tattoo inked on his body in backward lettering. Around the mirror are Polaroid photographs and post-it notes bearing enigmatic phrases. We understand that these things remind him why he was being chased, what he is trying to achieve. But seconds later he has forgotten, and will have to remind himself again.*

Christopher Nolan's (2000) film *Memento* graphically illustrates one kind of fantastical effect that can follow brain injury: the inability to form new narrative memories, a consequence which condemns the man to live a life composed from many thousands of successive, short, disjunctive present moments. Lacking all permanent narrative memory for anything that has occurred since he was shot in the head, the man occupies a bizarre temporal frame. His experiences are constituted only fleetingly from partial fragments of narrative, and structured by affects and material continuities that link them in ways he can only imperfectly comprehend. Nolan embeds this unusual condition within a particularly dramatic narrative: the man's quest to identify the person who killed his wife and then shot him. The narratives of most psychotherapy clients are not so overtly dramatic, and most do not have brain injuries. Nevertheless, the structures and functions of the brains of both therapists and clients are consistently as relevant to *their* narratives and experiences as the damaged brain of Nolan's character is relevant to his.

In this chapter, I will describe some of the ways in which neuroscience may be relevant to the discursive psychotherapies. Whilst conceptual clarity is vital to any such enterprise, the 'turn to language' (Harré 1992) with which these therapies are associated may make this clarity difficult to achieve. In the pragmatic situation of the therapeutic encounter conceptual issues are typically managed informally, but in the present context they must be squarely addressed. One issue is that theories and methods that prioritize language as the medium and fabric of human experience and social relations tend to ignore, downplay or occlude extra-discursive influences, including the body and its brain (e.g. Brown et al. 2009; Leder 1990; Shilling 2003; Stam 1998; Wendell 1996). Another is that, in their focus on language, these theories and methods may simultaneously go too far, and yet not far enough. In endowing language with a singular power of constitution and a seminal force of transformation, they may go too far; but in arbitrarily confining the practices and effects of socialization to the linguistic realm, they may not go far enough. Some preparatory framing is therefore needed, in order to develop a nuanced position that accords appropriate significances to both bodies *and* language.

Contemporary human and social science host manifold accounts of discourse and narrative (e.g. Crossley 2000; Fairclough 2005; Foucault 1977; Freeman 1993; Laclau and Mouffe 1985; Potter and Wetherell 1987) that together constitute a complex, interdependent, evolving field of knowledge. Ontologically diverse with respect to the relations they posit between discourse, materiality and the body, these theories nevertheless share a common preoccupation with the organising and/or constitutive power of language. Discursive psychotherapies take from the broadly poststructuralist stance shared by the majority of these theories a commitment to practising without recourse to notions of 'inner' selves and a liberating emphasis on the multiplicity of culturally-embedded narratives (White 1991, 2001). Contemporary neuroscience, too, is complex, specialized, and rapidly developing, a heterogenous assemblage of theories, technologies and practices interrogating the object frequently proclaimed as the most complicated in the known universe: the human brain. And neuroscience, similarly, contains significant diversity: its sub-disciplines variously emphasize the cognitive, affective, social, or computational aspects of neural activity (Gazzaniga 2009; Harmon-Jones and Winkielman 2007; Panksepp 1998; Trappenberg 2009), whilst its methods embrace real-time brain imaging techniques, animal experiments, lesion studies, and studies of behaviour. Following the explosion of research in the 1990s' 'decade of the brain', neuroscience is now also spawning applied sub-disciplines: for example, a relatively distinct subdiscipline of educational neuroscience seems to be currently emerging (Szucs and Goswami 2007). So both discursive and narrative theory and neuroscience are complex, heterogeneous and evolving: a comprehensive account of either, still less of the associations between them, is impossible here.

Moreover, any apparent simplification supplied by the focus upon psychotherapy is more chimerical than actual, since in psychotherapy the totality of the client's experience is at stake, and this totality never resides exclusively in language (Kenwood 1999). In psychotherapy the relevance of the extra-discursive—the subordinate or silenced story (White 2004), the unspoken and, perhaps, unspeakable—is something of which therapists must often be acutely aware. But the extra-discursive gains additional force here because the neural, the synaptic, the chemical, and the various fluctuating potentialities they supply, are so obviously not *just* matters of discourse: there are, for example, unassailable organic reasons why the man in Nolan's film is not a good candidate for narrative therapy. These issues are sharpened by the truism that people seeking psychotherapy are typically experiencing some form of distress. Whatever the particular complexion of their difficulties and regardless of how they are theorized by therapists, the experience of distress is always an embodied one, always played out within the concrete particulars of given social and material situations (Smail 2005): this, indeed, is the case for *all* experiences.

All this suggests that in order to sensibly relate discourse and narrative with neuroscience we need some appropriate ontology of what it is to speak. Whilst we need not close down the definition of either 'discourse' or 'narrative', for the purposes of the present discussion our understanding of the speech that carries them must include its simultaneous corporeal aspects. We need to recognize how speech is relationally interpellated, socioculturally organized by discourse, and enactive of multiple narratives; and simultaneously to recognize how it is enabled by multiple, interacting brain–body systems that imbue speaking with a visceral sense of the speaker's embodied intentionality. Some scholars of language have already begun to achieve this by considering the social significances of the lived, phenomenological body: Shotter (1993) argues that discursive interaction always relies upon a background of 'knowing of the third kind', an embodied form of 'sensual, practical-moral knowledge' by which we simultaneously apprehend and influence each other through our bodies as well as through our intellects. This embodied knowing consists primarily of feelings, which continuously inhabit and surround speech, giving it motive, force, intensity, valence, and nuance. Both in subjectivity and in social interaction, feelings and speech (including Vygotskian 'inner speech') operate in a dialectical, mutually transformative fashion, and there is a constant interchange and flux between the two (Cromby 2007b).

Psychotherapists work predominantly with meanings, but attempts to include bodies in meaning-making frequently founder upon restrictive readings of poststructuralism that artificially constitute language as some kind of pure autonomous realm (e.g. Hepburn 2003). These difficulties are neutralized by Ruthrof (1997), who articulates a poststructuralist semantics demonstrating that meaning is the product of multiple sign systems, and that these systems *always* include the embodied signs generated by our bodies. Embodied signs are experienced phenomenologically as feelings, and are enabled by the various biological systems with which our species is endowed: thermal, haptic, gustatory, visceral, kinaesthetic, etc. Ruthrof shows how the meanings of these embodied feelings are decreed by their intrinsic corporeal qualities as they arise, contingently with other signs, in the lived moments of experience. Whereas the meaning of linguistic signs is constituted through difference and deferral and decreed by (mutable) social convention, the meanings of embodied signs flow from their somatic textures and intensities as they signify, contingently, with the signs of language. The meanings of these embodied signs are therefore bound up with the meanings of words, but not reducible to them: a feeling of anxiety is already itself a meaningful sign, but its full meaning is contingent upon how it signifies alongside other signs, including (but not limited to) those of language.

Thus, meaning is not just socially constructed, it is *co-constituted*: on the one hand through the symbolic–conceptual–discursive register that discourse and narrative emphasizes, and on the other by the continual phenomenological experience of the moving, feeling body.

But there nevertheless remains a considerable distance between this phenomenological body and the empirically observable brain and body of neuroscience. Brain processes are of a different order to embodied experiences, whatever correspondences are drawn between them, and it is vital that this difference is marked. Here, I will follow Harré (2002) in characterizing brain processes and systems as characteristics of *organisms*: these neural functions supply affordances, orientations, capacities and tendencies that *enable*, but do not determine, the activity of *persons*. In Harré's account, persons—not organisms, or the molecules of which they are formed—are the primary unit of analysis, since only persons have intentions and moral accountability. Persons, not organisms, deploy narratives to position themselves with respect to others; persons, not organisms, seek to resolve their difficulties in therapeutic engagements with others. Nevertheless, persons depend upon and are influenced by their organismic capacities, just as they are also influenced by the causal powers of the molecules from which these organisms are constituted. Recognizing this, Harré also offers what he calls a 'taxonomic priority principle': simply put, this means that we can only meaningfully study the neural (organismic) and biochemical (molecular) bases of any given activity if the *person* can be meaningfully said to be actually engaged in that activity.

All this may seem like a particularly bloviatory way of introducing the substantive material that follows, but is necessary for various reasons. First, as has been intimated, there are frequent conceptual problems associated with attempts to reconcile language and the body. Second, proponents of discourse and narrative are often suspicious of neuroscience and sometimes reject it entirely. Engagement with neuroscience can work progressively to complement, rather than undermine, discursive and other social scientific perspectives (Cromby 2004; van Ommen 2005; Wilson 2004); nevertheless, real dangers remain. Third, there is widespread conceptual confusion regarding what neuroscience and its associated imaging techniques can actually tell us, and a climate of expectation which has sometimes led to neuroscience being mis-applied and over-sold (see for example Goswami 2004). Fourth, we inhabit a cultural moment where neuroscience (and the related disciplines of genomics and pharmacology) is enrolled within 'the politics of life itself' (N. Rose 2001; N. Rose and Rabinow 2006). Arguably, we are now becoming 'neurochemical selves' (N. Rose 2005) increasingly encouraged to understand our experiences in terms of brain chemistry and structure rather than social practice and relations. At a historical juncture when the politics of class, ethnicity, gender, and sexuality have blurred, becoming co-opted by other concerns, issues of longevity, reproduction and health gain renewed political significance: neuroscience both feeds into these concerns, and is freighted by them. And fifth, the field of psychotherapy is itself haunted by a particular neural spectre: Freud's 'Project for a Scientific Psychology', the abandoned attempt to relate neurological process to interpersonal meaning which is sometimes said to illustrate the impossibility of making coherent links between neural process and therapeutic work.

Yet neuroscience has changed profoundly since Freud, to the extent that there is now even a thriving subdiscipline of neuro-psychoanalysis (Solms and Turnbull 2002); some engagement with the literature relating neuroscience and psychotherapy is therefore appropriate. Both to contextualize the subsequent review and provide some essential basic concepts, the next section presents an extremely brief summary of what is currently known and taken to be largely uncontroversial about relevant brain structure and function, synthesized primarily from Beaumont et al. (1996), Damasio (1999), and S. Rose (1997). Just as a neuroscientist must necessarily accept certain initial tenets in order to engage sensibly with discourse theory, this information represents a minimal subset of neuroscientific findings and concepts necessary to enable productive engagement by discursive psychotherapists.

Neural basics

It is a matter of convention rather than anatomy that we place the boundary of the brain at the base of the skull. The nervous system, a seamless outgrowth of the brain, actually permeates the entire body, just as 'bodily' influences—sensory and kinaesthetic feedback, and a continuous wash of hormones, peptides, and other chemicals—flood continuously through the brain: as Damasio (1994) puts it, not only is the brain embodied, the body is 'embrained'. The average adult human brain contains about 100 billion neurons: nerve cells with extended bodies called axons that transmit electrical signals, and which communicate across the tiny gaps that separate them by releasing neurotransmitting chemicals (e.g. serotonin, dopamine). These neurotransmitters influence the probability that a receiving neuron will become active or 'fire', releasing its own neurotransmitters into the next synapse. The probability of this occurring is also modulated by other neurotransmitting chemicals, notably hormones and peptides. Whilst the number of connections between neurons varies hugely, one neuron is frequently connected to many thousands of others.

There is good evidence that some aspects of specific human abilities are enabled by neural activity localized to particular parts of the brain's gross structure, and that this organization is shared, with slight variation, by most individuals. For example, the limbic system is composed of the amygdala, hypothalamus, hippocampus, and other areas: this system is especially important for enabling affect, although the hippocampus also plays an important role in consolidating new memories (the man in Nolan's film probably had hippocampal damage). In most people language is largely specialized to left hemisphere systems (Gazzaniga 1998), whereas affective understandings are more associated with the right hemisphere (Borod et al. 1998). Brains nevertheless exhibit individual variation and significant plasticity, especially at the level of fine structure. Lesions to a specified area do not always have the effect that would be predicted, and regions usually specialized for one kind of function can get recruited for others: for example, in the brains of visually-impaired people, areas that usually process vision can be used for reading Braille (Roder and Neville 2003). Cromby (2007a) notes that one way of interpreting the many imaging studies that link changing patterns of brain activation to specific practices and activities, is that the brain itself is socialized, and Schore (2001) describes how social influences get built into the brain from the earliest stages of development onward; for example, how the organization and density of inhibitory and excitatory connections between limbic and cortical areas is influenced by early relationships. So although the brain's gross structure exhibits marked invariance, finer elements of structure and function exhibit significant plasticity. This understanding accords with critical analyses showing that many studies erroneously overstate genetic influence (Joseph 2003).

The staggering number of connections between its billions of neurons allows the brain to function as an extraordinarily complex 'system of systems' composed of multiple, parallel processes. These systems are distributed throughout the brain, contain multiple feedback loops, and are said to be organized into neural networks. Neural networks consist of neurons in different brain areas that fire synchronously: they are intrinsically complicated, and the connections between their neurons are usually multiple; moreover, individual neurons can be part of more than one network.

Relatively stable neural networks get formed when the same neurons fire repeatedly, because this strengthens the connections between them: in Hebb's (1949) terms, neurons that fire together, wire together. While some neurons in a network might enable processes that are available for introspective awareness, others may recruit subcortical tracts not available to consciousness: these elements of processing are sometimes described as unconscious, although it is potentially less confusing to describe them as *a*conscious. Further complexity arises because firing can serve to inhibit the activity of adjacent neurons in a network, as well as to activate them, and because networks frequently recruit affective areas that supply a-representational, visceral or sensuous elements of experience.

The operation of neural networks means that all but the very simplest tasks involve activity in more than one brain area: thus some areas—called association cortices—are notable for the way that multiple networks converge within them. Most abilities are therefore enabled by multiple elementary processes carried out in parallel. Remembering, for example, typically recruits affective systems in the limbic area as well as explicit, declarative (e.g. linguistic) systems in the neocortex. Additional areas get activated according to the specific content of the memory, and reflect the processing that occurred when it was formed: visual memories are partially enabled by areas of the occipital cortex, specialized for vision, whereas memories of sounds are partially enabled by the auditory cortices in the temporal lobes. Remembering, then, is always a reconstructive rather than a veridical activity, with the consequence that frequently activated memories bear the traces of subsequent activations, woven into the recalled particulars of the originary event (Le Doux 1999).

Neuroscience and psychotherapy

With this very basic description of neural structure and functioning as foundation, I will now describe some of the literature relating neuroscience and psychotherapy. The review is necessarily illustrative rather than comprehensive; moreover, most of the work reviewed refers to psychotherapy in general because there is very little that specifically addresses discursive therapies. The literature relates neuroscience to psychotherapy with individuals and with couples, and within a variety of therapeutic modalities; neuroscience is also used to re-work notions of distress, and to interrogate some of the processes that occur during therapy. Authors vary, both in their degree of enthusiasm for neuroscience to inform psychotherapy and in their assessment of its potentials, and some are markedly pessimistic. Manteufel (2005) places great emphasis upon the complexity and uncertainty involved in moving between psychotherapy and neuroscience. He warns of the dangers of reductionism, and notes that many imaging studies fail to move beyond the simple correlation of brain activation patterns with activities, leaving many of the questions of most interest to psychotherapists (for example, whether the brain activity was inhibitory or excitatory) unanswered. In contrast, Fonagy (2004) is unconcerned about reductionism but nevertheless sees neuroscience making only limited contributions to psychotherapy, by identifying (hypothetical) biological vulnerabilities to distress and providing 'objective' tests of therapeutic efficacy. However, the great majority of the work is both optimistic and enthusiastic, and some authors even use their engagement with neuroscience to make specific suggestions for therapeutic practice. Three interwoven themes with particular relevance for discursive psychotherapy can be drawn from this literature: the significance of affect, the character of memory, and embodied knowing.

The significance of affect

Language is primarily enabled by neocortical systems in the left hemisphere, a 'system of systems' that Gazzaniga (2000) calls 'the interpreter' and which, in his account, also provides the neural basis for Vygotskian 'inner speech' (Cromby and Harper 2009). By contrast, affects are enabled by multiple brain systems, primarily in the lower brain. Panksepp (1998) has identified a series of neural circuits, common to all mammals, which promotes different sensibilities and is associated with distinct regimes of feeling. These circuits originate in subcortical areas, and are postulated to be base elements of the neural systems that enable complex human emotions. Panksepp names these circuits using uppercase titles intended to capture their essential character whilst simultaneously avoiding confusion with everyday language. Thus, PANIC is a brain system associated with feelings of vulnerability, loneliness, and insecurity, which promotes the urge to seek security, company, and companionship. It is enabled by the action of corticotrophic-releasing factor in midbrain circuits including the periaqueductal grey. Similarly FEAR is associated with feelings of anxiety, and with escape and avoidance activities; it is enabled by circuits flowing through the periaqueductal grey and amygdala, and the release of glutamate and other excitatory neuropeptides.

Panksepp and others (e.g. Damasio 1999, 2003; Le Doux 1999, 2000) postulate that these affective systems are absolutely fundamental to our experience, providing much of the raw material of consciousness itself. Whilst it is obvious that language can drive affect (being told some news can make you happy, angry, or sad) there is also experimental evidence that affect can drive language. Working with split-brain patients (whose corpus callosum has been severed to control intractable epilepsy), Gazzaniga (2000) showed that when affective states were induced and their origins masked from the (linguistic) left hemisphere, patients spontaneously 'confabulated': they generated plausible, but demonstrably erroneous, explanations for how they felt. So the relations between affect and language are bi-directional, but the existence of separate systems for each means that they can also operate somewhat independently (how we feel does not always match what we say). Panksepp characterizes affect systems as 'basic operating system' circuits and argues that they have common features that distinguish them from other brain systems: these include a significant degree of genetic predetermination, the ability to promote diverse activities and alter the sensitivity of sensory systems, a tendency to outlast their precipitating circumstances, and the capacity (through conditioning) to come under the control of neutral stimuli.

The implications of this for psychotherapy recur constantly in the literature. For example, Cozolino's (2002) chapter on the 'narrative self' draws on Damasio to emphasize the inevitability of gaps in self-awareness and relates these to affective charges enabled by the somatic marker system—a system with a critical node in the prefrontal lobe, which calls out body-state profiles (feelings) associated with prior events and uses them to guide decision-making (Damasio 1994). Cappas et al. (2005) discuss the mutual dependency of cognition and emotion with reference to trauma, and in relation to the central significance of therapeutic relationships. Similarly, Folensbee's (2007) medicalized account sketches a 'big picture' model that identifies nine elements of neural function especially relevant to therapists: executive function (the ability to activate some systems and inhibit others), attention, sensation, integration, motor ability, arousal, affect, anxiety, and patterns (neural networks, and the connections between them). Folensbee suggests that every experience we have will, to varying degrees, activate each of these neural functions, and so it might be therapeutically useful to consider the relative contribution of each to different kinds of distress. For example, superficially similar impulsive activity may be due to hyperactive emotion systems, disorganized attention, over-arousal, or weak impulse control (executive function). Different psychotherapeutic strategies would follow from each, and in each the relation between affect and language appears somewhat differently.

Ecker and Toomey (Toomey and Ecker 2007, 2009; Ecker and Toomey 2008) place the relation between affect and language at the centre of their discussion of strategies of cognitive regulation which, they say, are most prominent in cognitive-behavioural and narrative therapies that promote explicit, conscious strategies of control, enabled primarily by the neocortex, in order to mediate affective responses enabled primarily by the amygdala and limbic areas. They argue that the universal applicability of this strategy depends upon the belief that amygdala learning is indelible, permanent, and incapable of modification. Countless studies of fear conditioning have shown that learned responses can be 'extinguished', but the readiness with which these extinguished responses can return suggests that conditioned fear learning involves permanent, immutable amygdala learning. However, they note, it has been recognized in recent years that there are some circumstances in which it seems that learned fear responses enabled by the amygdala *can* be transformed or 'reconsolidated'. This raises the possibility that therapeutic strategies might exploit this reconsolidation process, and they argue that their own 'coherence therapy' does this with its strategy of 'juxtapositioning': pairing present-moment emotional responses in therapy with explicit understandings of learned emotional responses from the past, in ways that disconfirm negative expectations. However, although they report clinical success with this treatment they present no independent evaluations, and nor do they have any neuroscientific evidence that juxtapositioning works in the amygdala in the way they suggest.

Atkinson et al. (2005) describe how their engagement with Panksepp's work led them to conceive of their couples therapy primarily as a matter of coaching clients in new affective habits: for example, suppressing tendencies to engage the RAGE system and replacing them with habitual tendencies to engage one of the more affiliative systems. They argue that once these basic systems are engaged: 'People often fail to think and act in needed ways because they find that they're not in the mood. They can't sustain needed attitudes or actions. The wrong brain state shows up, and they find themselves with attitudes and urges that take them in the wrong direction' (Atkinson et al. 2005, p. 7). Thus, they began to view therapy as being less about fostering insight or awareness, and more about training clients to engage the most functional affect system for their circumstances. Following the Hebbian principle that repetition develops new neural networks, they reasoned that therapy must deploy repetitive practice to succeed. Accordingly, they began making personalized audio tapes for clients and asking them to play these tapes at difficult moments, so that 'Clients didn't need to remember new ways of thinking when they were upset, they just needed to remember to turn on the tape recorder' (Atkinson et al. 2005, p. 9). They report that clients who used the tapes gradually began to experience changes in their affective states at moments of stress, and describe this as evidence that appropriate new neural connections had been formed.

Another therapeutic strategy informed by the relationship between affect and language is offered by Lipchik et al. (2005), who propose that neuroscientific information might be given to clients in therapy. They offer the example of a woman who experiences bouts of extreme rage, and whose therapist explained that simply trying to 'control' her anger would be unlikely to help 'because of the way the cognitive systems in the brain shut down when the emotional systems are over-stimulated' (p. 64). The woman was relieved by this—presumably because of its normalizing implication—and subsequently better able to experiment with methods for reducing emotional stimulation (exercise, relaxation, breathing techniques). Rather than holding the woman (person) accountable for her anger, Lipchik et al.'s alternative narrative placed responsibility with her organism (brain): a version of the 'externalizing' technique used in discursive therapy to separate person from problem and facilitate the construction of more adaptive narratives.

The character of memory

As we have seen, memories are enabled by multiple brain systems: some are explicit and declarative, others are implicit and affective, and the precise contribution each makes to a given memory will differ in accord with the nature of the event. The complex implications of this for psychotherapy are considered in almost all of the works reviewed here, with extended discussions provided by Cozolino (2002) and Folensbee (2007). In one of the few papers to invoke neuroscience that is concerned specifically with discursive psychotherapy, Beaudoin (2005) describes how discussions of the complexity of memory might facilitate clients coming to terms with trauma by helping them to better realize what agency they did and did not have. Similarly, Cappas et al. (2005) derive what they describe as seven 'principles' of brain-based psychotherapy, and emphasize how the role of multiple brain systems in the constitution of memories opens up retrieval to influence from the present context. They note that a frequent goal of narrative therapy is to work with this potential for contextual modification by rehearsing new narratives that emphasize positive memories or otherwise better serve current functioning.

The relations between memory and language are central to Seltzer's (2005) description of her method of pre-cognitive therapy—a way of working with unverbalized trauma that uses images, drawn by clients, to represent houses associated with different periods of their lives. She argues that many traumatic memories cannot be easily verbalized because they are enabled by the limbic system, and consist of affective (typically anxious) body-states associated with relatively diffuse, non-verbal symbolic content. Using a case study, she shows how pre-cognitive therapy successfully allowed a client to begin to name previously shadowy elements of her traumatic past and integrate elements of these 'silenced stories' into an explicit, coherent narrative.

Similarly, Toomey and Ecker (2009) discuss the potentials of reparative attachment therapy, which they say is supported by neuroscientific work exploring the consequences for brain development of dysfunctional early relationships characterized by non-attunement (caregiver failures to supply appropriate experiences of emotional regulation), abuse, and trauma. Such experiences impair the acquisition of coherent personal narratives that successfully integrate explicit memories containing cause-and-effect sequences—enabled predominantly by systems in the left-hemisphere neocortex—with implicit, affective memories enabled largely by right-hemisphere neocortical and limbic systems. Toomey and Ecker argue that for clients whose presenting symptom is both rooted in dysfunctional early experience *and* amenable to therapeutic change through new experiences of therapeutic interaction, reparative attachment might effectively re-integrate fragmented memories into coherent narratives (although they acknowledge that only small numbers of clients will meet both requirements).

Thus, implicit memories—memories that lack explicit, declarative, representational, symbolic, or linguistic content of the kind that discursive therapies work with—are largely affective in character: rather than being mystical 'body memories', they are enabled by subcortical, limbic, and right-hemisphere neural systems not dependent on language. The operation of these multiple systems is perhaps most obvious in the experience of 'flashbacks' for traumatic events, where sudden involuntary recall of an event in the form of a vivid image is accompanied by a powerful physical charge (Brewin 2001).

Embodied knowing

The area of neuroscience that has perhaps most excited the imagination of psychotherapists in recent years relates to mirror neurons: neurons which fire, both when an action or expression is performed, and when we see the same action or expression being performed by another (Gallese and Goldman 1998). Mirror neurons were first identified in the sensorimotor cortex of macaque monkeys, and a recent study now claims to have demonstrated their existence in humans (Mukamel et al. 2010). There is also evidence for networks that may function as human mirror neuron systems, and it has been proposed that these are the neural basis of empathy in everyday life (Haidt 2003).

Similar suggestions have been made about the possible role of human mirror neurons in psychotherapeutic empathy, because of their claimed potential to allow 'direct' access to (a version of) the embodied experience of others (Gallese et al. 2007). With particular reference to psychoanalysis, Gallese and colleagues further propose that experiences of projective identification (where therapist and client unwittingly act in ways that fulfil each other's unspoken fears) and counter transference (the therapist's feeling for the client in relation to her or his predicament) might be explained in terms of the operation of mirror neurons. Similarly, Lipchik et al. (2005) suggest that the mirror neuron system might enable what they call 'dual track thinking' (therapist monitoring of client's dysfunctional emotions and intentional stances) by providing therapists with a continuous flow of information about clients' embodied states, and Seltzer (2005) discusses the possible role of mirror neurons in enabling experiences of therapeutic resonance and empathy.

In a related discussion, Vivona (2009a) assesses the relevance for psychoanalysis of neuroscientific research on embodied language. She reviews a series of brain imaging studies suggesting various close and bidirectional links between language and the body, including sensorimotor and affective influences and associations with mirror neuron systems. She relates her review to psychoanalytic accounts of the relations between language and the body, arguing that neuroscience has the potential to inform their evaluation and that this would have both theoretical and clinical import. One specific potential she sees is for neuroscientific studies of embodied language to reveal something of the ways in which words and phrases can come to have particular *personal* connotations that overlay their normative meanings.

Problems and dangers

As demonstrated in the previous section, progress is being made toward identifying ways in which neural systems might both facilitate and impede psychotherapy: this is leading some therapists to experiment with new therapeutic strategies, and to understand their work in new and different ways. However, there are continuing difficulties associated with the deployment of neuroscience that are not always adequately recognised in this literature; it is to a consideration of some of these that we now turn.

Perhaps the most widespread and fundamental difficulty relates to the distinction between persons and organisms that Harré sees as necessary, and is a conceptual error that Bennett and Hacker (2003) describe as the 'mereological fallacy': a tendency in contemporary neuroscience to write about the brain as though it were simply identical to the person or mind. Mereology is the study of part-whole relationships, and Bennett and Hacker show that neuroscientists frequently attribute psychological activities (believing, interpreting, choosing, deciding, etc.) to brains (organisms, or parts thereof) when, logically, these activities can only be attributed to wholes—persons. This is mistaken because, whatever their character, neural systems alone cannot believe, decide and so on: these are human activities, not brain functions. As Bennett and Hacker put it:

> It is not that as a matter of fact brains do not think, hypothesise and decide, see and hear, ask and answer questions; rather, it makes no sense to ascribe such predicates *or their negations* to the brain. The brain neither sees, nor is it blind – just as sticks and stones are not awake, *but they are not asleep either*. The brain does not hear, but it is not deaf, any more than trees are deaf. The brain makes no decisions, but nor is it indecisive. Only what *can* decide can be indecisive. So, too, the brain cannot be conscious; only the living creature whose brain it is can be conscious – or unconscious. *The brain is not a logically appropriate subject for psychological predicates*
> (Bennett and Hacker 2003, p. 72, emphases in original).

Bennett and Hacker describe the mereological fallacy as a 'mutant' or 'degenerate' form of Cartesian dualism. Cartesian thinking applied psychological predicates to the mind, then secondarily to the human being: current neuroscience simply applies them to the brain. Their detailed examples of the mereological fallacy from the core fields of contemporary neuroscience (cognitive, affective, developmental, social, etc) show

how it is associated with errors of reasoning and interpretation and demonstrate its influence in the works of many of the major neuroscientists (e.g. Damasio 1994; Le Doux 1999) whose research informs the literature on psychotherapy and neuroscience. Perhaps unsurprisingly, then, the mereological fallacy sometimes permeates the literature reviewed here. For example, descriptions of symptoms were frequently juxtaposed with descriptions of the characteristics of neural systems, as though one were simply equivalent to the other. Similarly, therapeutic improvement was frequently re-described in neuroscientific language as the development of new (unspecified, unidentified) synaptic connections, or as hypothetical changes in relative activation between different brain systems and regions. But unless these moves to the language of neuroscience actually add explanatory force, this is mere neurobabble. Apart from the largely speculative character of these claims, the conceptual error is that we begin to imagine that neural change can simply be equated with therapeutic change, that it might somehow reveal its 'truth', perhaps independently of what people themselves can tell us. We see this in attempts to use imaging techniques as 'objective' outcome measures in psychotherapy (e.g. Linden 2006).

The mereological fallacy is also associated with dualism, reification, and biological reductionism. Treating the brain as though it has psychological characteristics creates the superficial appearance that mind–body dualism has been transcended, when in fact it simply pushes this dualism 'inside' the brain, throttling it down to the level of neurons and synapses—where it immediately re-appears as the 'hard problem' (Chalmers 1995) of how neural processes might be able to generate conscious state or qualia. Reification follows, because simply equating the brain with the person falsely shifts the full weight of explanatory attention to the neural level when it should also lie elsewhere. Similarly, equating the brain with the person is a form of reductionism that brackets off interpersonal and social explanations for psychological phenomena, rendering them entirely as context rather than constituent, and making emergent societal properties (Archer 1995) mysterious or invisible. In driving explanation down to the microscopic level, reductionism obliterates many of the nuanced distinctions persons effortlessly make in the conduct of everyday life. For example, even if we knew very much more about how brain processes enable the simple task of writing a signature, a *comprehensive* neural explanation would remain impossible because:

> no amount of neural knowledge would suffice to discriminate between writing one's name, copying one's name, practising one's signature, forging a name, writing an autograph, signing a cheque, witnessing a will, signing a death warrant, and so on … the differences between these are circumstance-dependent, functions not only of the individual's intentions but also of the social and legal conventions that must obtain to make the having of such intentions and the performance of such actions possible
>
> (Bennett and Hacker 2003 p. 360).

In the literature on psychotherapy and neuroscience reviewed here Folensbee's discussion of anxiety provides a good example of how the mereological fallacy leads to reification, reductionism and dualsim. Having reviewed evidence showing that anxiety functions as part of a monitoring system that 'scans' incoming stimuli for similarities with situations previously associated with negative experiences, he explains how this means that anxiety may also accompany new experiences, since novel stimuli cannot already be known to be safe. Then he goes on to claim:

> The connection between novelty and anxiety also helps explain why people feel 'at home' in maladaptive functioning and uncomfortable when functioning in new, more adaptive ways. It appears that the connection between novelty and anxiety can be so strong that remaining in abusive relationships is more bearable than taking steps to become more independent and therefore free of abuse
>
> (Folensbee 2007, p. 47).

We see here all of the interdependent problems that follow from taking a part (the anxiety system) for a whole (the person). This move reifies the complex and contingent fabric that constitutes contemporary human relationship choices (gendered power relations, life trajectories, interdependent relational meanings, social structures, material resources, legal and social conventions, moral codes, ethical practices, obligations, rights, responsibilities, etc.) as the outcome of a purely neural process. In substituting for this massive complexity (and the contingently interacting causal influences that flowing through it) the operation of a neural circuit, this reification is also a reduction. It erases the possibility of any explanation that includes both individuals and their social and material worlds, replacing it with a much abraded explanation solely at the neural level: consequently, it must ignore the fact that novelty is also frequently enjoyable. The explanation is also clearly dualistic: rather than exploring how the social and neural interpenetrate and are mutually co-constituted it simply replaces one with the other. It keeps the individual (neural systems) distinct from the social (relationships, conventions, commitments etc.), and in so doing potentially activates a series of other dualisms— between nature and culture, emotion and reason, and so on.

Vivona (2009b) provides a penetrating analysis of writings about the mirror neuron system and psychoanalysis that clearly shows how flawed reasoning can arise when neuroscientific work is allied to psychotherapy: although she does not draw upon Bennett and Hacker's work, her account evinces similar concerns with the errors that arise when we mistake parts for wholes. Noting the enthusiasm with which the concept of mirror neurons has been received, both within and outside of psychoanalysis, Vivona first cautions that human mirror neurons have still not been identified (her analysis was published before recent research that seems to confirm their existence (Mukamel et al. 2010)). Then she notes that, despite their name, mirror neurons do not actually 'mirror': they fire in response to a *range* of similar actions. Moreover, they only do so under certain conditions, and their firing is influenced by both development and context. Hence, the simplicity of the 'mirror' metaphor serves to mask important intentional and contextual complexity that this putative neural system alone could not contain (much as neural systems alone could not account for all of the possible variation in the meanings of writing a signature). Metaphors in neuroscience have great potential to mislead (Bennett and Hacker 2003, pp. 78-81).

Vivona describes how recent writings have popularized the idea that countertransference, projective identification, empathy, and unconscious communication might all be accounted for largely in terms of the operation of human mirror neurons, because 'the mirror neuron system enables an automatic, direct, accurate simulation of the other's experience' (Vivona 2009b, p. 530). She then identifies three assumptions that necessarily underpin this claim. First is the 'correspondence assumption': that brain activity is straightforwardly associated with mental activity, so that we can know what the mind is doing when we know what the brain is doing. Vivona argues that this assumption is empirically premature since many correspondences between brain activation and mental activities have yet to be established, and that all extant mirror neuron studies, including those with humans, measure brain activity but *not* mental activity. This necessarily means that 'a kind of circular reasoning is initiated, in which brain activity is taken as an empirical indication of a mental activity that has been inferred from it' (Vivona 2009b, p. 533). Thus, despite strong claims that human mirror neurons enable us to grasp the intentions of others and infer their goals, "cognitive processes such as 'grasping' and 'inferring' have not been assessed in mirror neuron studies with either humans or monkeys" (Vivona 2009b, p. 533).

The uptake of mirror neuron research in psychoanalysis also relies upon the 'shared experience assumption': that similar brain activity in two people, one of whom is observing the other, indicates similar internal experience. Yet Vivona observes that only one study (Schulte-Ruther et al. (2007)) has thus far assessed the extent to which observing the emotions of others induces similar emotions in observers, and its findings challenge the shared experience assumption. Participants were shown images of angry or fearful faces whilst subjected to fMRI (functional magnetic resonance imaging) scans; although the scans confirmed that putative human mirror neuron systems were being activated, participants frequently reported emotions incongruent with those they observed. Emotional responses to fearful expressions were either fearful or, alternately, compassionate; in response to angry expressions the majority of participants reported feeling 'attacked', 'uneasy', or 'uncomfortable'. Moreover, greater degree of emotional congruence in responding to the fearful faces were not accompanied by greater activation of the brain areas postulated to contain human mirror neurons.

The third assumption Vivona identifies in the psychotherapeutic uptake of mirror neuron research is the 'directness assumption': that the observer's brain activity provides direct access to the experience of the observed without any cognitive or linguistic mediation being needed. Challenging this, Vivona notes that there are studies showing that some degree of inference occurs when the mirror system is activated, and that for some neuroscientists this evidence is so strong that it 'inverts' the assumption of direct access and suggests that mirror neuron system activity is an outcome of understanding rather than its basis.

Thus, Vivona's analysis shows that there are problems with each of the three assumptions underpinning the simple equation of mirror neurons with psychotherapeutic empathy, countertransference and projective identification. Importantly, she is not opposed to neuroscience per se and remains convinced that information about the brain can and should inform therapeutic practice. Her analysis shows how the confusion of parts with wholes, persons with organisms, mirror neurons with intentional, aware, empathizing, co-present humans, produces errors with important implications for the ways in which mirror neuron research is taken up in psychotherapy. Whatever potentials neuroscience might hold for discursive psychotherapy, then, caution will always be needed.

Concluding thoughts

> 'I reckon that he is secretly sad about this' said Lucy, 'because I am sure that the wet patches I sometimes see on his pillow in the mornings are from tears.' I looked at Daniel, wondering whether or not he would confirm this. Suddenly I saw a tear surfacing at the corner of his eye. We all saw it. Daniel turned his head aside ... But things were never the same after this tear
>
> (White 2001, p. 3).

Speech is already embodied, feeling bodies generate meanings outwith linguistic representation, and—as this quotation shows—discursive psychotherapists do already recognise this in their practice. As we deploy discourses and construct narratives, our talking both recruits and is imbued with embodied meanings. In using discourses to position ourselves with respect to others, we enact moral stances and occupy discursive positions already bound up with regimes of affect; in using narratives to order our experience, we invoke layers of memory both explicit and implicit, both symbolic-discursive and affective-embodied. Speech is *always* the activity of embodied persons, continuously informed by the character, state and meanings of the body–brain system and thoroughly bound up with social relations and material influences; meaning is not just socially constructed, it is also co-constituted.

It has already been noted that the (predominantly) constructionist theories of discourse and narrative that underpin discursive psychotherapy largely fail to consider how extra-discursive influences contribute to the co-constitution of meaning and experience. The heated debate concerning relativism and discursive approaches in psychology (e.g. Edwards, Ashmore & Potter 1995; Hibberd 2001; McLennan 2001; Parker 1999) raised numerous concerns about the disregard of these influences, but did not resolve them; consequently, problems associated with their relative neglect continue to sporadically recur (e.g. Corcoran 2010; Potter 2010; Riley, Sims-Schouten & Willig 2007; Speer 2007). Their inadequate conceptualisation has already impacted upon discursive psychotherapeutic engagement with neuroscience: Beaudoin's (2005) narrative therapy paper about agency and choice following trauma references both Damasio and Cozolino, acknowledges the existence of multiple memory systems, and discusses both kinetic and sensory memory. Yet her discussion never develops these references in terms of the affective and embodied neural systems these two authors emphasise so strongly: consequently, sensory memories are treated predominantly as recall for *facts* about a traumatic event ("How many times did your body push him away?") and there is no consideration whatsoever of the affective, feelingful aspects of memory that are central to the work of both authors. Similarly, other narrative therapy accounts of the multiplicity of memory (e.g. White 2004) acknowledge autobiographical, semantic, procedural, episodic and short-term memories, but don't also grant recognition to memories that are felt and affective.

So it seems that a more sophisticated conceptualisation of speech, a move from social construction to co-constitution, is necessary for discursive psychotherapy to engage adequately with neuroscience. Making this move would yield the additional benefit of facilitating engagement with the other exciting intellectual developments that are currently occurring in relation to each of the themes discernable in the literature on psychotherapy and neuroscience. For example, with respect to embodied knowing there are numerous strands of contemporary scholarship foregrounding the contribution of the body to meaning, talking and thinking, and even cognitive psychologists are now beginning to engage with what are being called embodied, enactive or situated cognitive processes (Anderson 2003). Johnson (2007) provides an interesting recent account of embodied knowing that implicates sensori-motor processing, and Shotter's work has long emphasised the body's contribution to social life and meaning, as does my own recent work concentrating on feelings which—with relevance to psychotherapy—includes conceptualisations of both misery (Cromby 2004) and paranoia (Cromby & Harper 2009) as socially-induced feeling states.

Recent years have also seen the rise of memory studies, an interdisciplinary engagement with the social, cultural, political and technological aspects of remembering and forgetting. Some of this work is directly relevant to discursive psychotherapy. For example, Middleton & Brown (2005) present discursive analyses of remembering within a novel conceptual frame primarily derived from two sources: Bergson's account of memory as 'always on', always swelling and 'gnawing' into the present; and Halbwach's account of the ways in which memories are both localised and emplaced with respect to material objects and social settings. Their framework has been applied to memories of child abuse and trauma, both to analyse agency (Reavey & Brown 2007) and discuss the tensions between the veridicality of such memories, on the one hand, and the variability of their situated discursive deployment on the other (Reavey & Brown 2006).

Finally, with respect to affect interest is currently so sustained and widespread that in some quarters an 'affective turn' is being proclaimed (e.g. Athanasiou, Hantzaroula & Yannakopoulos 2008; Blackman & Cromby, 2007; Clough & Halley 2007). Whilst historically the human and social sciences have always been interested in the affective, what is currently distinctive is both the acceleration of interest in affect, emotion and feeling and their conceptualisation as co-constituted hybrids, neither simply biological nor wholly social. The affective turn is itself informed by neuroscience, but also mobilises concepts from psychoanalysis (Walkerdine 2010), Deleuzian philosophy (Massumi 1995) and Tompkins' emotion theory (Sedgewick 2003). In addition to the generic relevance for psychotherapy of engagement with feelings and emotions, recent scholarship associated with this emergent trend has discussed aspects of psychotherapeutic clinical work (Brennan 2004), presented analyses of trauma (Clough 2010; Walkerdine 2010), and explored the experiences of people given diagnoses of schizophrenia (Tucker 2010).

To conclude: discursive psychotherapy's future development would be enhanced by considering a more sophisticated notion of speech that explicitly conceptualises the felt, the affective and the embodied. This would facilitate an enriching engagement with multiple areas of relevant scholarship: not just neuroscience, but also memory studies, embodied meaning and cognition, and affect. Ultimately, this advance from social construction to co-constitution might produce a version of the discursive psychotherapies that comprehensively conceptualises both power relations and social and material influences (Smail 2005). It might enable therapists to conceptualise far more adequately the *totality* of distressing experiences: consequently, it would more effectively facilitate the generation of narratives that are both adaptive to the lived circumstances of clients and oriented meaningfully towards the futures that they might occupy.

References

Anderson, M. (2003). Embodied Cognition: a field guide. *Artificial Intelligence,* **149**(1), 91–130.

Archer, M. (1995). *Realist Social Theory: the morphogenetic approach.* Cambridge University Press, Cambridge.

Athanasiou, A., Hantzaroula, P., and Yannakopoulos, Y., . (2008). Towards a New Epistemology: the "affective turn". *Historein,* **8,** 5–16.

Atkinson, B., Atkinson, L., Kutz, P., et al. (2005). Rewiring neural states in couples therapy: advances from affective neuroscience. *Journal of Systemic Therapies,* **24**(3), 3–16.

Beaudoin, M. (2005). Agency and choice in the face of trauma: a narrative therapy map. *Journal of Systemic Therapies,* **24**(4), 32–50.

Beaumont, J. G., Kenealy, P. M., and Rogers, M. J. C. (1996). *The Blackwell Dictionary of Neuropsychology.* Blackwells, Oxford.

Bennett, M. R. and Hacker, P. M. S. (2003). *Philosophical Foundations of Neuroscience.* Blackwells, Oxford.

Blackman, L., and Cromby, J. (2008). Affect and Feeling. *International Journal of Critical Psychology,* **21,** 5–22.

Borod, J., Cicero, B., Obler, L., Welkowitz, J., Erhan, H., Santschi, C., et al. (1998). Right-hemisphere emotional perception: evidence across multiple channels. *Neuropsychology,* **12**(3), 446–58.

Brennan, T. (2004). *The Transmission of Affect,* Cornell University Press, Ithaca, New York.

Brewin, C. (2001). Memory processes in post-traumatic stress disorder. *International Review of Psychiatry,* **13,** 159–63.

Brown, S. D., Reavey, P., Cromby, J., Harper, D., and Johnson, K. (2009). Embodiment, Methodology, Process. In J. Latimer and M. Schillmeier (Eds.) *Knowing/Unknowing Bodies.* Blackwell, Oxford.

Cappas, N., Andres-Hyman, R., and Davidson, L. (2005). What psychotherapists can begin to learn from neuroscience: seven principles of a brain-based psychotherapy. *Psychology and Psychotherapy: theory, research and practice,* **42**(3), 374–83.

Chalmers, D. (1995). Facing up to the problem of consciousness. *Journal of Consciousness Studies,* **2**(3), 200–19.

Clough, P. (2010). Praying and playing to the beat of a child's metronome. *Subjectivity,* **3**(4), 349–65.

Clough, P. and Halley, J. (Eds.) (2007). *The Affective Turn: theorising the social.* Duke University Press, Durham NC.

Corcoran, T. (2010). What else life if not awkward? *British Journal of Social Psychology,* **49**(4), 679–84.

Cozolino, L. (2002). *The Neuroscience of Psychotherapy.* W.W.Norton, New York.

Cromby, J. (2004). Between constructionism and neuroscience: the societal co-constitution of embodied subjectivity. *Theory and Psychology,* **14**(6), 797–821.

Cromby, J. (2007a). Integrating social science with neuroscience: potentials and problems. *Biosocieties,* **2**(2), 149–70.

Cromby, J. (2007b). Toward a psychology of feeling. *International Journal of Critical Psychology,* **21,** 94–118.

Cromby, J. and Harper, D. (2009). Paranoia: a social account. *Theory and Psychology,* **19**(3), 335–51.
Crossley, M. (2000). *Introducing Narrative Psychology.* Open University Press, Buckingham.
Damasio, A. R. (1994). *Descartes Error: emotion, reason and the human brain.* London: Picador.
Damasio, A. R. (1999). *The Feeling of What Happens: body, emotion and the making of consciousness.* William Heinemann, London.
Damasio, A. R. (2003). *Looking for Spinoza: joy, sorrow and the feeling brain.* Harvest, Orlando.
Ecker, B. and Toomey, B. (2008). Depotentiation of symptom-producing implicit memory in coherence therapy. *Journal of Constructivist Psychology,* **21**(2), 87–150.
Edwards, D., Ashmore, M., and Potter, J. (1995). Death and furniture: the rhetoric, politics and theology of bottom-line arguments against relativism. *History of the Human Sciences,* **8**, 25–49.
Fairclough, N. (2005). Critical discourse analysis. *Marges Linguistiques,* **9**, 76–94.
Folensbee, R. (2007). *The Neuroscience of Psychological Therapies.* Cambridge University Press, Cambridge.
Fonagy, P. (2004). Psychotherapy meets neuroscience: a more focused future for psychotherapy research. *Psychiatric Bulletin,* **28**, 357–59.
Foucault, M. (1977). *Discipline and Punish.* Penguin, Harmondsworth.
Freeman, M. (1993). *Rewriting the Self: history, memory, narrative.* Routledge, London.
Gallese, V., Eagle, M., and Migone, P. (2007). Intentional Attunement: Mirror Neurons and the Neural Underpinnings of Interpersonal Relations. *Journal of the American Psychoanalytic Association,* **55**(1), 131–75.
Gallese, V. and Goldman, A. (1998). Mirror neurons and the simulation theory of mind-reading. *Trends in Cognitive Sciences,* **2**(12), 493–501.
Gazzaniga, M. S. (1998). Principles of human brain organisation derived from split-brain studies. *Neuron,* **14**, 217–28.
Gazzaniga, M. S. (2009). *The Cognitive Neurosciences* (4th ed.). MIT Press, Cambridge, MA.
Gazzaniga, M. S. (2000). *The Mind's Past.* University of California Press, Berkeley.
Goswami, U. (2004). Neuroscience and Education. *British Journal of Educational Psychology,* **74**, 1–14.
Haidt, J. (2003). The Moral Emotions, in RJ Davidson, K Scherer & H Goldsmith (eds). *Handbook of Affective Sciences*, Oxford University Press, Oxford, pp. 852–70.
Harmon-Jones, E. and Winkielman, P. (2007). *Social Neuroscience.* Guilford Press, New York.
Harré, R. (1992). The second cognitive revolution. *American Behavioural Scientist,* **36**, 3–7.
Harré, R. (2002). *Cognitive Science: a philosophical introduction.* Sage Publications, London.
Hebb, D. (1949). *The Organisation of Behaviour.* Wiley, New York.
Hepburn, A. (2003). *An Introduction to Critical Social Psychology.* Sage Publications, London.
Johnson, M. (2007). *The Meaning of the Body: aesthetics of human understanding.* University of Chicago Press, Chicago.
Joseph, J. (2003). *The Gene Illusion: genetic research in psychiatry and psychology under the microscope.* PCCS Books, Ross on Wye.
Hibberd, F. (2001). Relativism versus realism: all-but a specious dichotomy. *History of the Human Sciences,* **14**(3), 102–7.
Kenwood, C. (1999). Social constructionism: implications for psychotherapeutic practice. In D. J. Nightingale and J. Cromby (Eds.) *Social Constructionist Psychology: a critical analysis of theory and practice.* Open University Press, Buckingham.

Laclau, E. and Mouffe, C. (1985). *Hegemony and Socialist Strategy.* Verso, London.

Le Doux, J. (1999). *The Emotional Brain.* Phoenix, London.

Leder, D. (1990). *The Absent Body.* University of Chicago Press, Chicago, IL.

Linden, D. (2006). How psychotherapy changes the brain–the contribution of functional neuroimaging. *Molecular Psychiatry,* 11, 528–38.

Lipchik, E., Becker, M., Brasher, B., Derks, J., and Volkmann, J. (2005). Neuroscience: a new direction for solution-focused thinkers? *Journal of Systemic Therapies,* 24(3), 49–69.

Manteufel, A. (2005). Chromosomen non est omen: on the relationship between neurobiology and psychotherapy. *Journal of Systemic Therapies,* 24(3), 70–88.

Massumi, B. (2002). *Parables for the Virtual: movement, affect, sensation.* Duke University Press, Durham.

McLennan, G. (2001). 'Thus': reflections on Loughborough relativism. *History of the Human Sciences,* 14(3), 85–101.

Middleton, D. and Brown, S. D. (2005). *The Social Psychology of Experience: studies in remembering and forgetting.* Sage Publications, London.

Mukamel, R., Ekstrom, A., Kaplan, J., Iacoboni, M., and Fried, I. (2010). Single-Neuron Responses in Humans during Execution and Observation of Actions *Current Biology,* 20(8), 750–6.

Nolan, C. (Writer) (2000). *Memento.* Newmarket Films, USA.

Panksepp, J. (1998). *Affective Neuroscience.* Oxford University Press, Oxford.

Parker, I. (1999). Against relativism in psychology, on balance. *History of the Human Sciences,* 12(4), 61–78.

Potter, J. (2010). Contemporary discursive psychology: issues, prospects and Corcoran's awkward ontology. *British Journal of Social Psychology,* 49(4), 657–78.

Potter, J. and Wetherell, M. (1987). *Discourse and Social Psychology: beyond attitudes and behaviour.* Sage Publications, London.

Reavey, P. and Brown, S. D. (2006). Transforming Past Agency and Action in the Present: time, social remembering and child sexual abuse. *Theory and Psychology,* 16(2), 179–202.

Reavey, P. and Brown, S. D. (2007). The embodiment and spaces of memory: child sexual abuse and the construction of agency. *Journal of Social Work Practice,* 21(4), 213–29.

Riley, S., Sims-Schouten, W., and Willig, C. (2007). The Case for Critical Realist Discourse Analysis as a Viable Method in Discursive Work. *Theory and Psychology,* 17(1), 137–45.

Roder, B. and Neville, H. (2003). Developmental functional plasticity. In J. Grafman and I. Robertson (Eds.), *Handbook of Neuropsychology* (2nd ed.). Elsevier Science, Oxford.

Rose, N. (2001). The politics of life itself. *Theory, Culture and Society,* 18(6), 1–30.

Rose, N. (2005). Becoming Neurochemical Selves. http://www.lse.ac.uk/collections/sociology/pdf/Rose-BecomingNeurochemicalSelves.pdf [Accessed 4 December 2006.]

Rose, N. and Rabinow, P. (2006). Biopower Today. *Biosocieties,* 1, 195–217.

Rose, S. (1997). *Lifelines: life beyond the gene.* Oxford University Press, Oxford.

Ruthrof, H. (1997). *Semantics and the Body.* University of Toronto Press, Toronto.

Schore, A. (2001). The effects of early relational trauma on right brain development, affect regulation, and infant mental health. *Infant Mental Health Journal,* 22(1), 201–69.

Sedgewick, E. (2003). *Touching Feeling: affect, pedagogy, performativity.* Duke University Press, Durham.

Seltzer, W. (2005). Pre-cognitive therapy: a way to integrate neuroscience and psychotherapy. *Journal of Systemic Therapies,* 24(3), 32–48.

Schulte-Ruther, M., Markowitsch, H. J., Fink, G. R., and Piefke, M. (2007). Mirror neuron and theory of mind mechanisms involved in face-to-face interactions: A functional magnetic resonance imaging approach to empathy. *Journal of Cognitive Neuroscience,* **19**, 1354–72.

Shilling, C. (2003). *The Body and Social Theory* (2nd ed.). Sage Publications, London.

Shotter, J. (1993). *Conversational realities: constructing life through language.* Sage Publications, London.

Smail, D. J. (2005). *Power, interest and psychology: elements of a social materialist understanding of distress.* PCCS Books, Ross-On-Wye.

Solms, M. and Turnbull, O. (2002). *The brain and the inner world: an introduction to the neuroscience of subjective experience.* Other Press, New York.

Speer, S.. (2007). On recruiting conversation analysis for critical realist purposes. *Theory and Psychology,* **17**(1), 125–35.

Stam, H. (1998). The body's psychology and psychology's body. In H. Stam (Ed.) *The Body and Psychology*, pp. 1–12. Sage Publications, London.

Szucs, D. and Goswami, U. (2007). Educational neuroscience: defining a new discipline for the study of mental representations. *Mind, Brain and Education,* **1**(3), 114–27.

Toomey, B. and Ecker, B. (2007). Of neurons and knowings: constructivism, coherence psychology and their neurodynamic substrates. *Journal of Constructivist Psychology,* **20**(3), 201–45.

Toomey, B. and Ecker, B. (2009). Competing Visions of the Implications of Neuroscience for Psychotherapy. *Journal of Constructivist Psychology,* **22**(2), 95–140.

Trappenberg, T. (2009). *Fundamentals of Computational Neuroscience.* Oxford University Press, Oxford.

Tucker, I. (2010). Mental health service user territories: Enacting 'safe spaces' in the community. *Health,* **14**(4), 434–48.

van Ommen, C. (2005). Damasio's Subject: constructions of self in contemporary neuroscience. Paper presented at the International Society for Theoretical Psychology Conference, 20–24 June, Cape Town.

Vivona, J. (2009a). Embodied language in neuroscience and psychoanalysis. *Journal of the American Psychoanalytic Association,* **57**, 1327–57.

Vivona, J. (2009b). Leaping from brain to mind: a critique of mirror neuron explanations of countertransference. *Journal of the American Psychoanalytic Association,* **57**, 525–50.

Walkerdine, V. (2010). Communal beingness and affect: an exploration of trauma in an ex-industrial community. *Body and Society,* **16**(1), 91–116.

Wendell, S. (1996). *The Rejected Body: feminist philosophical reflections on disability.* Routledge, London.

White, M. (1991). Deconstruction and Therapy. *Dulwich Centre Newsletter,* **1**, 6–46.

White, M. (2001). Narrative practice and the unpacking of identity conclusions. *Gecko: a journal of deconstruction and narrative ideas in therapeutic practice,* **1**, 28–55.

White, M. (2004). Working with people who are suffering the consequences of multiple trauma. *International Journal of Narrative Therapy and Community Work,* **1**, 47–75.

Wilson, E. A. (2004). *Psychosomatic: feminism and the neurological body.* Duke University Press, Durham/London.

Chapter 17

Conversation and its therapeutic possibilities

Tom Strong

> To arrest the meanings of words once and for all, that is what Terror wants
> *Toward the postmodern*, Jean-Francois Lyotard (1993, p. 87).

At a conference in the early 1990s a speaker commented that, if one had problems with their car's functioning they should go to a mechanic, but if there were malfunctions with their thinking, feeling, or behaving they should come to see psychiatrists like him. The comment evoked many conflicting feelings I had about mental health practice at the time. Reassuringly and arrogantly, this psychiatrist articulated patients' complex problems with an easy to understand mechanical metaphor. Hopeless with machines myself, I had come to regard expert mechanics with amazement. Hearing an odd ping or a seemingly imperceptible timing issue, they seemed to know exactly what next to do, and, sure enough, I'd be back on the road. A recently graduated counselling psychologist, I wanted to be as helpful to my patients as these mechanics, and this psychiatrist told me that this was what he could do. Psychotherapy had become home to over 350 approaches to helping distraught patients. Surely, there was a parsimonious, if not correct, way to understand and help patients.

Part of the conflict I was having with what I'd heard was with the speaker's mechanic metaphor. A few years earlier I recall the cybernetician, Heinz von Foerster (1981), warning that social scientists too often had approached humans as if they were 'trivial machines'. However, the 1990s were also the 'decade of the brain' in North America, purportedly so that the brain's 'inner workings' could be expertly understood (as sophisticated machines?) and thus rendered therapeutically (mechanically?) modifiable. At the same time as this thrust in mental health was occurring, I joined many therapists who were being drawn to exciting new 'postmodern' ideas and practices. Narrative (see Chamberlain, Chapter 6), solution-focused (see Duffy, Chapter 9; Miller and McKergow, Chapter 9) and collaborative (see Levin and Bava, Chapter 7) approaches had become psychotherapy's 'third wave' as one prominent journal for therapists put it (O'Hanlon 1994). The premises and promises of these approaches were starkly at odds with the mechanic metaphor.

'Postmodern' has not been a helpful word in conveying what these new approaches to therapy are about. At their heart is a different view of how language use features in human problems and solutions than the view of the psychiatrist-as-mechanic above. Human problems were not seen as reducible to medically diagnosable and treatable symptoms or deficits, for starters. Conversations between therapists and patients took on seemingly new constructive and deconstructive potentials. How the concerns of therapy were named and understood was linked, in these approaches, to the stories, discourses and problem-organized conversations that had given and sustained their meaning. Therapists, accordingly, welcomed these lived meanings, stories, discourses, and conversations while inviting reflection upon them—as transformable forms of 'linguistic or discursive capture'. By linguistic or discursive capture, we refer to people conducting their lives within the taken-for-granted constraints of stories, discourses, or conversational patterns to which they have become accustomed or resigned. Thus, people don't just understand concerns in linguistic constructions, like words, stories and metaphors; their actions are typically informed by these constructions as if they were the only way to go forward. Pragmatically-oriented discursive therapists invite patients into conversations that transcend the limits of linguistically-fed understandings and discursively-patterned ways of interacting. Borrowing the pithy language of Wittgenstein (1958), they differently use language to help patients find new ways of 'going on'.

Just over a decade ago, the nearly forgotten Y2K problem confounded computer engineers, with dire predictions made for a planet that had increasingly come to rely on computers. This was a classic case of humans possibly becoming ensnared by their own constructions. Arguably, the most taken-for-granted human construction is language and how it gets put to use. Inside a particular story or discursive pattern one's lived experience is very real. Try telling a social democrat or conservative that their take on the world is incorrect. The discursive issue has been this binary of correct/incorrect understanding when evidence abounds that people get by just fine using very different languages—often for similar challenges in life, such as electing a government or conducting a spiritual life. In psychiatry or mental health this issue has been huge: is the field served best by a single language for representing patients' presenting concerns, such as the very controversial DSM-V (Frances 2010; Watters 2010); or many, culturally and phenomenologically sensitive languages? Again, the problem is with the binary implied by the last sentence's 'or'. The chief insight of the discursive approaches to therapy is that the languages used to represent our projects, experiences, and each other do more than inform; they animate those projects, experiences and characterizations in particularly human ways. What is postmodern about these therapeutic approaches is their struggle with the notion that the realms of human experience brought to therapy can be ultimately understandable in some language that is more than a social construction. What is discursive about these therapies is that they use conversational interaction to reflect upon and transcend the limits of language—the best language both therapist and patient can agree on, and collaborate from, without tying their dialogues to a 'correct' language.

There is a collaborative and pragmatic ethos evident in the conversations of most discursive therapists and patients (Anderson 1997; Levin and Bava, Chapter 7). A focus on collaboration can raise questions as to what is the nature of the expertise that therapists bring to such conversations (Strong 2002) if not to correctly name patients' concerns and direct their actions accordingly. Presumably, patients seek professional assistance for something they cannot come up with themselves. However, it would be a mistake to regard this kind of assistance-seeking as equating to patient assent to taking up a normal deferential role as provider of information so they can be directed by therapists. Discursive therapists, as we've seen, rely on patients to be shapers of the therapeutic process, inviting the patient's preferences and understandings, as they negotiate a shared therapeutic direction. This kind of therapeutic engagement, a kind of dialogic partnership, aims to flexibly catalyse the resources of both patient and therapist, as they talk new possibilities 'into being' (Heritage 1984). Differences occur between the therapeutic approaches over the extent to which the process needs to be structured in advance, in particular maps of practice (White 2007) or language games (de Shazer 1994), or more simply, in generative conversations unlike those the patient has been having with himself and others (Anderson 1997). Missing in each of these therapeutic conversations is a therapist prerogative for correctly diagnosing problems or prescribing interventions from such diagnoses. Instead, what makes these therapeutic conversations collaborative are the efforts to work from patient-agreed-to meanings in a customized and negotiated process.

Much of what discursive therapists say sounds well and good for that sizeable proportion of mental health patients who fit the category of 'worried well'. Where the harder questions arise is in considering patients who present with more severe concerns of a chronic or debilitating symptomatic nature. Regardless of the stance taken by therapists on the DSM-IV-TR or the ICD-10 psychiatric diagnoses, most therapists concede that some patient concerns are more intractable or incapacitating than others. It can be frustrating for newcomers to the discursive therapies to read of the work with little or no reference to the normal diagnostic categories central to most clinical case or efficacy studies. Similarly, the interventions of the discursive therapies do not conform with the normal manualized approaches one finds, for example, in studies involving use of cognitive therapy. This makes claims of helpfulness suspect to readers accustomed to randomized controlled trials. Indeed, as we read in the chapter by Chenail and olleagues (Chapter 13), evaluation of the discursive therapies is scant and very recent. Understandably, newcomers to the discursive therapies seek some assurance that discursive approaches to therapy can address recognizable forms of patient suffering, while being wary of where such approaches may be contraindicated. However, the expert diagnostic language that makes such suffering recognisable to many therapists is pretty much avoided by discursive therapists who prefer instead to work within patients' languages for problems and solutions. Such an approach poses similar challenges for person-centred therapists, though some now turn to rigorous case study evaluations of their work (e.g. McLeod and Elliott, 2011). Still, the non-discursive therapist can feel sceptical when reading Michael White's (1984) narrative family therapy case study in successfully overcoming 'sneaky poo' (i.e. encopresis). But, where is the proof that the discursive therapies make a difference in patients' lives beyond such case studies?

Some of this dearth of evaluation studies of discursive approaches to therapy relates to issues raised by Busch (Chapter 14) in his chapter on psychotherapy evaluation research. Discursive therapists often share a deep suspicion about scientific claims and research, particularly evaluative research that aims to control for the very conditions that resemble frontline clinical practice with varied patient concerns. A 'politics of evidence' (Larner 2004) has emerged over what should count as proof that therapy is helpful, as researchers grapple with questions like: can therapeutic interventions be evaluated for effectiveness in the same manner as drugs (Stiles and Shapiro 1989)? Excesses from the research side of the evidence-based practice movement have conveyed a sense that scientifically warranted therapy entails therapists' close adherence to diagnostic protocols; and (once a diagnosis is correctly obtained) similar adherence to intervention protocols (Gabbay and Le May 2011). Such a scripted approach makes therapy easier to evaluate in randomized clinical trials, but can encroach on the very elements of therapy that our contributors would describe as 'discursive'. Instead, discursive therapy tends toward a more improvised and unpredictable dialogue where the conversational and other resources of patient and therapist are pitted against patient concerns. However, such unpredictable dialogues using patient-preferred language defies what is conventionally required to rigorously evaluate discursive therapies as interventions. So, the evidence of their effectiveness remains slim.

A recent controversy for discursive and other therapists occurred when the Blair government in the UK announced it would adopt Lord Layard's cultural prescription for more economy-enhancing happiness by exclusively investing in increased cognitive-behavioural therapy (CBT) services (Layard 2006). This announcement was defended because only CBT had scientific evidence to support its use. However, a national outcry by therapists and mental health organizations arose, and a government retraction followed (Prime Minister's Office, May 7, 2008). While CBT is particularly well-suited for conventional psychotherapy effectiveness research and Layard's cultural prescription, various concerns follow for discursive and other therapists (e.g. House and Loewenthal 2009).

Health sociologist, Nikolas Rose (e.g. 1990) has ominously referred to such intersections of government policy and psychological knowledge and practice as the 'psy complex'. By such a Foucaultian view, psychological knowledge is translated into a cultural apparatus (Agamben 2007) for producing and ensuring the production of particular kinds of human beings and interactions. People's mental health, according to this managerialism, can be correctly understood, and from such correct understandings interventions and evaluative practices can be used to guide or restore them to mental health. This extends to people's appropriation of such knowledge to use in 'governing' themselves 'appropriately' (Rose 1990). Discursive therapists take issue with this view of being human and of mental health practice, and often invite patients to critically reflect upon how such forms of knowledge can play constraining roles on governing personal as well as therapeutic behavior (Parker 1999). Critical psychologists and psychiatrists (Ingleby 1981; Szasz 2007) have long taken up these themes in asking therapists to help patients look beyond merely adapting to what has been taken for granted in their lives. Discursive therapists, particularly social therapists (Holzman and Newman, Chapter 10) and narrative therapists (Chamberlain, Chapter 6), invite these kinds of political challenges into therapeutic dialogue, and do so by inviting critical reflection on what patients understood and act on as 'taken for granted'. At a minimum, many discursive therapists are concerned about being complicit in dominant social understandings practices, and they are often very active in contesting such practices inside the consulting room and beyond it (e.g. Maniapoto, Chapter 12; Waldegrave, Chapter 11).

Behind the rising popularity of the discursive therapies are some important conceptual resources that have largely been ignored in the dominant story of psychotherapy's development. Through a historical focus on the basic activity of therapy—conversations between therapists and patients—therapy's development can be recast in discursive terms (see Shawver, Chapter 2). However, the social constructionist, or discursive, psychotherapy story is quite recent and draws from sources as diverse as hermeneutics, linguistic philosophy, social phenomenology, postcolonial and feminist thought, ethnomethodology, and discourse theory (Lock and Strong 2010). It is the breadth and hybrid potentials of these conceptual resources that sees contemporary discursive therapies rapidly diversifying and innovating some of the more traditional approaches to psychotherapy, such as psychoanalysis (Stern 2009) or cognitive therapy (Lyddon 1995). McNamee (2004) referred, in jest, to this diversification and hybridizing as a kind of 'promiscuity'. While the most commonly recognized discursive therapies (narrative, solution-focused, collaborative and social therapies) are represented in this volume, none of them existed by their current names thirty years ago. And, these discursive therapies continue to innovate, by drawing from new conceptual resources, as in the case of Miller and McKergow's chapter (Chapter 9) that brings together solution-focused therapy with complexity theory, or in narrative therapy's adoption of 'positioning theory' (Chamberlain, Chapter 6). Resourceful horizons of conceptual and therapeutic possibility continue to emerge, each pointing to new ways of being (Badiou 2007).

A welcomed request from our editors at Oxford University Press was for us to include writing on developments in neuroscience and how these relate to the discursive therapies. Each new promising development in psychiatry seems to hold the potential of making therapeutic dialogue irrelevant. A growing literature has developed that equates brain parts and brain functions with particular human outcomes, positive and negative (e.g. Armstrong and Morrow, 2010; Beaudoin, 2010). Like earlier artificial intelligence (i.e. computer) metaphors for human cognition, one can feel brought back to the psychiatrist-as-mechanic mentioned at the start of this chapter. Verbs like processing and transmitting convey a metaphoric and Cartesian sense that human capacities and difficulties can best be understood in terms of functional brain processes and hardware. This is a very different conception of mind and meaningful engagement than that proposed by thinkers like Bateson (1980) or Heidegger (e.g. Bracken, 2002). Differences over what neuroscience has to offer psychology and psychological forms of help were recently subjected to a top-drawer philosophical debate (Bennett et al. 2007). Wittgenstein scholar, Peter Hacker, took the view that neuroscientists too often anthropomorphize parts of the brain in what he refers to as the 'mereological fallacy'—a predilection for equating brain part X with behaviour Y, as if X holds the intention and executive capacity to enact Y. In this book we've featured two chapters which examine the role that neuroscientific information might play in discursive therapist judgement (Cromby, Chapter 16; Duffy, Chapter 15). The gist seems less that the brain is a repairable machine, and more on what it takes to engage those aspects of brain functioning facilitative of change. Seldom would discursive therapists and social constructionists conflate the words mind and brain, however. Instead, they more typically relate notions of mind, and by extension, change, to socio-cultural processes (Harré and Gillett, 1994; Vygotsky 1978; Wertsch 1998; Williams 2002) that extend well beyond what occurs inside one's cranium. Very different notions of therapeutic engagement and change follow from adopting the view that brains are the problem than from viewing mind as a coordination of patient-relevant discursive, cultural, and phenomenological factors.

We are fortunate to have had three of the most important theoretical contributors to the development of the discursive therapies offer important chapters to this volume that extend that development well into the future. Rom Harré, John Shotter, and Ken Gergen have played key roles in not only integrating discursive ideas from thinkers as diverse as Wittgenstein, Goffman, Foucault, Bakhtin, and Gadamer; they have been calling into question the understanding of science that has grounded mainstream psychological thought for some time (e.g. Gergen 1973; Harré and Secord 1972; Shotter 1975). In some respects, today's approaches to the discursive therapies were made possible by the insights and critiques Gergen, Harré, and Shotter courageously brought to mainstream psychology. Their chapters here do far more than provide the conceptual underpinnings for the discursive therapies as we currently know them, they map out large new territories in which discursive practices can continue to develop, including into arenas like organizational development, international dispute resolution, and embodied relational practices. Each of these authors remains prolific in furthering the conceptual boundaries and resources discursive therapists can turn to in further developing their conversational practices (e.g. Gergen 2009; Shotter 2010; Tan et al. 2010).

Therapeutic conversation itself is seen in different ways compared to how it is regarded in most therapeutic approaches. The notion that therapist and patient are information-swappers and processors is replaced by a reflexive and participatory view of dialogue. Questions become interventions (e.g. Tomm 1988) for what they can bring forth as understandings and commitments to action—and for the understandings and actions they ignore. What matters to discursive therapists is how patients can be actively engaged in meaning construction, meanings that they are willing to take away and act on. Thus, considerable attention is given to how this conversational engagement can avoid therapist impositions or exclusions of meaning (e.g. Strong and Sutherland, 2007; Weingarten 1992). A greater focus is given to the rhetorical and relational performance of therapeutic dialogue; to the 'conversational realities' (Shotter 1993; Chapter 5) created from patient and therapist interactions. Discursive therapists want to use therapeutic discourse to intervene in the everyday problem-discourses patients present (Maranhao 1986), and they recognize that this involves close coordination of preferred conversational developments with patients.

Two of the animating principles guiding discursive therapists can be traced back to the 18th-century philologist, Giambattista Vico (1744/1999). Vico's writing presaged some key modern/postmodern debates in attempting to make clear the need for sciences of being human that did not fit the ascending Newtonian scientific paradigm. In particular, Vico wrote of a need for 'poetic wisdom'; to be mindful that many challenges in life required more than the kinds of formulaic response modern science could provide. A second and related principle is what Vico called, 'linguistic poverty'; circumstances where language comes up short for people who use it in naming their concerns and addressing them. The modern view that people's problems can be correctly named and addressed plays right into Vico's concerns. Had scientists continued to be guided only by the Newtonian paradigm, they and the rest of humanity would have failed to benefit from the kinds of conceptual and other resources afforded by the paradigmatic revolution brought on by Einstein (Kuhn 1962).

Implicit in the discursive therapies is a human and relational science that is playing catch-up, but it probably will be a science that won't deliver the kinds of knowledge the basic sciences supply to engineering. Concurrent with the increasing popularity of the discursive therapies has been a proliferation of new qualitative research methods, best illustrated in the near doubling of the field's most popular handbook (Denzin and Lincoln 1994, 2011). As with the growth of the discursive therapies, a postmodern and social constructionist impetus has driven the development of new research methods; each asking different questions, and seeking different kinds of answers than had been associated with most social science up until a generation ago (Crotty 1998). Indeed, there have been purposeful conflations of research methods and therapeutic or developmental intentions. The field of action research brings together similarly interested and concerned people in transforming the understandings and circumstances shaping their lives (Cooperrrider and Whitney 2005; Waldegrave, Chapter 11). This is a very different kind of 'science' than the kind that aims to objectively know a phenomenon first, so that the knowledge gained can be used in informing later change initiatives. What is to be made of the questions that discursive therapists or discursively oriented researchers ask people that invite previously unconsidered answers those people prefer and see themselves capable of acting on? What can the findings of discursive methods of research offer discursive and other therapists?

Discursive research seems to primarily cleave what transpires in people's communicative interactions in a fundamental way. On one side are those concerned with power and what gets marginalized in interpersonal and cultural dialogues, a macro-view of discourse in which the aim is to expose how particular discourses have dominated, so that consideration of alternative discourses is made possible. This view is central to the Foucaultian ideas informing narrative therapy (Chamberlain, Chapter 6; Madigan 1992) where the effects of dominant stories and narratives are linked to how problems are understood and enacted. Once such dominance is exposed then alternative choices of narratives and discourses become possible. This critical, deconstructive conversational work is done in therapy, but also features in critical discourse analyses where a focus on dominant cultural discourses invites consideration of more preferred and emancipating alternatives (e.g. Fairclough 1992). There is also, on the other side, a micro-focus on the pragmatics of people's turn-taking in conversation that informs conversation analysis and the production of, for example, solution-talk over problem talk (e.g. Gale and Lawless 2004). The micro-discursive focus is on the use of conversational practices for what they elicit or sustain, while the macro-discursive focus is on the cultural discourses and stories people use as resources for shared understanding and action. Until recently, these taken-for-granted dimensions of understanding and social interaction were largely ignored for two reasons. First, when the dominant belief has been that the world can be understood and talked about in a correct way, then alternatives to that correct way are distortions and best ignored. Second, if talking with someone is about information swapping and processing, then the rhetorical aspects of talking for social influence also becomes a distortion. Discursive research and therapy take their cue from the later Wittgenstein (1958): that a focus on correct language for understanding and interaction idealizes language in a particular way not reflected in the everyday uses people make of language in different forms of life. What matters are uses of language that help people get by when faced by the challenges of everyday life. Thus, both discursive approaches to therapy, and to research, focus on helping people 'go on', to overcome Vico's 'linguistic poverty'.

Inside the different discursive therapies, as with most other approaches to therapy, there are what Bakhtin (1981) referred to as centripetal and centrifugal tendencies. On the centripetal side are those who seek consolidation and standardization of the approaches, in maps (White 2007) or protocols (de Shazer 1988). On the centrifugal side, one finds hybrids (e.g. Ecker and Hulley 1995; Eron and Lund, 1994) and whole new approaches catalysed by the conceptual resources of the most common discursive therapies (e.g. Pollard 2008; Seikkula and Arnkil 2006). One prominent chronicler of family therapy's developments was so bold as to suggest that, with the advent of the postmodern or social constructionist approaches to therapy, the time had come to 'set aside the model in family therapy' (Hoffman 1998). Such a proclamation can be disconcerting for those new to, but interested in learning, the discursive therapies.

Throughout this book, we and our contributors have aimed to provide a variety of conceptual and conversational resources that could be useful to informing a discursive approach to therapy. The breadth of resources we have shared has been considerable but does share some themes which we feel map out a somewhat unique landscape for people concerned with helping people acquire new understandings and actions. The discursive approaches to therapy are now into their second generation; and the first compilations (e.g.; Friedman 1993; McNamee and Gergen 1992) showcased exciting and controversial new arrivals into mainstream mental health. The excitement has waned somewhat while increasing numbers of discursively oriented therapists engage patients in the kinds of dialogues readers of this volume should now find familiar. What has happened as the discursive therapies enter their second generation is a set of different challenges than those which gave rise to these therapies in the first place.

Now, much a part of the broader landscape of contemporary mental health, the discursive therapies are represented in the most common textbooks for graduate trained therapists (e.g. Corsini and Wedding 2008; Nichols and Schwartz, 2005), and are among the most commonly practised of therapies. Their 'legitimacy' or efficacy remains a question in these days of evidence-based practice. A challenge faces discursive therapists to demonstrate that their work can make important differences in patients' lives, and it has only been recently that such evidence has been coming forward (e.g. Chenail et al., Chapter 13). The reason such evidence matters comes with the practices third-party payers are willing to pay for, or publicly funded institutions are willing to endorse as appropriate. These payers and institutions typically adopt a medically-oriented discourse of symptom severity and approved treatment protocols, to administer frontline practice. Such an administrative discourse can present challenges, given how much at odds it can be with the discursive therapists' own discourse of engaging patients in naming problems (typically in non-symptom terms) and in co-developing interventions (Strong and Mudry, in press). These kinds of challenges are similarly faced by therapists who practice non-manualized and 'unsupported' therapies like psychoanalysis, existential, person-centred, and gestalt therapy. Small wonder, then, that the most commonly endorsed and practiced psychotherapy is CBT for having its scientific warrant. These challenges notwithstanding, the discursive therapies have continually grown in popularity among practicing therapists, since their introduction in the late 1980s and early 1990s.

The discursive therapies have become common within the array of therapeutic approaches individuals, couples and families can turn to for help, but the prevalence of their use by therapists and patients remains largely unknown (exception; Beaton et al. 2009). The 'postmodern' ideas that underpin these approaches continue to get a mixed reception among the lay public and academics–particularly for largely having originated, not from science, but from literary or text-based criticism (e.g. Cusset, 2008). The notion that there can be a politics over how to interpret and portray experience is hardly new (Habermas 1975; Ricoeur 1974), and a hermeneutic insight arose from efforts to interpret the Bible 'correctly'. Readers could not get inside the minds and intentions of its original authors, and could only bring their backgrounds of understanding to understand words and meanings from the very different historical and cultural backgrounds of the Bible's authors (Gadamer 1988). Science was, in part, an answer to conflicting interpretations; particularly authoritative interpretations that would govern personal and social interactions. However, a close examination within scientific fields of inquiry shows that science is not without its conflicting interpretations as well (Latour 1986). This is as much the case in mental health as it is in other spheres of scientific inquiry. Inevitably, what passes for scientific fact comes down to evaluative criteria and processes that humans socially use to determine them (Potter 1996). Whether seeking to best understand the Bible, or of some aspect of human life relevant to therapists, the postmodern or discursive challenge is one of accepting the word, authoritative, over 'correct'. 'Correct' presumes some ultimate understanding beyond human processes and criteria, while authoritative refers to the best and still contestable understandings that humans can rigorously and scientifically come up with.

Early in my training to become a psychologist I recall a joke, that the best indicator of therapeutic success was a patient's eventual fluency in the *therapist's* discourse. Nowadays, patients routinely present their concerns in psychiatric classifications, often having self-diagnosed while further reading up on the treatments websites suggest that they are supposed to receive. Discursive therapists tend to welcome any discourse patients present but don't stay 'there'. They typically don't translate what they are being told into their own expert discourse, from which they can offer a 'here is what is really going on and what can be done about that' discourse either. They work from a sense that any discourse affords certain possibilities for understanding and action while constraining other possibilities (Martin and Sugarman 1999). Thus, the conversations and language of discursive therapists tends to focus on generating meaningful and actionable possibilities while critically reflecting upon and talking beyond discursive constraints. But, when a particular discourse or way of interpreting things affords no such possibilities in the patient's view, it is time for a new discourse or meaning for the discursive therapist.

Why interpretation matters so much to discursive therapists—particularly in naming and addressing patient concerns—is hopefully, by now, obvious. Adopting Wittgenstein's (1958) terms, very different 'language games' follow from a stance that sees patient concerns as correctly diagnosable or treatable, than from a stance that sees patients as having become ensnared by a word or limiting self-narrative that can be deconstructed or alternatively co-authored (Shotter 1993). These are very different kinds of clinical conversation, and what matters to discursive therapists are dialogues that flexibly bring forth patient understandings, resources, and preferences. Considerable discursive flexibility is required to engage with patient discourses, invite critical reflection upon them, and negotiate the consideration of plausible and resourceful alternatives (Strong 2002). From an ethnomethodological standpoint (e.g. Heritage 1984), people in conversation are practically interpreting each other, negotiating their way forward in dialogue. Such practical interpreting involves not only making sense but conversationally working out the conversational focus and direction. While discursive therapists invite particular foci or directions (e.g. a solution-focused direction; de Shazer 1988), they see it as their conversational challenge to negotiate meanings and customize solutions from patients' responses. What matters, for discursive therapists, are meanings and actions patients invest themselves in by shaping how these are negotiated or co-constructed over the course of therapeutic dialogue. Of course, not just any co-constructed meaning or interpretation will do, as typically it must address realities beyond the therapeutic consultation.

'Resistance-informed' is one way of appreciating the work of discursive therapists (Wade 1997). Discursive capture was a concern of Foucault (1983), while the emancipatory focus of Deleuze and Guattari (1988) was on 'lines of flight' from any sense of discursive capture. This focus on resistance—even therapeutically inviting it as difference—can be an important animating aspect of discursive therapies. In many cases, patients have laboured under assumed meanings for their circumstance, but at least have opinions on, if not differences over, what those circumstances mean for them. Such differences, for Bakhtin (1981), were how the words of any dialogue could be brought to life, or 'peopled' with new intentions. Therapy can help such vital patient intentions get talked into being (Heritage 1984). What helps such intentions take flight are plausible ways to couple them with promising actions that break beyond those circumstances, as patients see those actions and circumstances.

Throughout this book the contributors have shared their ideas, practices, concerns, and enthusiasms. A diverse group of therapies were presented, and all take seriously the idea that the world as people know it is socially constructed through the different understandings and actions people come to construct through discourse, then adopt personally and interpersonally. Humans have an infinite capacity to use language and develop ways of socially interacting that open life possibilities while at the same time shutting others down. In the relatively recent history of psychotherapy there are many illustrations of well-intended therapists doing this as well (e.g. Cushman 1995; Hacking 1999). The modern idea that meaning for any phenomenon was determinable and that a phenomenon's scientific meaning could be finalized, is the 'terror' Lyotard (1993) was referring to in this chapter's opening quote. For Bakhtin (1981), there was no final resting place for the word; there can only be more responses in an unceasing chain of dialogue—unless we stop those responses with some monological insistence on certainty or some fetishized view on how things should be. Like Y2K, we humans are continuously brought back to our social constructions, with the language we use for understanding and informing action as our quintessential social construction. Each of our authors has had something to say about such potential constructive and deconstructive uses of language in therapy. Our hope in this book has been to bring together key voices from the discursive therapies, to invite further dialogue on discursive therapy's potentials.

References

Agamben, G. (2007). *'What is an apparatus'? and other essay.* Stanford University Press, Berkeley, CA.

Anderson, H. (1997). *Conversation, language and possibilities.* Basic Books, New York.

Armstrong, C. L. and Morrow, L. (Eds.) (2010). *Handbook of medical neuropsychology: Applications of cognitive neuroscience.* Springer, New York.

Badiou, A. (2007). *Being and event* (O. Feltham, Trans.). Continuum, New York.

Bakhtin, M. M. (1981). *The dialogic imagination. Four essays.* (M. Holquist, Ed.; C. Emerson and M Holquist, Trans). University of Texas Press, Austin, TX.

Bateson, G. (1980). *Mind and nature: A necessary unity.* Bantam, New York.

Beaton, J., Dienhart, A., Schmidt, J., & Turner, J. (2009). Clinical practice patterns of Canadian couple/marital/family therapists. *Journal of Marital and Family Therapy,* **35**, 193–203.

Beaudoin, M.-N. (2010). *The skill-ionaire in every child: Boosting children's socio-emotional skills using the latest in brain research.* Booklocker, Inc, Bangor, ME.

Bennett, M., Dennett, D., Hacker, P., and Searle, J. (2007). *Neuroscience & Philosophy: Brain, mind & language.* Columbia University Press, New York.

Bracken, P. (2002). *Trauma: Culture, meaning & philosophy.* Whurr Publishers, London.

Cooperrrider, D. and Whitney, D. (2005). *Appreciative inquiry: A positive revolution in change.* Berrett-Koehler Publishers, San Francisco, CA.

Corsini, R. J. and Wedding, D. (2008). *Current psychotherapies* (8th ed.). Thomson Brooks/Cole, Belmont, CA.

Crotty, M. (1998). *The foundations of social research: meaning and perspective in the research process.* Sage, London.

Cushman, P. (1995). *Constructing the self, constructing America.* Perseus Books, New York.

Cusset, F. (2008). *French theory: How Foucault, Derrida, Deleuze, & Co. transformed the intellectual life of the United States* (J. Fort, Trans). University of Minnesota Press, Minneapolis, MN.

Deleuze, G and Guattari, F. (1988). *A thousand plateaus: Capitalism and schizophrenia* (B. Massumi, Trans. and Foreword). University of Minnesota Press, Minneapolis, MN.

Denzin N. and Lincoln, Y. (1994). *The handbook of qualitative research.* Sage, London.

Denzin N.and Lincoln, Y. (Eds.) (2011). *The handbook of qualitative research* (4th ed.). Thousand Oaks, CA: Sage.

de Shazer, S. (1988). *Clues: Investigating solutions in brief therapy.* W.W. Norton, New York.

de Shazer, S. (1994). *When words were original magic.* W.W. Norton, New York.

Ecker, B. and Hulley, L. (1995). *Depth-oriented brief therapy: How to be brief when you were trained to be deep and vice versa.* Jossey-Bass, San Francisco, CA.

Eron J. W. and Lund, T. (1994). *Narrative solutions in brief therapy.* Guilford, New York.

Fairclough, N. (1992). *Discourse and social change.* Polity Press, Cambridge.

Foucault, M. (1983). Afterword: The subject and power. In H. L. Dreyfus and P. Rabinow (Eds.) *Michel Foucault: Beyond structuralism and hermeneutics*, pp. 208–26. University of Chicago Press, Chicago, IL.

Frances, A. (2010). It's not too late to save 'normal'. Opinion. *Los Angeles Times*, **1 March**. http://articles.latimes.com/2010/mar/01/opinion/la-oe-frances1–2010mar01

Friedman, S. (Ed.) (1993). *The new language of change.* Guilford Publications, New York.

Gabbay J. and Le May, A. (2011). *Practice-based evidence for healthcare: Clinical mindlines.* Routledge, New York.

Gadamer, H-G. (1988). *Truth and method* (2nd revised ed.) (J. Weinsheimer and D.G. Marshall, Trans.). Continuum, New York.

Gale, J., Lawless, J. and Roulston, K. (2004). Discursive approaches to clinical research. In T. Strong and D. Paré (Eds.). *Furthering talk: Advances in the discursive therapies*, pp. 125–44. Kluwer Academic/Plenum Publishers, New York.

Gergen, K. (1973). Social psychology as history. *Journal of Personality and Social Psychology,* **26**, 309–20.

Gergen, K. (2009). *Relational being: Beyond self and community.* Oxford University Press, New York.

Habermas, J. (1975). *Legitimation crisis* (T. McCarthy, Trans.). Beacon Press, New York.

Hacking, I. (1999). *Mad travelers: Reflections on the reality of transient mental illnesses.* Harvard University Press, Cambridge, MA.

Harré, R. and Secord, P (1972). *Explanation of social behavior.* Blackwell, Oxford.

Harré, R. and Giillett, G (1994). *The discursive mind.* Sage, London.

Heritage, J. (1984). *Garfinkel and ethnomethodology.* Polity Press, Cambridge.

Hoffman, L. (1998). Setting aside the model in family therapy. *Family Process,* **37**, 145–56.

House, R. and Loewenthal, D (Eds). (2009). *Against and for CBT: Towards a constructive dialogue.* PCCS Books, Ross-on-Wye.

Ingleby, D. (1981). *Critical psychiatry: the politics of mental health.* Penguin Books, London.

Kuhn, T. (1962). *The structure of scientific revolutions.* University of Chicago Press, Chicago, IL.

Larner, G. (2004). Family therapy and the politics of evidence. *Journal of Family Therapy,* **26**, 17–39.

Latour, B. (1986). *Science in action.* Harvard University Press, Cambridge, MA.

Layard, R. (2006). *Happiness.* Penguin, London.

Lock, A. J. and Strong, T. (2010). *Social constructionism: Sources and stirrings in theory and practice.* Cambridge University Press, New York.

Lyddon, W. J. (1995). Cognitive therapy and theories of knowing: A social constructionist view. *Journal of Counseling and Development,* **73**, 579–85.

Lyotard, J-F. (1993). *Toward the postmodern.* Humanities Press, London.

Madigan, S. (1992). The application of Michel Foucault's philosophy in the problem externalizing discourse of Michael White. *Journal of Family Therapy,* **14**, 265–79.

Maranhão, T. (1986). *Therapeutic discourse and Socratic dialogue: A cultural critique.* University of Wisconsin Press, Madison, WI.

Martin, J., and Sugarman, J. (1999). *The psychology of human possibility and constraint.* SUNY Press, Albany, NY.

McLeod, J. and Elliott, R. (2011). Systematic case study research: A practice-oriented introduction to building an evidence base for counselling and psychotherapy. *Counselling and Psychotherapy Research*, **11**(1), 1–10.

McNamee, S. (2004). Promiscuity in the practice of family therapy. *Journal of Family Therapy*, **26**, 224–44.

McNamee, S. and Gergen, K. (Eds.) (1992). *Therapy as social construction*. Sage, London.

Nichols, M. and Schwartz, R. (2005). *Family therapy concepts and methods* (5th ed.). Allyn & Bacon, Needham Heights, MA.

O'Hanlon, W. H. (1994). The third wave. *Family Therapy Networker*, **November/December**, 19–29.

Parker., I. (Ed.) (1999). *Deconstructing psychotherapy*. Routledge, New York.

Pollard, R. (2008). *Dialogue and desire: Mikhail Bakhtin and the linguistic turn in psychotherapy*. Karnac Books, London.

Potter, J. (1996). *Representing reality*. Sage, London.

Prime Minster's Office. (2008, **May** 7th). *Clarifying statement to the Government's Response to the Psychotherapy E-Petition*. Government of the United Kingdom. Statement available at http://www.number10.gov.uk/Page15454

Ricoeur, P. (1974). *The Conflict of Interpretations: Essays in Hermeneutics* (D. Ihde, Ed., W. Domingo et al. Trans.). Northwestern University Press, Evanston, IL.

Rose, N. (1990). *Governing the sou*. Routledge, London.

Seikkula, J. and Arnkil, T. (2006). *Dialogical meetings in social networks*. Karnac Books, London.

Shotter, J. (1975). *Images of man in psychological research*. Methuen, London.

Shotter, J. (1993). *Conversational realities*. Sage, London.

Shotter, J. (2010). *Social construction on the edge: Withness-thinking and embodiment*. Taos Institute Publications, Chagrin Falls, OH.

Stern, D. B. (2009). *Partners in thought: Working with unformulated experiences, dissociation, and enactment*. Routledge, New York.

Stiles, W. and Shapiro, D. (1989). Abuse of the drug metaphor in psychotherapy process-outcome-research. *Clinical Psychology Research*, **9**, 521–43.

Strong, T. (2002). Collaborative 'expertise' after the discursive turn. *The Journal of Psychotherapy Integration*, **12**, 218–32.

Strong, T. and Mudry, T. (in press). Motivational interview and solution focused counselling for problem gamblers: Considerations for meshing clinical and institutional discourses. *Canadian Journal of Counselling and Psychotherapy*.

Strong, T., & Sutherland, O. A. (2007). Conversational ethics in psychological dialogues: Discursive and collaborative considerations. *Canadian Psychology*, **48**, 94–105.

Szasz, T. (2007). *Coercion as cure: A critical history of psychiatry*. Transaction Publishers, Rutgers, NJ.

Tan, S-L, Pfordresher, P. and Harré, R (2010). *Psychology of music: From sound to significance*. Psychology Press, Hove, East Sussex.

Vico, G. (1744/1999). *New science* (3rd ed.) (D. Marsh, Trans.). Penguin, London. [First published in 1744].

von Foerster, H. (1981). *Observing systems*. Intersystems Publications, Seaside, CA.

Vygotsky, L. (1978). *Mind in society: The development of higher psychological processes* (M. Cole, V. John-Steiner, S. Scribner, and E. Souberman, Eds.). Harvard University Press, London.

Wade, A. (1997). Small acts of living: Everyday resistance to violence and other forms of oppression. *Contemporary Family Therapy,* **19**(1), 23–39.

Watters, E. (2010). *Crazy like us: The globalization of the American psyche.* Free Press, New York.

Weingarten, K. (1992). A consideration of intimate and non-intimate interactions in therapy. *Family Process,* **31**(1), 45–59.

Wertsch, J. V. (1998). *Mind as action.* Oxford University Press, New York.

White, M. (1984). Pseudo-encopresis: From avalanche to victory, from vicious to virtuous cycles. *Family Systems Medicine,* **2**, 150–60.

White, M. (2007). *Maps of narrative practice.* WW. Norton, New York.

Williams, M. (2002). *Wittgenstein, mind and meaning: Towards a social conception of mind.* Routledge, New York.

Wittgenstein, L. (1958) *Philosophical investigations* (3rd ed.) (G.E.M. Anscombe, Trans). MacMillan, New York.

Author Index

Abelson, R.P. 46
Acheson, Sir D. 204
Adam, B. 174
Adams, J.F. 41
Agamben, G. 311
American Psychiatric Association 3, 248, 259
American Psychological Association
  Presidential Task Force on Evidence-Based Practice 245–50, 252–62
  Task Force for Development of Practice Recommendations for Provision of Humanistic Psychosocial Services 245, 251, 253, 257, 260
  Task Force on Promotion and Dissemination of Psychological Procedures 249, 250, 251, 253, 255, 256, 259
Andersen, A. 179
Andersen, T. 87–8, 96–7, 117, 127, 136
Anderson, H. 18, 96, 127, 128, 129, 130, 131, 133, 135, 136, 137, 233, 234, 246, 248, 253, 303, 309, 310
Anderson, H. and Gehart, D. 127, 224, 235
Anderson, H. and Goolishian, H. 127, 233, 234
Anderson, H. and Levin, S.B. 126, 127
Andrews, J. 25, 235
Anti-Harassment Team of Selwyn College 114
Appleby, B.S. 154
Archer, M. 299
Armstrong, C.L. and Morrow, L. 312
Athanasiou, A., Hantzaroula, P. and Yannakopoulos, Y. 303
Atkinson, B., Atkinson, L., Kutz, P., et al. 295, 296
Augusta-Scott, T. and Dankworth, J. 233
Austin, J.L. 50, 92
Avidi, E. 262

Badiou, A. 312
Baker, G.P. 186
Bakhtin, M.M. 5, 16, 20, 88–9, 315, 317
Bandler, R., Grinder, J. and Satir V. 108
Bannink, F.P. 144, 146, 148
Barrionuevo, A. and Robbins, L. 273
Barry, D. 232
Barry, D. and Elmes, M. 232
Bateson, G. 88, 107–8, 112, 117, 120, 312
Baucum, D. 35
Baum, F.L. and Denslow, W.W. 146
Bava, S. 128
Bava, S. and Levin, S. 126, 128

Bavellas, J.B., McGee, D., Phillips, B. and Routledge, R. 167
Bazeman, J. 4
Beard, G.M. 27–8
Beaton, J., Dienhart, A., Schmidt, J. and Turner, J. 316
Beaudoin, M. 296, 302, 312
Beaumont, J.G., Kenealy, P.M. and Rogers, M.J.C. 291
Beck, A.T., Rush, A.J., Shaw, F.B. and Emery, G. 253
Behbehani, A.M. 1
Bellah, R., Madsen, R., Sullivan, W., Swidler, A. and Tipton, S. 202
Bennett, M.R., Dennett, D., Hacker, P.M.S. and Searle, J. 312
Bennett, M.R. and Hacker, P.M.S. 298, 300
Benzeval, M., Judge, K. and Whitehead, M. 198, 204
Beran, E. 60, 62–3
Berg, I.K. 18, 143
Berg, I.K. and Cauffmann, L. 143, 144
Berg, I.K. and De Jong, P. 227
Berg, I.K. and Dolan, Y. 143
Berg, I.K. and Miller, S.D. 143, 144
Berg, I.K. and Steiner, T. 143
Bergson, H. 90, 94, 303
Bermudez, J.M. and Bermudez, S. 232
Berne, E. 108
Besa, D. 231
Beutler, L.E. 250, 256
Beyebach, M.M., Rodriguez Sanchez, M.S. and De Miguel, J.A. 229
Bilham, R. 273
Blackman, L. and Cromby, J. 303
Blair-Broeker, C.T. 35
Block, M. 1
Bograd, M. 200
Bohart, A.C. 253
Bohart, A.C., O'Hara, M. and Leitner, L.M. 251
Bohr, N. 151
Boje, D.M., Alvarez, R.C. and Schooling, B. 232
Boje, D.M., Rosile, G., Dennehy, B. and Summers, D. 232
Borod, J., Cicero, B., Obler, L., Welkowitz, J., Erhan, H., Santschi, C., et al. 292
Boscolo, L. and Bertrando, P. 108
Boscolo, L., Cecchin, G., Hoffman, L. and Penn, P. 108
Bott, D. 24
Bowen, M. 108, 109

Boyatzis, R.E. 262
Boyers, R. and Orrill, R. 107
Bracken, P. 312
Brennan, T. 303
Breuer, J. 16
Brewin, C. 297
Briggs, L. 14
Brinkmann, S. 49
Brody, N. and Oppenheim, P. 152
Brown, L. 128
Brown, R. 59–60
Brown, S.D., Reavey, P., Cromby, J., Harper, D. and Johnson, K. 288
Bruner, E. 111
Bruner, J. 111, 117
Burke, K. 51, 53, 174
Burr, V. 247, 257
Busch, R. 262
Butler, J.S. 33

Calhoun, A. 14
Cameron, D. 8
Campbell, C. 33
Cappas, N., Andres-Hyman, R. and Davidson, L. 294, 296
Capra, F. 107
Carlson, M. 128
Carlson, T.D. 233
Chalmers, D. 299
Chamberlain, K. 255, 311
Chamberlain, S. 111
Chambless, D.L., Baker, M.J. and Baucom, D.H. 255, 256, 259
Chambless, D.L. and Hollon, S.D. 249, 251, 252, 253, 255, 256, 259
Chambless, D.L. and Ollendick, T.H. 259, 260
Chang, J. 236
Chapman, A.H. 37
Chwalisz, K. 252
Cilliers, P. 164, 169, 171, 172, 179, 180
Clanon, T.L. 27
Clough, P. 303
Clough, P. and Halley, J. 303
Cockburn, J.T., Thomas, F.N. and Cockburn, O.J. 228
Collins, Billy 154–5
Collins, J.A. and Fauser, B.C.J.M. 225
Combs, G. and Freedman, J. 106
Connie, E. and Metcalf, L. 227, 228
Conoley, C.W., Graham, J.M. and Neu, T. 229
Cook, D.J., Mulrow, C.D. and Haynes, R.B. 231
Cooper, A.B. 13, 33
Cooperrider, D. and Whitney, D. 314
Corcoran, J. and Pillai, V. 229
Corcoran, T. 84, 229, 302
Corsini, R.J. and Wedding, D. 315
Coué, E. 29
Coulehan, J.L. 1
Coulehan, R., Friedlander, M.L. and Heatherington, L. 231

Cowley, G. and Springen, K. 230, 231
Cozolino, L. 197, 270, 283, 294, 296
Crits-Christoph, P., Wilson, G.T. and Hollon, S.D. 255
Crocket, K. 232
Croll, S. and Bryant, R.A. 276
Cromby, J. 68, 271, 290, 291, 292, 303
Cromby, J. and Harper, D. 294, 303
Cromby, J. and Nightingale, D. 271
Crossley, M. 289
Crotty, M. 314
Cruz, J. and Littrell, J.M. 228
Cushman, P. 317
Cusset, F. 316

da Costa, D., Nelson, T.M., Rudes, J. and Guterman, J.T. 232, 233
Dalgleish, T., Rolfe, J., Golden, A.-M., Dunn, B.D. and Barnard, P.J. 276
Dallos, R. 233
Damasio, A.R. 270, 291, 292, 294, 299
Danziger, K. 254, 255
Darmody, M. and Adams, B. 229
Davies, B. 51, 53, 247, 250, 255
De Cock, K.M. 1
de Decker, A., Hermans, D., Raes, F. and Eelen, P. 276
De Haene, L. 225
De Jong, P. 18
De Jong, P. and Hopwood, L.E. 228
de Shazer, S. 16, 18, 108, 163, 164, 165, 224, 229, 310, 315, 317
de Shazer, S. and Berg, I. 143, 227
de Shazer, S., Berg, I. and Lipchik, E. 227
Dedaic, M.N. 56
Deleuze, G and Guattari, F. 317
Denborough, D. 106, 120, 230
Denborough, D., Freedman, J. and White, C. 106
Denzin, N.K. 128
Denzin, N.K. and Giardina, M.D. 245, 246, 255
Denzin, N.K. and Lincoln, Y. 314
Derrida, J. 111, 170, 173
DeSocio, J.E. 233
Disbury, P. 248, 262
Dolan, Y. 144
Donald, A. 251
Donohue, B., Allen, D.N. and Romero, V. 253
Donovan, M. 179
Draucker, C.B. 232, 233
Drewery, W. and Winslade, J. 247, 260
Drewery, W., Winslade, J. and Monk, G. 246, 260
Dreyfus, H. 15
Dubois, P. 27
Duncan, B.L., Miller, S.D. and Sparks, J. 263
Durgin, W.A. 28
Durie, M. 201
Durkheim, E. 109

Eakes, G. 144
Ecker, B. and Hulley, L. 315
Ecker, B. and Toomey, B. 295
Edwards, D. 72
Edwards, D., Ashmore, M. and Potter, J. 302
Ehrenreich, B. 29
Elkaim, M. 181
Emerson, R.M. 168
Epston, D. 15, 106, 109, 230, 263
Epston, D. and White, M. 106, 110
Ericksen, K. 41
Erikson, E. 197
Eron, J.W. and Lund, T. 315
Eschbich, C. 14
Esping-Andersen, G. 202
Etchison, M. and Kleist, D.M. 231

Fairclough, N. 289, 314
Farson, F.E. 35
Faul, M. 274
Feldman, N. and Silverman, B. 185
Fernandez, E., Cortés, A. and Tarragona, M. 235
Fish, S. 71
Fleischman, R.K. 250
Folensbee, R. 295, 296, 300
Folse, H. 152
Fonagy, P. 293
Fortun, M. and Bernstein, H.J. 270
Foucault, M. 8, 25, 106, 109, 111, 115, 249, 258, 259, 289, 317
Fox, N.J. 263
Fraenkel, P., Hameline, T. and Shannon, M. 232, 233, 236
Frances, A. 309
Frank, A.W. 168
Frankl, V.E. 107
Franklin, C., Streeter, C.L., Kim, J.S. and Tripodi, S.J. 144, 228
Fredman, G. 24
Freedman, J. and Combs, G. 106, 109, 113, 230
Freeman, M. 289
Freud, S. 13, 16, 29–30
Friedan, B. 205
Friedenberg, J.E. 272
Friedman, S. 315
Fromm, E. 32
Fromm-Reichmann, F. 32, 38
Frosh, S., Burck, C., Strickland-Clark, L. and Morgan, K. 262
Frydman, B., Wilson, I.M. and Wyer, J. 128
Fulford, K.W.M. 2, 20

Gabbay, J. and Le May, A. 311
Gadamer, H-G. 78, 316
Gale, J. 167
Gale, J., Lawless, J. and Roulston, K. 314
Gale, J. and Newfield, N. 167
Gallese, V., Eagle, M. and Migone, P. 297
Gallese, V. and Goldman, A. 297

Gardner, P.J. and Poole, J.M. 232, 233
Garfield, S.L. 41, 251
Garfinkel, H. 49, 72, 89
Gazzaniga, M.S. 289, 292, 294
Geertz, C. 110, 111, 120, 135, 247, 249
Gehart, D.R. 235, 236
Gehart, D.R. and Lucas, D. 236
Gehart, D.R., Tarragona, M. and Bava, S. 126, 236
Gehart-Brooks, D.R. and Lyle, R.R. 235
Gell-Mann, M. 169
Gergen, K.J. 5, 17, 65–6, 76, 127, 129, 130, 179, 225, 313
Gergen, M. 65
Gerhardt, S. 197
Gibson, J.J. 84
Gilbertson, A. and Filkins, D. 271
Gill, J.H. 165
Gilligan, C. 205
Gilman, A. 59–60
Gingerich, W.J. and Eisengart, S. 227, 228, 229
Gladding, S.T. 246, 253
Glaser, B.G. and Strauss, A.L. 262
Goffman, E. 53, 109, 111, 128
Goldner, V. 200
Goldstein, J.E. 25
Goodman, N. 101, 170, 171
Goolishian, H. 18, 126–7
Goolishian, H. and Anderson, H. 127
Gordon, C. 247, 248, 249
Goswami, U. 291
Graham, G. 2
Greenberg, L. 257
Greer, G. 205
Greimas, A.J. 46, 51, 53
Griffin, D. 164, 179, 180
Guba, E.G. and Lincoln, Y.S. 247, 248
Guilfoyle, M. 233
Guillain, G. 14
Guynn, R.W. 33

Habermas, J. 199, 316
Hacking, I. 13, 317
Haidt, J. 297
Haley, J. 107, 108
Haley, J. and Hoffman, L. 108
Handel, G. and Hewson, D. 108, 116
Hare-Mustin, R.T. 127
Harmon-Jones, E. and Winkielman, P. 289
Harper, D., Mulvey, M.R. and Robinson, M. 252
Harré, R. 5, 17, 51, 54, 288, 289, 298
Harré, R. and Gillett, G. 313
Harré, R. and Secord, P. 313
Harvey, A.G., Bryant, R.A. and Dang, S.T. 276
Haydon, M. 24
Hebb, D. 293
Heinroth, J.C. 25–7
Henderson, D., Hargreaves, I., Gregory, S. and Williams, J.M.G. 276

Henderson, V.L. 276
Heneghan, C. and Badenoch, D. 224, 226
Henry, W.P., Strupp, H.H.,
  Butler, S.F., Schacht, T.E. and
  Binder, J.L. 253, 254
Hepburn, A. 290
Heritage, J. 163, 167, 168, 310, 317
Herman, J. 200
Hewson, D. 116
Hibberd, F. 302
Higgins, D. 3
Higgins, R. 220
Hochschild, A. 206
Hoffman, L. 23, 24, 108, 315
Hogan, B.A. 232, 233
Holzman, L. 18, 185, 186, 189, 190, 246, 248, 261, 311
Holzman, L. and Mendez, R. 185
Holzman, L. and Newman, F. 187
Hood [Holzman L.] and Newman F. 192
Hooks, B. 205
Horewitz, J.S. 108
Horney, K. 32
Horsfall, D. 128
House, R. and Loewenthal, D. 311
Howarth, D. 8
Hoyt, M.F. 143, 153
Hull, A.M. 275
Hume, D. 271

Ingleby, D. 311
Ingram, C. and Perlesz, A. 233

Jackson, P.Z. and McKergow, M. 173
Jacobs, S., Kissil, K., Scott, D. and Davey, M. 235
James, W. 90–2, 98, 100, 102
Jantsch, E. 169
Jarvinen, M. and Miller, G. 168
Jaspers, K. 19
Jenner, E. 1
Jensen, P. 96
Johnson, L.D. and Miller, S.D. 144
Johnson, M. 303
Joiner, T.E., Van Orden, K.A., Witte, T.K. and Rudd, M.D. 133
Jones, F. 206
Jörvinen, M. and Miller, G. 168
Joseph, J. 292
Jourdan, A. 33

Kamsler, A. 200
Kangas, M., Henry, J.L. and Bryant, R.A. 276
Kawachi, I. and Berkman, L.F. 198, 204
Kawachi, I. and Kennedy, B. 198
Kazdin, A.E. 245
Keeling, M.L. and Nielson, L.R. 232, 233
Kendall, P.C. and Chambless, D.L. 257
Kenwood, C. 289
Kim, J.S. 143, 144, 228, 229

Kim, J.S. and Franklin, C. 228
Kimmel, M.S. 28–9
King, N.J. and Ollendick, T.H. 252
Kirmayer, H. 14
Kirschenbaum, H. 32, 33
Kirven, J. 233
Kiser, D. 227
Kitanaka, J. 14
Kitson, A. 258
Kitwood, T. 46
Koch, R. 1
Koplow, D.A. 1
Kraepelin, E. 2, 25
Kral, R. 144
Kropf, N.P. and Tandy, C. 233
Kuehlwein, K.T. 41
Kuhn, T.S. 72, 314
Kurtz, R. 41
Kuyken, W. and Brewin, C.R. 277
Kvarnes, R.G. 37, 38

L'Abate, L., Ganahl, G. and Hansen, J.C. 108
Laclau, E. and Mouffe, C. 289
Laing, R.D. 107
Laing, R.D. and Esterson, A. 107
Langellier, K.M. and Peterson, E. 168
Langer, S.K. 15
Larner, G. 311
Larner, W. 250
Latour, B. 72, 316
Launer, J. 24
Laws, M. 12
Layard, R. 311
Le Doux, J. 293, 294, 299
Leder, D. 288
Lee, M.Y., Greene, G.J., Uken, A., Sebold, J. and Rheinscheld, J. 228
Lessa, I. 8
Letiche, H. 180
Leupnitz, D.A. 108
Levant, R.F. and Hasan, N.T. 252, 253
Levin, S. 126, 130, 135, 235
Levinson, S.C. 166
Levitt, H.M., Neimeyer, R.A. and Williams, D.C. 256
Lewin, R. 169
Lewis, C.S. 282
Lewis, D. and Cheshire, A. 114
Lewis, T., Amini, F. and Lannon, R. 269, 277, 279
Li, S., Armstrong, M.S., Chaim, G., Kelly, C. and Shenfeld, J. 228
Lincoln, Y.S. and Guba, E.G. 247
Lindauer, R.J.L., Booij, J. and Habraken, J.B.A., et al. 275
Linden, D. 299
Lindforss, L. and Magnusson, D. 144, 228
Linley, P.A. 284
Lipchik, E. 127, 144
Lipchik, E., Becker, M., Brasher, B., Derks, J. and Volkmann, J. 296, 297

Lobman, C. 185
Lock, A.J. 101
Lock, A.J. and Strong, T. 312, 315
London, S. 136
London, S. and Rodriguez-Jazcilevich, I. 126
Love, C. 197
Lundblad, A.M. and Hansson, K. 228
Lyddon, W.J. 312
Lyotard, J.F. 23, 24, 115, 172, 308, 317

McAuliffe, G. 41
McCollum, E.E. and Trepper, T.S. 144
Macdonald, A. 144, 227, 228, 229
McDonough, M. and Koch, P. 235
McGee, D. 41
McGee, D., Vento, A.D. and Bavelas, J.B. 177
McGoldrick, M., Anderson, C.M. and Walsh, F. 108
McGoldrick, M. and Gerson, R. 108
McGregor, R., Ritchie, A., Serrano, A., Schuster, F. and Goolishian, H. 126
McHale, B. 3
McHugh, R.K., Murray, H.W. and Barlow, D.H. 252
MacIntyre, A. 5
Mackenbach, J. 198, 204
McKergow, M. 169
McKergow, M. and Korman, H. 172
McLennan, G. 302
McLeod, J. and Elliott, R. 310
MacMartin, C. 167
McNally, R.J., Lasko, N.B., Macklin, M.L. and Pitman, R.K. 276
McNally, R.J., Litz, B.T., Prassas, A., Shin, L.M. and Weathers, F.W. 276
McNamee, S. 312
McNamee, S. and Gergen, K. 127, 315
Madigan, S. 314
Madill, A. and Barkham, M. 262
Mahoney, M.J. 270
Main, M. 282
Maines, R.P. 148
Mandanes, C. 108
Manteufel, A. 293
Maranhäo, T. 313
Marmot, Sir M. 198, 204
Marshall, J.C. 14
Martin, J. and Sugarman, J. 316
Marx, K. 185
Marx, K. and Engels, F. 185
Maslow, A. 202
Massad, S. 185
Massumi, B. 303
Matos, M., Santos, M., Goncalves, M. and Martins, C. 232
Mattingly, C. and Fleming, M.H. 164
Maurial, M. 214
Maynard, D.W. 167
Mead, H. 220
Mead, S.M. 220

Mehl-Madrona, L. 231
Merleau-Ponty, M. 95, 99–100
Merry, U. 164, 169
Messmore, C. 235, 236
Metcalf, L. 144
Meyer, D. 29
Meyerhoff, B. 117
Micale, M.S. 13, 14
Middleton, D. and Brown, S.D. 303
Miller, G. 163, 164, 167, 168
Miller, G. and de Shazer, S. 168, 180
Miller, G., de Shazer, S. and DeJong, P. 143, 172, 230
Miller, S.D., Duncan, B.L. and Hubble, M.A. 263
Miller, S.D., Duncan, B.L., Sorrell, R. and Brown, G.S. 230
Ministry of Social Development (2009) 198, 203, 204, 205, 206
Minuchin, S. 108
Minuchin, S. and Fishman, H.C. 108
Mitchell, S.W. 28–9
Monk, G., Winslade, J., Crocket, K. and Epston, D. 106, 231, 232
Morgan, A. 230
Mukamel, R., Ekstrom, A., Kaplan, J., Iacoboni, M. and Fried, I. 297
Münsterberg, H. 30
Murray, C.E. and Murray, T.L. 144

Napier, A.Y. and Whitaker, C. 108
Nathan, P.E. and Gorman, J.M. 252
National Equality Panel (2010) 198
National Health Committee (1998) 198, 204
Ncube, N. 120
New Zealand Ministry of Justice (2001) 221
Newman, F. 18, 185–9, 191–4
Newman, F. and Holzman, L. 185, 186, 187, 189
Newsome, W.S. 144
Nicholls, D.A., Walton, J.A. and Price, K. 249
Nichols, M. and Schwartz, R. 315
Nicholson, S. 106
Nightingale, D.J. 68, 271
Nolan, C. 288
Norcross, J.C. 35, 41, 251, 253, 257
Nussbaum, M. 85

O'Connell, B. 246, 247
O'Connor, T.S., Davis, A., Meakes, E., Pickering, R. and Schuman, M. 233
O'Connor, T.S., Meakes, E., Pickering, M.R. and Schuman, M. 231, 233
Office for National Statistics (2005) 203
O'Hanlon, W.H. 308
Ormerod, P. 169
Owusu-Bempah, K. and Howitt, D. 201

Panksepp, J. 289, 294
Parker, I. 68, 302, 311
Parloff, G.H. 37
Pelias, R.J. 128

Peller, J. and Walter, J. 144
Penn, P. 235
Pere, R. 213
Perry, H.S. 32
Petticrew, M. and Roberts, H. 225, 226, 237
Pichot, T. 144
Pichot, T. and Dolan, Y. 144
Pinel, P. 25–6
Pitkin, H.F. 165, 166
Pizzey, E. 200
Polanyi, M. 94
Pollard, R. 315
Pomerantz, A. 167
Posner, M.I. and Rothbart, M.K. 197
Potter, J. 72, 302, 316
Potter, J. and Wetherell, M. 289
Prime Minister's Office 311
Prince, M. 60–2
Prochaska, J.O. 35, 41
Propp, V. 53

Quintana, S., Aboud, F., Chao, R., et al. 197

Rabinow, P. 119
Rabinow, P. and Rose, N. 246, 248
Rampage, C., Goodrich, T.J., Halstead, K. and Ellman, B. 127
Rauch, S.L., van der Kolk, B.A. and Fisler, R.E., et al. 275
Ray, F.K. 179
Ray, I. 27
Reavey, P. and Brown, S.D. 303
Reik, T. 31
Reil, J. 2
Reynolds, D. 24
Richardson, K.A., Cilliers, P. and Lissack, M. 170
Richert, A.J. 230
Ricoeur, P. 58, 316
Riedel, S. 1
Rieff, P. 30
Riley, S., Sims-Schouten, W. and Willig, C. 302
Riley, W.T., Schumann, M.F., Forman-Hoffman, V.L., Mihm, P., Applegate, B.W. and Asif, O. 252
Roder, B. and Neville, H. 292
Rogers, C. 18, 31–8
Rorty, R. 5
Rose, N. 246, 247, 250, 291, 311
Rose, N. and Rabinow, P. 291
Rose, S. 291
Rosenau, P.M. 171
Rosenhan, D. 2
Ross, M. 201
Roth, K. 24
Roth, P.A. 168
Roth, S., Becker, C., Herzig, M., Chasin, L. and Chasin, R. 127
Rothschild, P., Brownlee, K. and Gallant, P. 233
Roy-Chowdbury, S. 167

Royal Tangaere, A. 213
Rutgers, B.C.C. 252
Ruthrof, H. 290
Rycroft-Malone, J., Seers, K., Titchen, A., Harvey, G., Kitson, A. and McCormack, B. 246, 258
Ryle, G. 94

Sabat, S. 51
Sabo, K. 185
Sackett, D.L., Rosenberg, W.M.C., Gray, J.A.M., Haynes, R.B. and Richardson, W.S. 224, 252
Sackett, D.L. and Strauss, S. 252
Sacks, H. 166, 167
Sadler, J.Z. 259
Salit, C.R. 185
Sampson, E. 201
Sapir, E. 32
Sapyta, J., Riemer, M. and Bickman, L. 230
Sasz, T. 2
Satir, V. 108
Saussure, F. de 5
Sawrikar, P. and Hunt, C. 213
Scaer, R. 272, 273
Schank, R.C. 46
Schechner, R. 128
Schore, A. 270, 292
Schwartz, A. 14
Scull, A. 25
Sedgewick, E. 303
Seeling, B.J. 14
Seelye, K.Q. 271
Seidel, A. and Hedley, D. 228
Seikkula, J. 85–8, 90, 91, 98, 101
Seikkula, J. and Arnkil, T. 315
Selekman, M.D. 144
Seltzer, W. 296
Selvini Palazzoli, M.S., Cecchin, G., Boscolo, L. and Prata, G. 108
Senge, P. 97
Seymour, F.W. and Epston, D. 233
Sharry, J. 144
Shaw, P. 164, 172, 180
Shawver, L. 23, 24, 39–40
Shilling, C. 288
Shin, S.K. 228
Shonkoff, J. and Phillips, D. 197
Shorter, E. 13
Shotter, J. 4, 5, 17, 72, 90, 91, 103, 130, 131, 172, 290, 313, 317
Siegel, D.J. 270, 281, 282
Silver, E., Williams, A., Worthington, F. and Phillips, N. 231
Simon, D. 145, 152
Simon, R. 33
Smail, D.J. 303
Smedslund, J. 45
Smits, A.J., Powers, M.B., Berry, A.C. and Otto, M.W. 252

Smock, S.A., Trepper, T.S., Wetchler, J.L., McCollum, E.E., Ray, R. and Pierce, K. 228
Snow, C.P. 3
Solms, M. and Turnbull, O. 291
Sparks, J.A. and Muro, M.L. 235
Speer, S. 302
Spence, D. 79
Spring, B. 246
Stacey, R. 169, 170, 172, 178
Stacey, R., Griffin, D. and Shaw, P. 164
Stam, H. 288
Stams, G.J., Dekovic, M., Buist, K. and de Vries, L. 228
Stein, D.L. 169
Stephansson, J.G. 14
Stephens, R., Waldegrave, C. and Frater, P. 206
Stern, D.B. 312
Stiles, W. and Shapiro, D. 311
Stoddart, K.P., McDonnell, J., Temple, V. and Mustate, A. 228
Stow, C. 120
Stronach, I. 245
Strong, T. 23, 24, 101, 254, 261, 309, 317
Strong, T., Busch, R. and Couture, S. 262
Strong, T. and Lock. A. 254, 258
Strong, T. and Mudry, T. 316
Strong, T. and Pare, D. 224
Strong, T. and Sutherland, O. 180, 313
Sue, D.W. and Sue, D. 197, 201
Sullivan, H.S. 32–8
Sundet, R. 234
Sutherland, O. 154
Sween, E. 106, 111
Swim, S., George, S.A.S. and Wulff, D.P. 179
Szasz, T. 107, 135, 311
Szucs, D. and Goswami, U. 289

Tamasese, K., Peteru, C., Waldegrave, C. and Bush, A. 197
Tamasese, K. and Waldegrave, C. 201
Tan, S-L, Pfordresher, P. and Harré, R. 313
Tanenbaum, S. 243, 245, 246, 248, 251, 258
Tau, T. 217
Tawney, R.H. 202
Taylor, C. 203
Thorn, B.E. 245
Thornton, T. 2
Thorslund, K.W. 228
Throgmorton, J.A. 171
Timmermans, S. and Berg, M. 250
Todes, S. 103
Tomm, K. 16, 106, 109, 313
Tomori, C. and Bavelas, J.B. 177
Toomey, B. and Ecker, B. 295, 297
Torrance, H. 245
Torres, S. and Guerra, M.P. 232, 233
Trappenberg, T. 289
Trepper, T.S., McCollum, E.E., De Jong, P., Korman, H., Gingerich, W. and Franklin, C. 143, 153, 227

Tseng, W. 14
Tucker, I. 303

Unoca, Z. 60, 62–3

Valsiner, J. 45, 49
Van der Kolk, B.A. 272, 274, 275
Van der Kolk, B.A., Roth, S., Pelcovitz, D., Sunday, S., Spinaola, J. 273
van der Merwe, W.L. and Voestermans, P.P. 186
van Ommen, C. 291
Van Orden, K.A., Witte, T.K., Gordon, K.H., Bender, T.W. and Joiner, T.E. 134
Varela, F. 271
Vassallo, T. 233
Vico, G. 101, 313, 315
Vivona, J. 298, 300, 301
Voloshinov, V.N. 5, 6
von Foerster, H. 308
Vromans, L.P. and Schweitzer, R.D. 225, 231, 232, 233
Vygotsky, L.S. 85, 89, 95, 111, 120, 185, 186, 187, 189, 190, 191, 313

Wade, A. 284, 317
Wagner, J. 126, 235
Walach, H., Falkenberg, T., Lewith, G. and Jonas, W.B. 224, 227
Waldegrave, C. 196–211
Waldegrave, C., Stephens, R. and King, P. 198
Waldegrave, C., Tamasese, K., Tuhaka, F. and Campbell, W. 196
Waldegrave, C. and Waldegrave, K. 197
Waldrop, M.M. 164, 169
Walker, L. and Hayashi, L. 228
Walker, R. 219, 220
Walkerdine, V. 303
Walrond-Skinner, S. 108
Walsh, J.J. 29
Walter, J.L. and Peller, J.E. 149
Walters, M., Carter, R., Papp, P. and Silverstein, O. 108
Wampold, B.E. 262
Wampold, B.E., Goodheart, C.D. and Levant, R.F. 251, 253, 257, 259
Wampold, B.E., Lichtenberg, J.W. and Waehler, C.A. 251, 254, 257, 259
Watters, E. 14, 15, 309
Watzlawick, P., Weakland, J. and Fisch, R. 18, 108
Weakland, J. 151
Weber, M. 202
Weber, M., Davis, K. and McPhie, I. 233
Weeks, G.R. and L'Abate, L. 108
Weingarten, K. 106, 109, 313
Weiten, W. 199
Wendell, S. 288
Wertsch, J.V. 313
Wessel, I., Merckelbach, H. and Dekkers, T. 277

Westen, D., Novonty, C.M. and Thomson-Brenner, H. 259
Weston, H.E., Boxer, P. and Heatherington, L. 231
Whitaker, C.A. and Bumberry, W.M. 108
White, C. 109, 115
White, C. and Denborough, D. 106, 119
White, M. 15, 106, 116, 277, 279, 280, 284, 289, 310
White, M. and Epston, D. 106, 109, 127, 224, 230, 231, 232, 248, 261, 279
Whorf, B. 14
Wickman, S.A. 33
Wile, D.B. 128
Wilkinson, R. and Pickett, K. 198, 204
Williams, J. 217
Williams, J.M.G., Barnhofer, T. and Crane, C., et al. 276

Williams, J.M.G. and Broadbent, K. 276
Williams, M. 313, 315
Wilmshurst, L.A. 228
Wilson, E.A. 291
Wirtz, H. and Harari, R. 233
Wittgenstein, L. 67, 83, 85, 87, 92, 94, 99, 130, 131, 163–83, 186, 315, 317
Wolf, F.A. 149
Woollams, S. and Brown, M. 108
Worden, M. 108
Wyatt, R.C. 252, 254

Young, K. and Cooper, S. 232, 233
Young, S. and Holdore, G. 144

Zimmermann, T.S. 144

Subject Index

Aboriginal language 7
'abuse', meanings 200
activity and performance
  discourses 187–94
  in social therapeutic method 184–94
affect
  and language, cognitive regulation 295
  significance of 294–6
American Psychological Association (APA)
  evidence-based practice (EBP) 245–68
  see also Task Force
anger
  alternative action 87–8
  fear and 114–15
  'fighting' 15, 16
attachment therapy, consequences of dysfunctional early relationships 297
auditory hallucinations 155

Beard, G.M., on mental illness 27–8
bipolar disorder 155–9
body 269–87
  an outside-in phenomenon 273–4
  improving understanding and communication 281
  and language, reconciliation 291
  and narrative approaches to healing 269–87
  returning from war 271
brain
  basic neuroscience 292–3
  development of dysfunctional early relationships 297
  'mereological fallacy' 298–9, 312
  neurophysiology of trauma 274–6
  significance of affect 294–6
brain injury, *Memento* (film) 288
Brief Family Therapy Center 163
brief therapy *see* solution-focused brief therapy (SFBT)
bullying 113–15
  fear and anger 114

circumstantial evidence 224–40
clients
  'adjusting people to poverty' 199
  assumptions of the dominant culture 203
  as authors of their problems and failures 199
  as isolated entities 108
  more severe chronic concerns 310
  'thin' and 'thick' contextualizations of experience 247

cognitive questions 3–4
cognitive-behavioural therapy (CBT) services, govt. investment in 311
collaboration 109–10, 127, 128–9, 130, 139–40
collaborative therapy 18, 126–142
  connecting through uncertainty 136–7
  conversational partnership 132–3
  couples 128
  development 233–4
  history and discourse 126–7
  Houston-Galveston Institute 126–7
  language, listening, hearing, and reflecting 130–1
  opening conversations 129–30
  performing client–therapist relationships 131–2
  performing collaboration 128
  philosophical stance 129
  research 234–6
  suicide 132–9
communal 65–6, 201–2
communication
  as collaborative action 72–7
  'language' vs 'discourse' 5
complex systems 169–70
complexity theory 164–78
  description as a process of change 173
  'narrative emergence' 164
  possible futures 179–81
  in SFBT 169–74
  unpredictable and improvisational aspects of social interaction 173
  see also solution-focused brief therapy (SFBT)
context
  contextualization (knowing-from-within) 99–103
  see also clients; empirically-supported treatment (ESTs); evidence-based practice (EBP); 'just therapy' approach; mental illness; narrative therapy; psychotherapy; qualitative importance of social context; social constructionism; social context; talking to listen
conversation and its therapeutic possibilities 308–21
  language usage 309
  legitimacy question 316
  mechanical metaphor 308
  psy complex 311
  psychotherapy evaluation research 310–11
  see also discursive therapists

SUBJECT INDEX

conversion disorders, incidence 14
Coué, E., new kind of 'suggestion' 29
Counseling and Psychotherapy (Rogers) 33
counselling models 113–14
'crossroads' or 'road-forks' 96
cultural 13–15, 31–2, 198–203, 207
  dopes 47
  frameworks 219–20
  identity 213–18
  psychology 45, 49
  refuseniks 48
  see also Māori people
culture 3–5, 190–1, 197–203; *see also* Māori people

deconstruction 114–15
  deconstructive move 85, 87, 88, 91
depression and anxiety
  clinical presentation 14–15
  recent concept 76
dialogue, diffuse multi-dimensional nature 88–90
dialogic 88–90, 126
'discourse' 7–8
  vs 'language' 5–7
discursive therapies research 16–20, 314–15
  circumstantial evidence 224–40
  narrative review 226
  narrative therapy 15, 230–1
  qualitative research methods 314
  SFBT 226–30
  social constructional aspects 225
  'systematic narrative review' 225–7
discursive therapy 308–21
  centripetal and centrifugal tendencies 315
  collaborative and pragmatic ethos 309–10
  comparisons with biblical interpretations 316
  evaluation studies 310–11
  Foucaultian ideas 314
  insights and critiques providing mainstream psychological thought 313–14
  interpretation 317
  patients with more severe chronic concerns 310
  resistance informed 317–18
diseases
  elimination 1
  mental illness 2
DSM-IV-TR, on mental illness 3
Dulwich Centre 109, 115, 117–18, 230
duties and rights 46–50

embodied knowing 297–8
empirically-supported treatment (ESTs) 245, 249, 252
  consequences, possibilities, and questions 261–3
  FDA efficacy criteria 256
  outcome at expense of wider social context of client 256

Special Task Group (STG) on evaluation 257
thin contextualizations
  experimental methodolatry 254–5
  manuals vs relationship 252–4
  medical objectification 259–61
empirically-validated treatments (EVTs) 249
  concept change 251
  Division 12 Task Force report 251
ethics 179–80
  of solution-focused brief therapy 152
ethnomethodology 72, 312
externalizing the problem 15–16, 114, 120
evidence-based practice (EBP) 245–68
  qualitative importance of social context 247
  Task Force (APA) promotion 250–5
evidence-based practice in psychology (EBPP)
  development 251
  manualization 254
  paradoxical, problematic stance 254
  'qualitative research used to describe subjective, lived experiences' (Task Force) 258
  randomized controlled trial (RCT), as EBPP gold standard 246, 255, 258

facts and values 68
family
  basis of gender identification and role expectations 197
  belonging 197–9
  two-income, as societal norm 206
Food and Drug Administration (FDA)
  efficacy criteria 256
Foucaultian ideas
  conversation and its therapeutic possibilities 314
  governmentality 246
freedom vs imprisonment, pregnancy and (2 cases) 9–12
Freud, S., single standard tiotol 29–30

Gabriela's story of trauma 278–84
gender equity, and feminization of poverty 205–6
gender roles, transformation 205
governmentality, Foucaultian perspective 246
grief, C.S. Lewis on 282–4

Hamletmachine (Müller) 188
healing 269–85
  Māori expressions of healing 217
Hebbian principle, repetition develops new neural networks 295–6
Heinroth, J.C., on 'moral treatment' 25–7
Houston-Galveston Institute 126–7
humanities, vs sciences 3
hysteria, definition 13, 14

identity 197–8
  see also cultural identity; Māori people
ideology 68, 71, 112

SUBJECT INDEX   333

imprisonment vs freedom, pregnancy and (2 cases) 9–13
improvisation 18, 128, 173, 178, 189–90
indexicality 60
inner dialogues 85–8
intellectual attitude
  and difficulties of the will 94–6
  disadvantages 90–4
interactional event 167
intersubjective 77, 81, 245
intrapersonal positioning 60

just therapy approach 196–211
  assumptions of the dominant culture 203
  context and meaning 196–7
  critical role in post-industrial and secular states 204
  cultural, gender, and socioeconomic influences of meaning 198–9
  definition 198
  development 198
  gender equity and feminization of poverty 205–6
  Māori expressions of healing 212, 217–23
  practise and application 207

'knowing-from-within' 99–103

language 6–7
  act of greeting 17
  and the body, reconciliation 291
  conversations 17
  dealing with meanings 6
  'language games' 67, 165–8, 193
  and memory 296
  vs 'discourse' 5–7
'linguistic poverty' 313
listening
  non-directive listening 32
  'reflective/active' 35
  Rogers' and Sullivan's practices 35–6
  to hear the Unconscious 31
'lunatiks' 25–7

Māori people 212–23
  cultural frameworks 219
  cultural identity development 214
  expressions of healing, just therapy approach 212–23
  lack of a strong cultural identity 213
  Mana and Tapu 221
Marx, development of social therapy 185
meanings
  bridging the gap 79–80
  continuous transformation 79
  cultural, gender, and socioeconomic influences 198–9
  liberating 199–200
  subject to continuous reinterpretation 74–5
  subject to continuous transformation 79–80

'mechanical metaphor' 308
medical history 1–2
medical objectification 259–61
Memento (film), effect of brain injury 288
memory
  character of memory 296–7
  and language 296
mental illness 2
  clasification 2
  compassion towards patients 25–7
  historical context 24–9
  metaphor of ecological niche 13
  recent constructions 14
'mereological fallacy' 298–9, 312
  Cartesian dualism 298
metaphors with a systemic focus 199
methodolatry 254–5
methodological fetishism 254
Milan Therapy, circular questioning 41
'Miracle Question' 41
mirror neuron system 297–301
Mitchell, S.W., on neurasthenia 28–9
Multiple Impact Therapy (MIT) 233
multiple personality syndrome 60–3
  narratological analysis 61
Münsterberg, H., inappropriate tiotol 30

narrative, discourse, and psychotherapy 288–307
  embodied knowing 297–8
  neural basics 292–3
  problems and dangers 298–301
  significance of affect 294–6
  with trauma victims 269, 277–9
narrative review 226
narrative therapy 15, 16–17, 106–25, 230–1
  challenge to dominant structures and discourse of power 110–11
  collaboration 109–10
  as collaborative action 75–6
  community practice 118–21
  controlled studies 232
  counselling models 113–14
  discursive therapies research 15, 230–1
  dominant ideology and structures of power 112
  integration with other models of therapy 233
  separating issues from persons 111–12
  therapeutic context 106–8
national health services, health status from perspective of inequalities 204
neural networks, new, Hebbian principle 295–6
neuro-psychoanalysis 291
neuroscience
  basics 292–3
  conversation and its therapeutic possibilities 312–13
  discursive and other social scientific perspectives 291
  interpersonal 269

neuroscience (*cont.*)
  'mereological fallacy' 298–9, 312
  mirror neuron system 297–301
  neural and biochemical bases of a given activity 291
  neurophysiology of trauma 274–6
  and psychotherapy 293–4
  relation to discursive therapists 312

objectivity, as ideology 68
orthodoxy, current 3

performance 128, 132, 184–94
person's not the problem 111, 120
Pinel, Philippe, compassionate treatment of lunatiks 25–6
'politics of life' 171
positioning discourse 48
positioning theory 45–63
  clusters 49–50
  indexicality 60
  multiple personality syndrome 60–3
  speech-acts and other social meanings 50–1
post-cognitive questions 3–4
postmodern 234–5
  therapeutic approaches 309–10, 316
  new qualitative research methods 314
postmodernism 171
poverty
  adjusting people to 199
  feminization 205–6
  health services, health status from perspective of inequalities 204
  'linguistic poverty' 313
  public policy settings and therapeutic responses 203–5
power, dominant ideology and structures of power 112
practice-based evidence (PBE) 229, 233, 234, 263
practice-based research (PBR) 263
pregnancy, for/against freedom or imprisonment 9–12
pronoun analysis in discursive therapy 60–3
pronoun grammars, as psychologically relevant schemata 59–60
'psy complex' 311
The Psychiatric Interview (Sullivan) 37
'psychiatrist-as-mechanic' metaphor 308
psychological science
  norms 4
  'postmodernism' 4
psychotherapy 30
  discursive therapies 246
  evidence-based practice (EBP) 245–68
  'just' context in therapeutic process 207–9
  medical vs discursive contextualization 19–20
  narrative, discourse, and 288–307
  relevance of the extra-discursive 289
  skilled coordination 77

psychotherapy evaluation of practice 19
  3 criteria 249
  contemporary historical context 249–50
  as a governing activity 248–50
  'new managerialism' 250
  research 310–11
public policy settings, and therapeutic responses 203–5

qualitative importance of social context 247, 258
qualitative research methods 314
questioning
  circular 41
  'Miracle Question' 41

radical relationalism 65
RAGE system 295
randomized controlled trial (RCT), as EBPP gold standard 246, 255, 258
reflecting teams 117, 226
relational
  relational meaning 88, 300
  relational practices 128, 313
reproductive rights 12
  for/against freedom or imprisonment 9–12
  involuntary sterilization 12
resources
  conceptual resources 312–15
  discursive resources 7, 14–15, 45
responsive 84, 86–102
'rest home' 28
rhetorical 167–8
rights and duties 46–50
Rogers, C.R., attitudes of problem children 31–8
rules 46–8

schizophrenia
  history 2
  treatment 19
sciences
  norms 4
  'postmodernism' 4
  vs humanities 3
  see also neuroscience
selective serotonin reuptake inhibitors (SSRIs) 14
SFBT *see* solution-focused brief therapy
smallpox 1
social constructionism 65–81
  centrality of discourse 67
  collaborative therapy 18, 126–142
  communication as collaborative action 72–7
  completely bias-free researcher 236
  context of a social ecology 83–105
  individual utterances possess no meaning 72–3
  meanings 73–5
  objectivity as ideology 68
  ontological 83–105
  the real and the good 65

realist assumption 70
and SFBT 148–51
social lodgment of knowledge 65–7
strategic assumption 71–2
subjectivist assumption 70–1
therapeutic communication in question 69–70
therapy as collaborative action 75–6
traditions of coordination 74
transformation of therapeutic practices 80–1
social context
evidence-based therapy evaluation practice/ governance 244–68
qualitative importance 247
social ecology 83–105
'inner dialogues' 85–6
social justice and human rights 118
social practice 247
social sciences, status of superiority 199–200
social therapy 184–95
defined 187
development 18, 184–5, 187–8
as performance 184
therapists 18
solution-focused brief therapy (SFBT) 18, 143–62, 163–83
as an interactional event 167
applications and overview 144–5
beginnings 143–4
bipolar disorder 155–9
case studies 174–6
common questions asked 145
complexity perspective 169–70
complexity theory 164, 171–4
developers of brief therapy 143
discursive therapies research 226–30
problems and solutions as language games 165–6
reflections on SFBT and the discursive traditions 153–4
and social constructionism 148–51
solution-building as complex processes 177–8
solution-building as discursive processes 176–7
underlying assumptions 147
Wittgensteinian understanding 165–8
sparkling moments 114–15
stepfamily 54–9
'suggestion' 29
suicide
collaborative therapy 132–9
reflecting on the therapist's uncertainty 137–8
'safe' to discuss 135
terminal medical illnesses 136
therapist–client relationship 133
Sullivan, H.S., on anxiety 32–8

Sunday Star-Times case 10–12
symptom pools 13

'talking cure' 16
talking to listen 23–44
historical context 24–36
Taos Institute 127
Task Force (APA)
Empirically-Supported Therapy Relationships 257
Evidence-Based Practice, produces hierarchy of evidence criteria 258
increased recognition of demonstrably effective psychological treatments 252
on Promotion and Dissemination of Psychological Procedures (1995) 256
promotion of EVTs 251
The Timaru Herald case 9–10
therapeutic discourse, traditional vs solution-focused (table) 146
'tiotol' 24
domino 29
future of the practice 41
Rogers' style 36–7
stupid tiotol 39–40
Sullivan's practice 37–9
trauma 269–87
construct of trauma 271–3
embodied language and neuroscience 298
establishing emotional resonance with therapist 279–80
experiences that might be shared 284–5
finding a position of safety 280–1
'flashbacks' 297
Gabriela's story 278–84
grief, C.S. Lewis on 282–4
incorporating into ones's autobiography 282
moved by the body 271
and narrative approaches to healing 269–87
narrative approaches to therapy with victims 269, 277–9
neurophysiology 274–6
paradox of memory and traumatic stress 276–7

unique outcomes 113–15, 230

verbs, 'achievement' and 'task' verbs 94
violence and safety 200–3

will
attitude to and difficulties with 94–6
new ways of acting 96–9
'worried well' 310

zone of proximal development 190